BASIC SLEEP MECHANISMS

CONTRIBUTORS

DENISE ALBE-FESSARD

PER ANDERSEN

FREDERIC BREMER

M. BRUNELLI

MICHAEL H. CHASE

CARMINE D. CLEMENTE

WILLIAM C. DEMENT

M. DESCHENES

ALBERT GRAMSBERGEN

J. Y. HALLE

MICHEL JOUVET

WERNER P. KOELLA

HANS-GERD LENARD

F. MAGNI

DAVID R. METCALF

JAMES G. MINARD

MERRILL M. MITLER

GIUSEPPE MORUZZI

D. MUSUMECI

IAN OSWALD

OLGA PETRE-QUADENS

DOMINICK P. PURPURA

LOUIS W. SANDER

JOHN D. SCHLAG

FRANZ-JOSEF SCHULTE

MIRCEA STERIADE

MAURICE B. STERMAN

LUDO VAN BOGAERT

JAIME VILLABLANCA

P. WYZINSKI

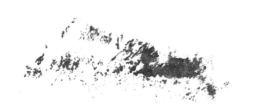

BASIC SLEEP MECHANISMS

Edited by

OLGA PETRE-QUADENS

Department of Developmental Neurology
Born-Bunge Research Foundation
Antwerp, Belgium

JOHN D. SCHLAG

Department of Anatomy
School of Medicine
University of California, Los Angeles
Los Angeles, California

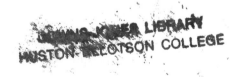

ACADEMIC PRESS   New York and London   **1974**

A Subsidiary of Harcourt Brace Jovanovich, Publishers

QP425
N3
1971

ACADEMIC PRESS, INC.
111 Fifth Avenue, New York, New York 10003

United Kingdom Edition published by
ACADEMIC PRESS, INC. (LONDON) LTD.
24/28 Oval Road, London NW1

Library of Congress Cataloging in Publication Data

NATO Advanced Study Institute, Bruges, 1971.
    Basic sleep mechanisms.

    Based on a symposium held June 24-30, 1971.
    Bibliography: p.
    1.   Sleep—Congresses.   I.   Petre-Quadens,
Olga J., ed.   II.   Schlag, John D., ed.   III.   Title.
[DNLM: 1.   Sleep—Congresses.   2.   Sleep disorders—
Congresses.   WL108 N101b 1971]
QP425.N3 1971   612'.821   73-2071
ISBN 0–12–552950–3

Contents

NEUROCHEMICAL MECHANISMS OF SLEEP

List of Contributors

Numbers in parentheses indicate the pages on which the authors' contributions begin.

PER ANDERSEN (127), Institute of Neurophysiology, University of Oslo, Oslo, Norway

FREDERIC BREMER (3), Unité de Recherches sur le Cerveau, Faculté de Médecine, Brussels, Belgium

M. BRUNELLI (33), Institute of Physiology of the University and CNR Laboratory of Neurophysiology, Pisa, Italy

MICHAEL H. CHASE (249), Departments of Anatomy and Physiology, University of California School of Medicine, Los Angeles, California

CARMINE D. CLEMENTE (83), Department of Anatomy, University of California School of Medicine, Los Angeles, California

WILLIAM C. DEMENT (271, 317), Department of Psychiatry, Stanford University School of Medicine, Stanford, California

M. DESCHENES (143), Laboratoire de Neurophysiologie, Université Laval, Québec, Canada

ALBERT GRAMSBERGEN (339), Department of Developmental Neurology, University Hospital, Groningen, The Netherlands

J. Y. HALLE (143), Laboratoire de Neurophysiologie, Université Laval, Québec, Canada

MICHEL JOUVET (207), Department of Experimental Medicine, School of Medicine, Lyon, France

WERNER P. KOELLA (237), Ciba-Geigy Ltd., Basel; University of Basle, Basle; and University of Berne, Basle, Switzerland

HANS-GERD LENARD (381), Department of Pediatrics, University of Göttingen, Göttingen, West Germany

F. MAGNI (33), Institute of Physiology of the University and CNR Laboratory of Neurophysiology, Pisa, Italy

MERRILL M. MITLER (271), Department of Psychiatry, Stanford University School of Medicine, Stanford, California

GIUSEPPE MORUZZI (13, 33, 415), Institute of Physiology of the University and CNR Laboratory of Neurophysiology, Pisa, Italy

D. MUSUMECI (33), Institute of Physiology of the University and CNR Laboratory of Neurophysiology, Pisa, Italy

IAN OSWALD (297), Department of Psychiatry, University of Edinburgh, Edinburgh, Scotland

OLGA PETRE-QUADENS (355), Department of Developmental Neurology, Born-Bunge Research Foundation, Antwerp, Belgium

DOMINICK P. PURPURA (99, 335), Department of Anatomy and the Rose F. Kennedy Center for Research in Mental Retardation and Human Development, Albert Einstein College of Medicine, Yeshiva University, Bronx, New York

FRANZ-JOSEF SCHULTE (381), Department of Pediatrics, University of Göttingen, Göttingen, West Germany

MIRCEA STERIADE (143), Laboratoire de Neurophysiologie, Départment de Physiologie, Faculté de Médecine, Université Laval, Québec, Canada

MAURICE B. STERMAN (83), Veterans Administration Hospital, Sepulveda, California; and School of Medicine, University of California, Los Angeles, California

LUDO VAN BOGAERT (xiii), Burn-Bunge Research Foundation, Antwerp, Belgium

JAIME VILLABLANCA (51, 317), Department of Psychiatry, Mental Retardation Program, NPI, University of California, Los Angeles, California

P. WYZINSKI (143), Laboratoire de Neurophysiologie, Université Laval, Québec, Canada

Foreword

When Dr. Petre-Quadens first suggested that I devote a course of the NATO Advanced Study Institute to the study of basic sleep mechanisms, I was immediately enthusiastic, since the topic was related to some of my long-time interests. In addition, the project provided us with the opportunity to honor our colleague, Professor Bremer, one of the great pioneers in the study of the physiology of sleep.

The conference was entirely conceived by Dr. Petre-Quadens and her colleagues. The high quality of both the presentations and the discussions attests to the fact that the topic deserves to be approached from a broad viewpoint. The exchanges between the fields of clinical phenomenology and modern physiology were extremely fruitful.

During the first decades of this century the problem of sleep appealed little to neurologists and even less to neuropathologists: They were satisfied with the idea that some "center" was impaired. The attitude of physiologists was quite different.

Clinicians, for their part, had disclosed a few interesting facts. For instance, it was known that some epileptic patients had only night seizures, sometimes at the same hour—such seizures being possibly replaced by nightmares, by sleep—walking automatisms, or else by short-lasting oneiric bursts. Stressing the role of sleep as an activator of certain paroxysms, as illustrated by these observations, remains, however, to the credit of physiologists who discovered particular features in the night sleep of certain patients when a comparison was made with their own day sleep. In such epileptic states, phases of degradation and then of return to consciousness with sharp alterations of affective behavior were clinically evident. Besides, for a long time the feeling of "*déjà vu*" had been noted in certain epilepsies, particularly temporal or following temporo-occipital lesions.

Up to the surge of von Economo's epidemic encephalitis in 1918–1920, we had never seen such a variability, such an intrication of disturbances of the states of wakefulness, sleep, and dreaming associated with affective disorders and occurring sometimes with a nycthemeral rhythmicity, at other times with a periodic recurrence which is not yet well understood today. This disease reinstated the problem of sleep as one of the major neurological concerns by reason of the presence of insomnias, hypersomnias, oneiric states, hypnagogic or even real hallucinations.

Unfortunately, the diffuseness of mesencephalic lesions in this condition was very disappointing—all the more so since one could have expected, for the first time, a precise localization of the sleep and wakefulness centers, thanks to this disease. Indeed, certain observations extracted entire fragments of memories, dreams, and visions from the patient's subconscious with such vivacity that it would not have been permissible to ignore their significance. Hence, willingly or not, clinicians found themselves confronted with this subconscious domain which normally surrounds our states of wakefulness; a domain to which different psychological schools started to pay attention at that time. From anatomical studies came also another notion: that certain cerebral levels are more frequently affected. To the frequently changing clinical disorders corresponded small, diffuse lesions, dispersed preferentially through the whole mesencephalic sector. Thus specified, the problem had direct relations with some of the questions approached by neurophysiologists at about that time.

Surprisingly—I could even have said anticipatively—these hypnic and oneiric disturbances were accompanied by fugacious and constantly variable alterations of ocular motility and orientation, and of tonic cardiorespiratory, vegetative, and sexual functions while often such disturbances occurred with a non-nycthemeral rhythmicity.

For the notion of "sleep center" was substituted that of a manifold of interrelated structures extended from the pontomesencephalic level to the hypothalamus and the orbital frontal area. Already in 1968, in a Lyon symposium on *"Rêve et Conscience,"* I had pointed to the necessity of postulating a hierarchy of functional systems in accordance with a Jacksonian mode of organization.

It also became easier to understand that a normal subject, while going from a state of arousal to sleepiness and from sleep to waking, is passing through a series of phases illustrated, almost in a caricatural way, by the observation of chronic or acute lethargic encephalitic cases. Indeed, beside the disorder—or more correctly the inversion—of the sleep rhythms, one could detect disruptions of vigilance characterized by states of lucid anxiety with vegetative phenomena simultaneously involving the cardiac, metabolic, and respiratory rhythms and positive or negative paroxystic modifications of tonus. To these states of "trances" were sometimes associated obscene or scatologic speeches and always strongly erotic images but without concomitant deficits of consciousness or memory. The association of sleep bursts with polypneic periods, interrupted by short apnea with or without premonitory oneirism, was a fact that caught our attention.

The association of tonic postural lapses, affective reactions, and sleepiness could also be seen in narcolepsies. Such patients sometimes showed cyclical postural changes, accompanied or substituted by hallucinations of an hypnagogic type, particularly rich and often leading to sleep. Periods of transitory apnea without tonic alterations could be followed by very short periods of sleepiness. The hallucinations sometimes evolved into a wakeful dream not dissimilar to epileptic oneiric states except for the memorization. For these patients, the transition from wakefulness to night sleep could be experienced as a difficult and sometimes frightening period. Some of them even proceeded through this transitional period with an almost obsessional ceremonial designed to counteract the anxiety for their hypnagogic hallucinations, the content of which was often transferred in their night dreams. Hypnagogic-like hallucinations could exceptionally occur without sleep and without tonic modifications. Certain narcoleptics could also pass directly from wakefulness to sleep without half-sleep visions.

In the course of these clinical observations, one could realize how it might be difficult to distinguish a true sleep from a postcritical state, or to determine the beginning or even the reality of an hypersomnia, or to make sure that certain encephalitic patients had insomnia instead of a rapid succession of short periods of sleep interspersed with bursts of anxiety.

Neurologists have probably been much more interested in sleep than in dreams. This is no longer the case. There is a consensus to regard both as heterogenous states and, from this viewpoint, the contributions to this conference throw light on a number of phenomena that we, neurologists, could not understand previously.

Today you are approaching the study of these phenomena, one by one, with methods adopted from the natural sciences. Your work has given to the problems of vigilance, sleep, and dreams a privileged status in modern neurophysiology. Nowadays this field extends broadly beyond the frame in which it was believed that it would remain contained.

If your work has not sufficiently permeated the neurological way of thinking, it must be because the abstract notions derived from neurophysiology and used to describe its experimentation are not readily applicable to the complex phenomena which correspond to human neurological states.

It is this difference in methodological approach which fills us simultaneously with admiration and anxiety. While we marvel at the precision and the relative constancy of your experimental results, yet we are unable to use them as they are in our phenomenology.

We cannot ignore the gap remaining between the acquisitions provided by the natural sciences and the possibility of their application to explain human phenomena. The fact that experimental discoveries, dependent on a strict organization and technical control, cannot directly find their place in our neurology of the states of wakefulness and vigilance, does not diminish their usefulness. On the contrary: No one knows what new data—even if they are far remote from clinical research—may mean sooner or later for the interpretation of changes affecting man. Any new data, even if they are in contradiction with the apparently inexpugnable theories issued from those natural sciences which are the furthest away from neurology, deserve to be tested in the domain of the human sciences. For us in this Occidental world, a fight spread over a millenium has been devoted to protect the human significance and dignity of our freedom of believing, thinking, and acting. Any research which is not based on this principle, even if it leads to great material progress, does not really enrich us much. Any extrapolation remains valid as long as one does not regard it as a demonstrated conclusion. Extrapolation often is at the origin of fruitful progresses in research. One does not realize enough the consequences brought about in science by errors carried on as intangible truths until some active mind started to question them. Correcting errors has sometimes made possible the disclosure of new and more valuable data.

There is a tendency, in the financing of research as well as in education, to split human sciences, i.e., those which consider the human being as a thinking creature, from natural sciences where technology dominates all problems. I believe that all researches which accept this destructive division, whatever material progress they provide, are neither complete nor satisfying from a human point of view.

The motivation of this conference seems to me to be the expression of both this differentiation and this complementarity.

Much to the credit of the participants, this ensured the value of this conference.

Ludo van Bogaert

Preface

Progress in the various disciplines of sleep research has been so fast during the recent years that it has become difficult to achieve an integrated overview of our knowledge in this field. On June 24–30, 1971, a NATO Advanced Study Institute was convened at the Castle of Male, Bruges, Belgium, for the purpose of provoking dialogues between specialists and, thereby, of attempting a synthesis of the material. Formal presentations by an international group of neurophysiologists, neurochemists, neuropharmacologists, and clinicians mainly served to introduce seminars and open discussions which occupied most of the time of the conference.

The success of this formula was such that all participants agreed to repeat their joint effort and produce a published up-dated review. This book is the result of a continued exchange of new facts and ideas about basic mechanisms of sleep. Throughout the whole text, it will be felt that all authors have been eager to communicate with each other as they did in Bruges. They had to face questions of more general interest than those pertaining to their individual subspecialties. They questioned the relevance of animal-model studies to the understanding of human sleep. For one of the first times, they attempted a comprehensive discussion of data on neurohumoral agents involved in sleep and their role in terms of the changing electrical patterns of neuronal activity. Thus, several basic theories originated earlier by some of the participants were put to test.

In the past three decades, many nervous structures, from the lower level of the brain stem to the cerebral cortex, have been attributed particular functions in the induction, maintenance, or interruption of sleep. As most of the proponents of these hypotheses were present at the meeting, the ensuing discussion, enriched by more recent arguments, provides a critical confrontation of older and current views. Experimental data were also appraised in the light of observations on neonates and pathological human cases. The participation of clinicians was invaluable in constantly raising the leading questions and stressing the relevant aspects of basic researches.

O. Petre-Quadens
J. D. Schlag

Acknowledgments

Acknowledgment is made to the NATO Scientific Committee, whose support and sponsorship of the Conference made this publication possible. We wish to thank particularly Dr. Ludo van Bogaert and many other persons for their efficient help in organizing the Conference. The authors of the chapters and discussions have made considerable efforts to up-date their presentations and comments and to deal with the new problems raised in the controversies and we express our gratitude to each of them. Finally, we want to thank most warmly Mr. W. De Cock who has so generously aided us in the preparation of this volume.

NEUROPHYSIOLOGICAL MECHANISMS OF SLEEP

CHAPTER ONE

Historical Development of Ideas on Sleep

FREDERIC BREMER

To draw a sketch of the evolution of the ideas concerning a scientific problem is a perilous task for one who, rightly or wrongly, believes that his work has had some influence on this evolution. It is difficult for him to avoid a bias resulting in a distortion of the correct perspective. There is also the obvious danger, of which I am all too well aware, of boring one's audience by the recall of known stories. However, returning to the sources and following the tortuous path already climbed toward a provisory truth may be a rewarding exercise.

As is known, the first anatomo-clinical documents dealing with the neurophysiological determinism of sleep were published in the last third of the nineteenth century by Gayet (1875) in France and by Mauthner (1890) in Austria. They indicated the importance of a rostral mesencephalic lesion for the pathogeny of lethargic syndromes. Interest in the sleep problem was stirred in 1920 by the revelation of the disorders of sleep characterizing the viral encephalitis that raged at that time all over the world. The study of its pathology led von Economo (1929) to the description of two opposite syndromes: the one of hypersomnia, the other of sleeplessness, and to the recognition of their correlation with two distinct localizations of the degenerative encephalitic processes. In the case of the lethargic patients the predominant

3

site of lesions was in the mesencephalic tegmentum and in the posterior hypothalamus, while in the insomniac ones, the lesion affected mainly basal forebrain and adjacent striate structures. Today, these conclusions appear as prophetic. But at the time of their formulation the diffusion of the encephalitic lesions in the brain justified a legitimate scepticism as to the alleged physiological significance of the two distinct loci. Although the same criticism could not be made of the conclusions of papers by Fulton and Bailey (1929) and by Marinesco and others (1929), who a little later described the association of a lethargic condition with various lesions having in common their situation at the base of the brain, a recourse to animal experimentation was obviously necessary.

Ranson and his associates (1939), who inaugurated anatomo-clinical experimentation on cats and monkeys, in 1938, came to about the same conclusion as von Economo (1929) concerning the posterior hypothalamus situation of lesions followed by a lethargic syndrome, and thus they located a waking mechanism in this region. Yet, by their experiments, they were unable to confirm von Economo's conclusions (1929) as to the existence of a preoptic hypnogenic locus. Another important work on the same lines was performed by Nauta (1946). In a paper the publication of which was delayed by the war, Nauta described the effects of various brain lesions on the sleep–waking cycle of the rat. The particular value of this work lies both in the accurate histological study of nervous degeneration following the experimental lesions and in a lucid discussion of the physiological bearing of the results. Nauta (1946) agreed with von Economo (1929) and Ranson's (1939) conclusions concerning the situation of a waking "center" (he carefully put the terms between quotation marks) at the mesencephalo-hypothalamic junction, and he agreed with von Economo's statement as to the existence of a hypnogenic structure in the basal preoptic area. The destruction of this area was indeed followed by a complete insomnia and by a motor agitation which eventually led to the death of the rat after a few days. The combined destruction of the two antagonist structures allowed the maintenance or the restoration of an approximately normal waking–sleep balance.

At that time, Hess (1944) had already published the results of his pioneer electrical stimulation experiments with a cat, which had led him to infer the existence, in the thalamic *massa intermedia*, of a region whose electrical stimulation with progressive slope pulses at a low frequency induced a state of drowsiness or sleep having all the behavioral characteristics of spontaneous sleep. Hess's interpretation of his experimental data was, however, not accepted by Ranson and his school. Their disagreement led to bitter controversy. Hess finally refuted the criticisms aimed at his stimulation method, while Monnier *et al.* (1960) confirmed the authenticity of the sleep syndrome which followed the low-frequency stimulation of medial thalamic nuclei. But, they did not solve the difficulty resulting from the thalamic location of the critical structure, in consideration of the fact, recently confirmed again by Andersen and Andersson (1968) and by Angeleri and others (1969), that its destruction is not followed by insomnia.

If, forgetting the chronological hiatus, one considers Nauta's paper (1946) together with von Economo's (1929) and Ranson's (1939), the problem faced by the sleep researcher at that time was to understand how a relatively small lesion at the base of the brain so severely perturbated the functioning of the telencephalon and prevented the maintenance of its activity at the level which is necessary for the correct behavioral performances characterizing what Claude Bernard called *la vie de relation*. The waking "center" having been given a posterior hypothalamic and anterior mesencephalic location, its arousal properties were attributed by von Economo (1929) and by Ranson (1939) to a corticipetal reverberation of the neurovegetative influences it exerts primarily at the periphery—a concept recalling, *mutatis mutandis*, William James's theory of emotions. A similar idea was included in Hess's conception, who saw an explanation of the waking–sleep alternation in the opposition of an "ergotropic" and a "trophotropic" system. Except for a fugitive allusion by Ranson, the possibility of ascending arousal impulses reaching the telencephalon directly was apparently not considered at that time.

This is where brain-stem transection experiments proved to be of help. When I performed them in 1935, my motivation was an unprejudiced curiosity. Having adopted a technique of decerebration in the cat that left the forebrain *in situ* after a mesencephalic transection immediately caudal to the IIId nerve nuclei, I wished to know what the brain structures thus separated from the rest of the neuraxis would become functionally, as one likes to know what happens behind a curtain, the curtain being here the plane of the intercollicular section. The circumstances were favorable for attacking this problem. A few years before, Alex Forbes had introduced electronic amplification in neurophysiological technique. Faithful electromagnetic oscillographs, pending the imminent introduction of the CR oscilloscope, had replaced the Lippman electrometer and the string galvanometer. These technical advances had just allowed the confirmation and extension by Adrian and Matthews of Hans Berger's startling discovery of the human alpha rhythm and of its blocking by sensory stimulations alerting the subject.

When I contemplated the ocular syndrome of the isolated forebrain (i.e., the complete immobility of the eyes and the fissurated pupils) and its electrocorticogram of 6–10 Hz regular amplitude modulation, its highly synchronous potential waves and its endless monotony, contrasting with the labile fast electrocorticogram of the alert cat, I had the shock which one experiences in the face of a new natural phenomenon.

It was soon found in controlled experiments that a high spinal section did not significantly modify the ocular behavior and the cortical electrogenesis observed in the intact animal. If I had been more anatomically minded, I would have concluded that, between the planes of a spinal section at the level of the first cervical segment (C1) and a mesencephalic transection, lies a neural structure that is necessary for the maintenance of the waking condition of the diencephalon and telencephalon. Instead, I attributed the sleeplike ocular and electroencephalographic characteristics of the isolated forebrain to its extensive deafferentation, depriving it of the minimal flow of ascending sensory impulses apparently necessary for the central "tone" of its neuronal populations. The synchronizing EEG effect of optic nerve bilateral sections in the *encéphale isolé* cat, performed in my laboratory by Elsa Claes (1939), as well as my cortical undercutting experiments, gave apparent support to this interpretation. I would have been still more convinced of its truth if I had known of the hypnogenic effect, to be found 20 years later by Anne Roger and her associates (1956), that a bilateral section of the Vth nerve exerts on the *encéphale isolé*.

These facts can now be easily incorporated into the activating reticular concept which Moruzzi and Magoun deduced in 1949 with their discovery of the arousal effect of electrical stimulation of the mesencephalic reticular tegmentum and of its similarity with sensory arousal, and from the demonstration of the contrasting behavioral and electroencephalographic consequences of selective lemniscal and brain-stem core sections performed by Magoun and his associates (1963). These complementary sets of data established that the ascending impulses energizing the diencephalon and telencephalon are not in the main the sensory ones reaching these structures directly but that the arousing impulses are emitted by a population of nerve cells with rostrally projecting axons, embedded in the brain-stem core among the reticular neurons whose descending axons were long known by neurologists.

During the decade which followed these fundamental achievements, the histological features of the ascending reticular system were established by Nauta's and Brodal's degeneration studies, by the Scheibels' Golgi impregnation pictures (1958), and by the electrophysiological tracking experiments of Jasper (1949–1958), extending the pioneer work of Morison and Dempsey (1942). The electrophysiological, biochemical, pharmacological, and psychophysiological exploration of the system revealed a number of facts of great importance for the elucidation of the biological background of conscious experience and for the understanding of the mechanisms of general anesthesia. Among these notions some should be mentioned on account of their psychophysiological implications. One is the reciprocity of the relations between the activating reticular system and the cerebral cortex, with the revelation of the functional importance of corticoreticular influences. Another is the strong facilitatory effect which is exerted by a discharge of ascending reticular impulses on synaptic transmissions at thalamic and cortical levels as well as on the speed of perceptual operations depending from these transmissions. Finally, there is the relation of this facilitatory process to the effective antagonism exerted by the barrage of ascending reticular impulses on the intrathalamic autogenic inhibitory processes which have been disclosed by the work of Andersen and Eccles (1962) and of Purpura (1969).

The arousing power of the ascending reticular impulses led logically to the idea that an essential factor in the determinism of sleep in mammals is the dampening of the activating reticular system—a dampening thought to result either from a functional depression, by fatigue or intoxication of neuronal populations—or from a critical reduction of the afferent support of their tonic activity, or by a combination of the two factors. This explanation did not exclude the possibility of a cooperation of active inhibitory mechanisms in the process of sleep induction. An essay which I wrote in 1954 ended with the following conclusions:

> In the process of neuronal de-activation which culminates in sleep, the functional slackening of the brain-stem reticular formation, by reason of the latter's central situation in the nervous apparatus of arousal, plays without doubt an essential role. The hypothesis of an hypnogenic center cooperating with the waking apparatus in the regulation of sleep is a logical assumption, but one whose adoption still raises theoretical and technical difficulties [Bremer, 1954, p. 158].

Many things have happened since I wrote these lines. But, I still believe that the passive and active determinisms of sleep—more precisely of ordinary, slow-wave sleep—are complementary notions which should not be regarded as conceptually opposed.

Initially, the notion of the participation of inhibitory mechanisms in the sleep induction process was based only on electrical stimulation experiments. The situation completely changed in 1959, when a group of physiologists in Moruzzi's laboratory conclusively demonstrated the existence of a region in the cat's caudal brain stem which could legitimately be called a hypnogenic structure. They showed that, contrasting with the lethargic condition of the brain isolated by a mesencephalic intercollicular transection, the forebrain disconnected from the bulbar reticular formation by a midpontine pretrigeminal section revealed an almost permanent alert waking condition, betrayed both by typical electrocortical arousal signs and by the striking attentive behavior of the eyes. The same arousal symptoms were observed when the caudal brain stem was paralyzed by local narcosis. Stimulation and focal destruction experiments led to the designation, as the responsible hypnogenic structure, of a reticular territory in the neighborhood of the nucleus of the fasciculus solitarius, a nucleus known as the site of convergence of various visceral afferents. These connections probably account for the fact that the hypnogenic structure can be put in action reflexly, sometimes with an astounding rapidity, by mechanical stimulation of sino-carotidian baroreceptors (the Koch-Dell experiment), and by electrical stimulation of thick afferent fibers in the vago-sympathetic trunk (the Padell-Dell experiment, 1964).

Among the possible explanations of these hypnogenic effects, one which has the advantage of logical strategy and parsimony postulates an active inhibition of the ascending arousal reticular system by impulses issued from the bulbopontine brain stem. Experiments by Marthe Bonvallet and her associates (1963–1966) supported this interpretation. Furthermore, they suggested the possibility of a negative feedback relationship between the two reticular territories, aiming at the stabilization of the waking level.

But, in 1962, the matter was complicated by the demonstration in the cat, of another hypnogenic structure located in the same basal preoptic area which had been already postulated as having such a role by von Economo (1929) on the basis of his anatomo-clinical observations and by Nauta (1946) on the basis of his experiments on the rat. In Sterman and Clemente's experiments (1962 a,b) and also in Hernández-Peón and Chavez-Ibarra's studies (1963), the feline preoptic structure was activated by electrical stimuli which were effective, i.e., hypnogenic, even at high frequency. The sleep effect could also be obtained by a sensory stimulation that had been associated with the electrical one in a classical conditioning paradigm. The bilateral destruction of the preoptic focus was followed by the same lasting insomnia and motor agitation that Nauta (1946) had described as a result of the same lesion in the rat. The determinism of the sleep effect observed in the preoptic stimulation experiments seemed to involve, here also, an active inhibition of the mesencephalic arousal system by impulses conveyed to it by a pathway still to be identified. In experiments performed on the *encéphale isolé* cat I found electrophysiological evidence of this inhibitory preoptic–reticular mechanism, which is also indicated by recent microphysiological observations performed by Siegel. It would be associated with the inhibition of the postural tone of the antigravity musculature observed by Clemente and Sterman (1967).

The coexistence of two different, and apparently anatomically, unrelated hypnogenic structures would create a conceptual difficulty if we did not know the richness of nature's creative imagination. Besides, the multiplicity of hypnogenic structures could be explained by the notion of several sleep-inductive reactions, each one related to a particular behavioral situation and having its own afferent and central circuitry.

Up to now I have commented on the evolution of the concepts concerning the neurophysiological determinism of the hypnic phenomenon as if mammalian sleep was a unitary state, with only degrees in its depth. But, an important development occurring in 1958 forced us to abandon this comfortable unitary position and to admit the fundamental dualism of sleep states. It was the discovery, by Dement (1958) in Kleitman's laboratory of "low voltage fast electroencephalogram patterns during behavioral sleep in the cat." The discovery was soon extended to human sleep by Dement and Kleitman (1957) and the phenomenon was experimentally analyzed in the cat notably by Jouvet (1967–1970) and by Rossi et al. (1961).

While ordinary sleep is characterized by a regular relatively slow frequency EEG, implying a diffuse synchronization of the thalamo-cortical electrogenesis —hence its designation as slow-wave sleep or synchronized sleep—during the brief hypnoid phases discovered by Dement and Kleitman (1957), the cortical electrogenesis, both in its spontaneous and in its reactional manifestations, shows a paradoxical similarity with the arousal EEG—hence the categorization as paradoxical, or activated, or desynchronized sleep phases. Another label—rapid eye movement sleep or REM sleep—alludes to the ocular behavioral aspect, while the label deep sleep (which, in my opinion, should be abandoned) connotes the fact that the arousal threshold has been found to be distinctly higher during these sleep periods than during slow wave sleep.

The symptomatology of REM sleep is not exhausted by these characteristics. Among other features are the so-called PGO spikes recorded in the cat and monkey from the pontine reticular formation, the lateral geniculate nucleus, and the occipital cortex; the sudden disappearance of postural, especially cervical, muscle tone; diffuse muscle twitching; and various neurovegetative phenomena including a fall of blood pressure. If we add, last but not least, to this already impressive list, the demonstrated coincidence of REM episodes with dream episodes of sleep in man, one can understand the perplexity of the physiologist facing such an intriguing symptomatology. One should not be surprised if the central determinism of such a complex phenomenon has proved to be a most difficult problem whose complete solution is far from being found. Except for the pontine location of the tegmental reticular region which triggers the parasleep episodes, the neural circuitry of the phenomenon is still largely uncertain. It has been shown that this triggering normally requires a preliminary stage of slow wave sleep. Another notable fact is that the artificial suppression of the sleep phases during a few days results, both in animal and in man, in a debt of that hypnic state which is paid by an increase of total circadian duration, proportional to the length of the suppression period. These two facts together suggest the processing of a chain of metabolic events in the transition between slow wave sleep and parasleep, a hypothesis which is still the theme of much experimental work.

The various behavioral accompaniments of REM sleep are also currently under study. Work by Pompeiano (1967a) has been especially devoted to the causal analysis of the ocular symptoms and of the paralytic spinal mechanism. The determinism of the latter suggests an analogy with the "apparent death" syndrome of lower vertebrates, as if an archaic inhibitory apparatus in the course of evolution had been utilized by nature for the protection of the dreamer against the dangerous consequences of his dream phantasms, had they been realized. In this context is should be recalled that the sleep of lower vertebrates is entirely of the slow wave type; that parasleep appears in birds in the form of very brief episodes; and that, in higher mammals where it is fully developed, the aptitude for parasleep—revealed by its rhombencephalic symptomatology—unexpectedly precedes in ontogeny the aptitude for slow wave sleep, as if the brain–stem mechanism responsible for the behavioral symptoms of parasleep took a momentary advantage from the immaturity of the higher nervous structures which will inhibit it later, except for short periods.

The latest development in sleep research has been the sudden impact of the biochemical approach, especially in explaining the role played by the anabolism and catabolism of biogenic monoamines in the determinism of the two states of sleep. This far-reaching advance has its histochemical basis in the work of Falck and his colleagues (1962), Dahlstrom, Falck and Fuxe (1964), revealing by selective fluorescence techniques the presence in the brain stem of neurons containing either 5-hydroxytryptamine (5-HT, serotonin) or noradrenaline. These histochemical data have been skillfully used by Jouvet and his followers (1967–1970), which also called on all the resources of biochemical pharmacology. Among the strategies employed, one may mention the administration, not of the monoamines themselves but of their immediate precursors which can cross the blood–brain barrier; the use of reserpine, which by the mobilization of the amines from their cellular binding sites leads to their enzymatic destruction and ultimately to their tissular depletion; the inhibition of monoamine oxidase, resulting in a rise of the amine concentration in blood and tissues; and the pharmacological blocking of their synthesis.

Important facts have been thus established. They have shown that a correlation exists in the cat between the percentage of serotonin in the brain and the daily percentages of the two types of sleep; that, in agreement with the histological data presented by the Swedish authors, the main source of the cerebral indolamine lies apparently in the raphé nuclear system of the brain stem, for an extensive destruction of this group of midline nuclei was followed by an almost total insomnia in Jouvet's experiments, while its partial destruction resulted in a reduction of slow wave sleep proportional to the reduction of cerebral serotonin; and that, after a reserpine injection, the restoration of the serotonin level by an injection of 5-hydroxytryptophan, the metabolic precursor of the monoamine, led to the reappearance of slow sleep, while the restoration of the catecholamine level by an injection of dihydroxyphenylalanine (dopa), acting apparently as the precursor of catecholamines, resulted in the reappearance of the muscular symptomatology of parasleep. On the other hand, the study of the effects of the administration of a potent monoamine oxidase inhibitor suggests that the transition from slow wave sleep to parasleep depends on a complex interplay of indoleamine and catecholamine influences at the neuronal level in the brain-stem reticular formation.

Yet, in the interpretation of these intricate causal relationships many uncertainties still persist, which will, I hope, stimulate useful exchanges of views. One of them concerns some disturbing discrepancies between clinical and animal experimental results. On the other hand, how can the humoral data be conciliated with the electrophysiological and lesional information concerning the neural circuitry involved in the mechanisms of ordinary, slow wave sleep? Should the monoamines implicated in the sleep determinism be considered as operational synaptic transmitters, or do they represent neurohormones ensuring a modulatory neuronal control of instinctive affective behaviors, whose perturbation leads indirectly to hypnoid disorder? What is the functional, homeostatic, significance of ordinary slow wave sleep, a question which Evarts (1970) and Kety (1961) have recently submitted to a critical, perhaps too negative, reexamination? And what about the still more enigmatic functional significance of REM sleep? Are the pontogeniculate spikes instrumental in its determinism or are they merely electrical epiphenomena of the functional condition of the brain at that time? Is cortical dream activity a simple by-product of the paradoxical hypnoid phases, or has it a functional *raison d'être* in its own right? Does a dream reveal a hidden psychic activity laden with Freudian subconscious complexes? Or, to quote the conclusions arrived at recently by Frederic Snyder (1970) repeating an opinion formulated 80 years ago by Mary Calkins "Is the outstanding feature of dream settings their commonplaceness?" These are, among many others, some of the problems and difficulties still to be solved.

CHAPTER TWO

Neural Mechanisms of the Sleep–Waking Cycle

GIUSEPPE MORUZZI

The theme of the present report is neither sleep nor wakefulness, but the problem of the alternation between these two states, the sleep–waking cycle. The theories on passive and active mechanisms of sleep, the classical experiments which are usually quoted in support of either point of view— Bremer's *encéphale isolé*, Hess's induced sleep—are known to everybody. They may be regarded as the silent introduction to our report, indeed to all the modern neurophysiology of sleep.

For reasons of space, only the results obtained on the chronic decerebrate cat and on the chronic *cerveau isolé* will be reported and discussed. An attempt at an interpretation will be made at the end.

1. The Chronic Decerebrate Cat

An alternation of activity recalling the sleep–waking cycle is already present in the extremely simplified conditions provided by a chronic decerebrate cat. Of course we are concerned here neither with true sleep nor with true wakefulness. These observations definitely show, however, that there is an alternation of the postural and motor aspects of sleep and waking behavior. There is little doubt that, at least under these experimental conditions, only structures lying within the brain stem may be responsible for the rhythm.

The literature on the "waking" and "sleep" behavior of the chronic decerebrate cat has been extensively reviewed (Moruzzi, 1972). Bazett and Penfield (1922) and Head (1923) observed that extensor rigidity occasionally decreased in their chronic preparations, only to reappear again following stimulations which exert an arousing influence on the normal animal. Rioch (1954) pointed out that such phenomena were likely to be related to cyclic changes of posture recalling sleep. Jouvet (1962b, 1967a) showed that these cataplexic episodes of the decerebrate cat were associated with an atonia of the antigravity muscles, similar to that which characterizes the paradoxical sleep episodes of the normal animal. Both Jouvet (1962b) and Hobson (1965) presented convincing evidence that the collapse of extensor rigidity could occur also in the absence of the cerebellum, provided the pons and the medulla remained connected to the spinal cord.

In the present report only the results of chronic precollicular decerebration will be reviewed at length, since only in these experimental conditions can postural changes be related to ocular behavior. There are two fundamental papers, by Bard and Macht (1958) and by Villablanca (1966a). In this detailed account we are going to draw extensively from a recent review (Moruzzi, 1972).

Bard and Macht (1958) are responsible for an important technical advance. They left an isolated hypothalamic island connected with the hypophysis and obtained in this way a long survival period, with good regulation of the diuresis. Two precollicular cats, which lived for 31 and 154 days, "slept" in a crouched portion, marked by loss of rigidity and drooping of the head. They responded to slight auditory stimuli by raising their heads, standing, and even walking.

Villablanca (1966a) published in 1966 an important study on the behavior of chronically decerebrate cats, which he followed for a mean time of 485 days. Three levels of decerebration were utilized: (1) precollicular sections, rostral to the third nerve nuclei (high mesencephalic cats); (2) rostral mesencephalic sections, damaging or destroying these nuclei; (3) postcollicular sections. The long survival was made possible by the technique of the diencephalo-hypophyseal island (Bard and Macht, 1958). The observations made after 15–20 days in the high mesencephalic cat are particularly important for sleep physiology.

The waking behavior was described as follows:

> In prolonged observation a high mesencephalic cat could be found crouching, sitting, attempting to walk or engaged in iterative climbing if suddenly stopped by a wall. These postures included a variable degree of hyperextension of the neck as a residual manifestation of decerebrate rigidity. The eyelids were open, the nictitating membranes retracted, and pupils were widely dilated so that, at times, the iris was hardly visible. The eyeballs either were motionless in the center of the orbit or exhibited slow conjugated movements. At this stage the animal would respond to sudden noises with rotation of the head toward the source of noise and was able to display defense reactions to nociceptive stimuli [Villablanca, 1966a, p. 563].

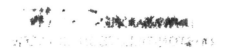

The "waking" behavior of the pupils is shown in Fig. 2.1A. Villablanca (1966a, p. 573) rightly emphasized that the mydriasis observed in a state of "wakefulness" in the chronic precollicular cat was surprisingly similar to that of the free-moving, unanesthetized animal at the moment of the arousal from sleep or during the waking state. Pupillary dilation, in fact (1) occurred as integrated patterns of ocular signs of wakefulness; (2) could be evoked by auditory stimuli; (3) was present after preganglionic sympathectomy. Hence the effect was mainly due to inhibition of the Edinger–Westphal nucleus.

Villablanca (Fig. 2.1C) recognized that the precollicular cat exhibited periods in which the pattern of pupillary behavior was similar to that of the normal animal during sleep with EEG synchronization. He called this period the "variable myosis stage" (VMS). To quote:

> If a chronic, "waking" high decerebrate cat was left undisturbed, its motor activity decreased; the waking posture tended to collapse and the animal lay down in a random position. The eyelids and nictitating membranes closed and the pupils exhibited fluctuating myosis. The eyeballs exhibited slow and often dissociated movements tending toward

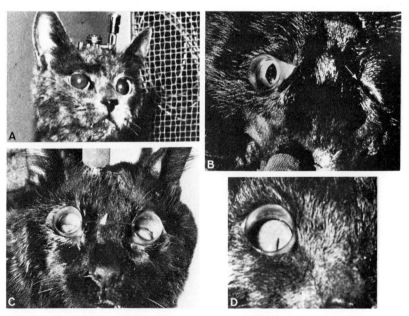

Fig. 2.1. Pupillary and ocular responses during "wakefulness" and "sleep" of the chronic precollicular cat. A. Wide-open eyelids and mydriasis during "wakefulness." B. Variable myosis stage, corresponding to light (synchronized) sleep. C–D. Extreme myosis stage, corresponding to deep (desynchronized) sleep characterized by relaxed nictitating membranes (C), inward rotation of the eyes, and fissurated myosis (D). [From Villablanca, 1966a]

an inward and downward rotation. At this stage of sleep the brainstem electrical patterns did not change significantly. Spontaneously or following exteroceptive stimuli the pupils would widen, the nictitating membranes and eyelids retract and the eyeballs would quickly revert to a symmetrical central position. If sufficiently intense, the stimuli would result in postural and EMG arousal. Auditory stimuli were very effective in causing arousal in the chronic animal, with weak sounds evoking marked, although usually short lasting, pupillary dilation. The stimulus intensity required to produce the reversal of the ocular sleep pattern was higher when the pupillary diameter was small and had been maintained for a longer time [Villablanca, 1966a, pp. 565–566].

The postural (Fig. 2.2A) and ocular (Figs. 2.1B; 2.3) signs of the VMS in the chronic precollicular cat are similar to those which accompany the phase of sleep with EEG synchronization in the normal cat (see Berlucchi *et al.*, 1964b). As could be expected, the typical integrated behavior that occurs in the normal cat during the phase immediately preceding the onset of sleep is not seen in the chronic precollicular preparation. Only ocular and postural fragments of sleep behavior are observed. Indeed, although patterns of sexual and of fear behavior can still be observed in the precollicular cat (Bard and Macht, 1958), they are always fragmentary and incomplete. Complete patterns of behavior are observed only when the cerebrum, or at least the hypothalamus, is connected to the brain stem.

The relationship between the VMS of the chronic precollicular preparation and the ocular and somatic manifestations of sleep with EEG synchronization of the normal cat is suggested more by the sequence of events in the decerebrate preparation, than by individual behavioral similarities, whose significance might be controversial. Periods characterized by pupillary dilation, clearly related to the mydriasis of the waking cat, were followed by episodes of VMS, *in the absence of any fall of extensor tonus*. Since the cataplexic episodes occurred later and were characterized by another typical pupillary behavior (the extreme myosis stage, EMS, to be described below), Villablanca's hypothesis appears

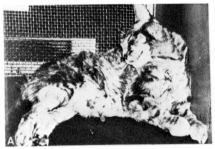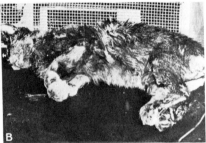

Fig. 2.2. Bodily manifestations of light (A) and of deep (B) sleep in the chronic precollicular cat. [From Villablanca, 1966a]

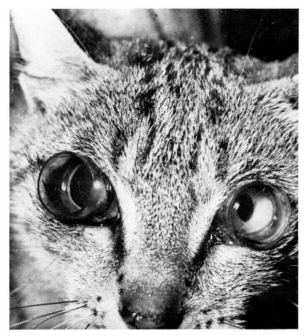

Fig. 2.3. Pupillary manifestations of light sleep in the chronic precollicular cat, 72 days after decerebration, 18 hr after right cervical sympathectomy. [From Villablanca, 1966a]

as a likely one. The VMS is related neither to arousal nor paradoxical sleep, but rather to an intermediate stage in the temporal sequence of events. In the normal cat this intermediate stage is actually sleep with EEG synchronization. This conclusion is of course strengthened by the behavioral similarities described above.

Such a hypothesis is supported by the fact that the VMS is followed by the extreme myosis stage (EMS), which clearly corresponds to the cataplexic episodes of the chronic rostropontine preparation:

> If the cat was not disturbed during VMS both ocular and body sleep patterns tended to become accentuated. At any moment the myosis could become extreme (*"extreme myosis stage"*; EMS) and the muscular tonus would decrease (dropping of the head, relaxation of the perioral muscles and lowering of the whiskers), down to complete limb and body atonia. Neck muscles EMG became silent as soon as pupils reached maximum constriction. Simultaneously brief bursts of clonic muscular activity appeared in any part of the body, but particularly in the face where contraction of the extrinsic muscles of the eyes gave rise to rapid eye movements (REM's) [Villablanca, 1966a, p. 566].

These postural (Fig. 2.2B) and ocular behavioral patterns (Fig. 2.1C,D) recall those of the normal cat during sleep with EEG desynchronization (see Berlucchi *et al.*, 1964b). They are in fact associated with the electrophysiological pontine manifestations, which are always present when this phase of sleep occurs in the normal animal (see Jouvet, 1967a). The duration of the EMS episodes might be as long as 20–25 min, and could be interrupted by natural or reticular stimulations. The threshold of arousal was much higher during EMS than during VMS, an observation recalling similar differences between the episodes of sleep characterized, respectively, by synchronized and desynchronized EEG (Jouvet, 1967a).

In summary, cyclic changes of behavior, clearly related to the physiological alternation of sleep and wakefulness of the normal animal, may be found in the chronic decerebrate preparation, a conclusion fitting the observations made on human cases of anencephaly (Gamper, 1926, see Jovanović, 1969, p. 67, for the literature). However, these rhythmic changes of brainstem activities are affected by the chronic decerebration in at least three ways.

1. We have seen that the cataplexic episodes of the decerebrate preparation occur throughout the nychthemeron (Jouvet, 1967a), while the paradoxical sleep episodes occur, in the normal animal, only when it is behaviorally asleep. A likely explanation is that the outbursts of pontine activity responsible for the paradoxical episodes (see Jouvet, 1967) are blocked by the cerebrum during the waking state; although their total duration, probably related to local neurochemical factors, is approximately the same (Jouvet, 1967a).

2. The extreme myosis stage, corresponding to the paradoxical episodes of the normal cat, appears during the first 10 days after decerebration, while the variable myosis stage, corresponding to sleep with EEG synchronization, appears only after 10–15 days. Hence the brain stem mechanisms underlying the paradoxical episodes are less severely affected by decerebration.

3. Even in very long-term chronic experiments, slow synchronous waves ("spindles") never appear in the truncated brain stem, while they are constantly present in the normal animal (see Jouvet, 1967a). These electrical manifestations are driven by the cerebrum, probably through pyramidal (Adrian and Moruzzi, 1939) or corticoreticular (von Baumgarten *et al.*, 1954; see Moruzzi, 1954) connections. Their absence represents a major difference between sleep manifestations in the normal and in the decerebrate animal.

Summing up, the experiments on the chronic decerebrate cat show that an alternation of postural and ocular behaviors, recalling the states of sleep and wakefulness of the intact animal, may occur when only the brain stem is available.

A distinction should be made, from the beginning, between experimental data and hypotheses. It is an experimental observation that some neural mechanisms underlying the sleep–waking cycle are potentially present in the brain stem. If we take into consideration the physiological observation alone—the neurochemical and neuropharmacological findings will be discussed later, and will be reviewed by Jouvet (Chapter 9, this volume)—we have no right, however, to assume that rhythmicity arises in the brain stem also when the cerebrum is present. This is simply a hypothesis, one that undoubtedly deserves the greatest consideration. We definitely know that heart rhythmicity arises in the sinoatrial node, and that the atrioventricular node becomes the pacemaker only when the sinus node is destroyed or cooled. Our knowledge with respect to the neural mechanisms responsible for sleep regulation, however, is by far less precise. We do not have yet physiological data which justify the statement that the primary pacemaker of the sleep–waking cycle is located in the brain stem. Even if the rhythm arises in the brain stem of the normal animal, it is likely to be modified by the ascending and descending connections with the cerebrum.

II. The Chronic *Cerveau Isolé* Cat

Here again the reader is referred to a recent, extensive review (Moruzzi, 1972) for the literature on the *cerveau isolé*. Genovesi *et al.* (1956) made the unexpected observation that when the final outcome of multistage lesions was a complete intercollicular interruption of the brain stem, sparing only the pes pedunculi bilaterally, the cat could appear awake according to the usual ocular and EEG criteria. This study led to the conclusion that a state of alertness might be present in a cerebrum completely isolated from the ascending flow of impulses, via spinal cord and brain stem.

In subsequent experiments, complete midbrain transection was carried out in a single operation, and the animals were followed for longer periods of time. Also in these chronic *cerveau isolé* preparations, behavioral and EEG signs clearly showed that after some time the animals were able to maintain a state of wakefulness.

Batsel (1960) reported his studies on *cerveau isolé* dogs, which he had been able to follow for several weeks. The survival period lasted up to 73 days, a remarkable achievement which was mainly due to a new surgical technique of transection. He noted that with the passage of time there was a tendency for EEG spindles to diminish in number and frequency, until spontaneous desynchronization began to appear, followed by cycles of alternating synchronization and desynchronization. His sections were practically precollicular, so that ocular behavior could not be controlled, and occasionally even the caudal diencephalon had been encroached upon. The spontaneous desynchronization occurred in these high *cerveau isolé* cats even after section of the optic nerves. Olfactory EEG arousal could not be produced when the EEG was spontaneously synchronized.

We are not going to review Batsel's experiments on the low *cerveau isolé*, since the midbrain had remained attached to the cerebrum. In this experimental situation, EEG and behavioral signs of wakefulness might be due to the midbrain reticular formation which had remained connected to the cerebrum.

The chronic *cerveau isolé* cats of Villablanca (1962, 1965) had been transected at rostral midbrain or precollicular levels. In five animals the operation was combined with photocoagulation of the optic disks and ablation of the olfactory bulbs. Spontaneous periods of EEG desynchronization (Fig. 2.4), often lasting several hours, appeared 7–10 days after the brain stem section, even in the completely deafferented cerebrum. The periods of EEG synchronization occupied 35–50% of the total recording time.

After precollicular section, the experimenter may rely only on EEG recording. Behavioral observations on eyes can obviously be made only in the low *cerveau isolé*. Because of its importance, Villablanca's study (1966b) on pupillary behavior will be briefly reported although it is concerned with the low *cerveau isolé*.

In order to eliminate the changes produced by photic reflexes, the optic disks were photocoagulated, thus reproducing the experimental situation of the sleep studies made by Berlucchi *et al.* (1964b) on the free-moving cat. Extreme myosis was present in these visually deafferented preparations during

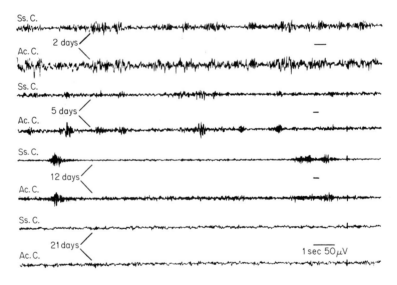

Fig. 2.4. Reappearance of desynchronized patterns in the chronic *cerveau isolé*. Lengthening of the interspindle lulls as chronicity progresses; full activation after 3 weeks. [From Villablanca, 1965]

2. NEURAL MECHANISMS OF THE SLEEP–WAKING CYCLE

the first postoperative week, when EEG synchronization was complete, confirming the original findings of Bremer (1935, 1937, 1938c). As lapses of EEG desynchronization began to appear, the myosis became less marked. The chronic *cerveau isolé* cats were followed for quite long periods of time, 15–72 days. Eventually, cycles of desynchronization–synchronization reappeared. They were accompanied by corresponding changes in the pupillary diameter, similar in sign to those observed during sleep and wakefulness in blinded cats by Berlucchi *et al.* (1964b). At the onset of the EEG synchronization, olfactory stimulation produced EEG arousal and pupillary dilation; however both effects disappeared, and the pupils became fissured as synchronization progressed. The pupillary dilation occurring during EEG arousal was less marked than in the free-moving, blinded cat (Berlucchi *et al.*, 1964b), and the remarkable difference remained after sympathetic preganglionic denervation. The inhibition of the parasympathetic pupillary tone produced by arousal is thus apparently less strong after postcollicular section, an observation confirming Zbrozyina and Bonvallet's conclusions (1963) on the tonic inhibitory influence exerted by the medulla on the Edinger–Westphal nuclei.

Summing up, the experiments on the chronic, high *cerveau isolé* show that a cerebrum completely separated from the brain stem may present a clear-cut alternation of EEG patterns, recalling those observed in the cycle of synchronized sleep and wakefulness of the intact animal.

Here again, a distinction should be made between experimental observations and hypotheses. It is an experimental fact that the mechanisms underlying some basic aspects of the sleep–waking cycle are potentially present in the cerebrum. Of course we have no right to assume that rhythmicity arises within the cerebrum also when neural connections with the brain stem have not been interrupted. At any event, even if it is conceded that a sleep cycle arises in the cerebrum, when all ascending and descending connections are intact, this rhythm is likely to be modulated by the brain stem.

III. The Hypothesis of the Brain-Stem Origin of the Sleep–Waking Cycle

We are going to consider only the alternation between wakefulness and synchronized sleep. The problem of paradoxical sleep has been extensively reviewed by Jouvet (1967, 1972).

The hypothesis that the sleep–waking cycle arises in the brain stem implies (1) the existence of antagonistically oriented systems which might be located anywhere between the lower medulla and the upper mesencephalon, and (2) the possibility that interaction of these systems occurs at brain stem levels, so that either the structures inducing wakefulness or those inducing sleep gain the upper hand.

The physiological evidence in favor of two antagonistic, tonically active systems, is very substantial. The waking structures are represented by the activating reticular system (Moruzzi and Magoun, 1949), while the works on the midpontine pretrigeminal cat (Batini *et al.*, 1958, 1959) have led to the localization in the lower brain stem of antagonistically oriented, EEG synchronizing and sleep-inducing structures. Stimulation experiments led Magnes *et al.* (1961) to the conclusion that these structures were localized in the region of the solitary tract. Other lines of evidence (see Bonvallet, 1966; Dell, 1971) strongly supported such an assumption. Furthermore, lesion experiments carried out in the late 1960s led Jouvet (see Jouvet, 1967a; 1972) to the conclusion that these sleep-inducing structures are mainly localized in the raphe nuclei. As pointed out by him (1972), about two-thirds of the raphe system is situated caudally to the midpontine transection; moreover, the selective lesion of the raphe caudally to a midpontine level gives rise to an insomnia similar to that of the pretrigeminal preparation. Recent investigations by Puizillout and Terneaux (1971) have shown that structures of the lower brain stem endowed with an EEG synchronizing influence are located also outside the raphe. In fact, EEG synchronization and myosis may still be elicited by stimulating vago-aortic fibers after destruction of the raphe nuclei. Summing up, both structures localized in the region of the solitary tract, which are driven by baroceptive volleys (see Bonvallet *et al.*, 1954), and the raphe nuclei are responsible for the deactivating influence of the lower brain stem.

A complete surgical separation between the activating and deactivating systems is impossible, for obvious anatomical reasons, but there is little doubt that a midpontine level of the section provides the best results. In fact, most of the activating system remains above this section, while most of the deactivating structures are localized caudally.

Jouvet's monoaminergic theory (1972) suggests that the sleep–waking cycle arises in the brain stem of the animal with an intact cerebrum. The impressive amount of neuropharmacological and neurochemical evidence on the chemical mediators of the two antagonistic systems of the brain stem will be reviewed by him in Chapter 9 of this book. In short, we know that monoamines are the neurotransmitters of both the activating and deactivating systems. The sleep-inducing neurons of the raphe system contain 5-hydroxy-tryptamine, which is probably released from several endings located in the ponto-mesencephalic reticular formation and in different structures of the cerebrum. Perikarya containing noradrenaline are localized in the lateral part of the brain stem tegmentum. Several lines of converging evidence show that the monoamines which are synthesized within the perikarya by specific enzymes are transported through the axons to the terminals, where they are stored and eventually released and interact with receptor sites. While the enzymes are always produced by the somata, it seems that the endings may take up the precursor molecules and that the synthesis of the neurotransmitter occurs also (and probably mainly) there. This is certainly true for the peripheral noradrenergic neurons. Alterations of either the 5-HT or NA systems, produced in several ways, have opposite effects. On the whole, the core of Jouvet's monoaminergic theory is that release of 5-hydroxytryptamine at central serotoninergic synapses is responsible for the onset of sleep, while the maintenance of alertness is due to local release of catecholamines.[1]

To sum up, we know that in the brain stem there are two systems exerting opposite influences on the sleep–waking cycle. Both of them are tonically active, but phasic effects occur at the onset of sleep and at the moment of arousal. We know, moreover, that the sleep–wakefulness inducing systems synthesize, store, and release, respectively, 5-hydroxytryptamine and noradrenaline; and that the neurotransmitters act at the receptor sites of serotoninergic and noradrenergic synapses, corresponding to the terminals of ascending and descending pathways. We know, finally, that in the chronic decerebrate preparation an alternation between the two types of activity occurs with purely brain-stem mechanisms, an effect that can be explained only with the existence of reciprocal influences between the two antagonistic systems.

The point to be discussed is whether the sleep–waking cycle also arises in the brain stem when it is normally connected to the cerebrum.

The experiments on the chronic decerebrate cat show, in fact, only a potential rhythmic behavior. All the results obtained along the neurophysiological, neurochemical, and neuropharmacological lines would also fit the hypothesis that the two opposite systems simply modulate the activity of a sleep–waking cycle arising, say, within the hypothalamus.

In fact, only the demonstration that stored 5-hydroxytryptamine increases while stored noradrenaline decreases during physiological wakefulness, and that opposite events occur during physiological sleep, would provide evidence in favor of the monoaminergic doctrine of the sleep–waking cycle.

In the adult rat there is an increase of endogenous catecholamines during the day, when the rat tends to sleep. This would appear to fit the monoaminergic doctrine. However, the same trend is observed also for 5-hydroxytryptamine, an observation that would seem to conflict with the hypothesis. Nevertheless, Jouvet (1972) has rightly pointed out that changes in endogenous levels are difficult to interpret without the parallel determination of the turnover of the amines.

The other lines of evidence gathered by Jouvet and his colleagues (see Jouvet (1972) are very important for the identification of the physiological significance of the noradrenergic and serotoninergic brain-stem neurons, for

---

[1] We want to thank Professor Jouvet for permission to read the manuscript of his report (Chapter 9, this volume) and to quote from it.

the study of their neurochemical properties; and, finally, for explaining the action of certain drugs and the possible mechanisms underlying some types of insomnia. However, only the existence of a clear and consistent relationship between the physiological sleep–waking cycle on the one hand, and the changes in the synthesis, storage, and release of the neurotransmitters on the other, might provide the experimental proof of the monoaminergic theory of brain stem rhythmicity.

IV. The Hypothesis of the Cerebral Origin of the Sleep–Waking Cycle

The first point to be discussed is whether there is a true sleep–waking cycle in the cerebrum of the chronic *cerveau isolé*. In fact, when the alternation between periods of EEG synchronization and desynchronization cannot be related to behavioral signs—as in the high *cerveau isolé*—the point may be raised that the EEG desynchronization is not necessarily an index of a state recalling the wakefulness of the normal animal. Episodes of paradoxical sleep are, in fact, characterized by desynchronized EEG patterns. This objection is refuted by the following data, reported and fully discussed by Villablanca (1965, p. 583).

1. All EEG and behavioral signs of desynchronized sleep are related to, and probably produced by, neuronal discharges arising in the pons (see Jouvet, 1962, 1967), therefore caudally to any collicular section:
2. In the low *cerveau isolé*, i.e., after postcollicular section, one observes only the rapid eye movements produced by the discharge of the VIth cranial nerve neurons, which are caudal to the transection (Villablanca, 1966b).
3. The episodes of spontaneous EEG desynchronization may continue for hours (Villablanca, 1965), while the episodes of paradoxical sleep occuring in the free-moving cat last only 15–20 min (see Jouvet, 1967a).
4. EEG and pupillary signs of activation may be produced by olfactory stimulation, which in the intact cat causes only arousal, never paradoxical sleep (Villablanca, 1965).

Since behavioral tests are impossible in the high *cerveau isolé*, it might be advisable to control these conclusions with Tönnies automatic EEG interval spectrum analysis, since it has been shown with this technique that in normal man the EEG features of desynchronized sleep are in fact different from those characterizing the state of arousal (Tönnies, 1969).

If we conclude that in the chronic *cerveau isolé* there is an alternation between states corresponding, respectively, to synchronized sleep and wakefulness of the normal animal, the next step is to see whether the cycle is neurogenic in nature.

This was the conclusion Villablanca (1965) drew from his experiments, when he stated that "the isolation of the forebrain from neural influences has revealed what appears to be an autochtonous mechanism, which operates in a cyclical pattern alternating from electrocortical desynchronization and electrocortical synchronization [1965, p. 585]."

An alternative explanation has recently been put forward by Jouvet (1972). He states that in the chronic *cerveau isolé* preparation, sensory stimulations may activate the ascending noradrenergic pontomesencephalic systems. He suggests that "either catecholamines or their metabolites may be taken up by the blood and activate effectors situated rostrally to the transection, which might be in a state of postsynaptic supersensitivity [1972a, p. 262]." This suggestion had been put forward by Villablanca himself in an earlier paper (1962). The reader is referred to Jouvet's review (1972a,b) for the literature on humoral transmission in sleep.

The neuropharmacological basis of this hypothesis should first be discussed. Several synapses of the ascending noradrenergic systems are located above the midbrain transection, and the corresponding receptors might give rise to EEG desynchronization when combined with the specific mediator. The main difficulty is represented by the fact that the mediator does not cross the blood–brain barrier. In fact, no EEG arousal is obtained by intracarotid injections of noradrenaline (Capon, 1959; Mantegazzini *et al.*, 1959), which does not cross the blood–brain barrier. Mantegazzini and Glässer (1960) have shown that the EEG of the acute *cerveau isolé* cat is reversibly desynchronized by intracarotid injection of L-dopa (Fig. 2.5); however, 3,4-dihydroxyphenylal-anine (L-dopa), a precursor of noradrenaline, crosses the blood–brain circulation.

The implications of Jouvet's hypothesis deserve careful consideration.

1. Precursors of noradrenaline which are able to cross the blood–brain barrier may flow into the systemic circulation from noradrenergic neurons lying within the truncated brain stem, when either the ponto-midbrain arousing systems or the executive pontine mechanisms of the paradoxical episodes become active. Dopa would be of course the likely candidate. The quantities involved should be quite large, for the reasons stated below, and therefore might be detected in the arterial blood of the chronic *cerveau isolé* cat during the periods of EEG activation.

2. Only a tiny fraction of the precursors reaching the left ventricle would attain the cerebrum through the carotid route. These molecules would be taken up either (1) by the degenerated NA terminals (an unlikely hypothesis) and by the endings of sprouting catecholinergic axons or (2) by the perikarya of nor-adrenergic neurons lying above this transections.[2] In both cases the precursor

---

[2] See Jouvet (1972) for references.

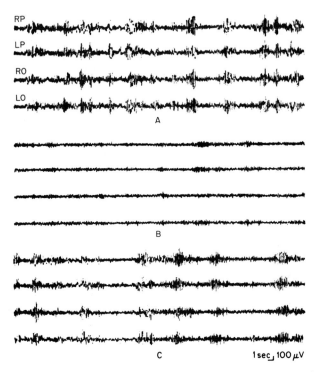

Fig. 2.5. Reversible suppression of synchronous patterns by intracarotid injection of dopa. A. Spindles and interspindle lulls (EEG synchronization) in the acute *cerveau isolé* cat. Parietal (P) and occipital (O) left (L) and right (R) leads. B. EEG desynchronization, 5 min after intracarotid injection of 10 mg of dopa. C. Synchronized pattern 2 hr after B (and 5 min after intravenous injection of 10 mg of dopa). The effect of the intravenous injection (slight increase of the interspindle lulls) is much smaller than that of the intracarotid injection. [From Mantegazzini and Glässer, 1960]

should be transformed, locally, into the noradrenaline mediator. Concerning hypothesis (1), two objections may be raised: (a) Where do the synthesizing enzymes come from, when axons are no longer connected with the soma? (b) How are mediators released in the absence of nerve impulses? On the whole, only noradrenergic neurons lying above the section are likely to be involved.

3. Only a very marked denervation hypersensitivity could explain how these tiny amount of mediator may produce EEG arousal. While the existence of denervation hypersensitivity is well demonstrated at the peripheral synapses (Cannon and Rosenblueth, 1949), its existence is doubtful for the central nervous system (see Krnjević *et al.*, 1970). It has been suggested (Krnjević *et al.*, 1970) that the increase of the receptive area after denervation—the main cause

of hypersensitivity at the peripheral synapses—can hardly occur on the postsynaptic membrane of central neurons, which in normal conditions is already profusely covered by *boutons terminaux*.[3]

The main evidence against the humoral mechanism of the reappearance of sleep–waking cycle in the chronic isolated cerebrum has been provided by Villablanca (1966a). He has indeed shown that the brain-stem structures involved in the onset of the synchronized and desynchronized episodes of sleep and of the periods of wakefulness of the normal cat may present a rhythmic alternation in their activity even after precollicular decerebration, once the preparation has reached a critical stage of longevity. Hence the two noradrenergic systems of the brain stem which are responsible, respectively, for arousal and for paradoxical episodes may show periodic signs of activation and deactivation after chronic precollicular section. Since several endings of both systems and also noradrenergic neurons are located above this section, we have *qualitatively* the neuropharmacological and neurochemical conditions for a humoral correlation between brain stem and cerebrum. This humoral correlation, however, is not supported by Villablanca's observations on the time distribution (1) of the cataplexic episodes arising in the brain stem and (2) of the periods of synchronization and desynchronization of the chronically isolated cerebrum (Fig. 2.6). Cataplexic episodes occur also in fact when the EEG is synchronized, and the synchronous patterns are by no means disrupted by this event, an observation showing that release of neurotransmitters or of their precursors by the pontine structures responsible for the paradoxical episodes is inadequate, *quantitatively*, to desynchronize the EEG pattern.

It might be maintained that humoral transmission occurs only during spontaneous activation of the waking structures of the brain stem. This hypothesis

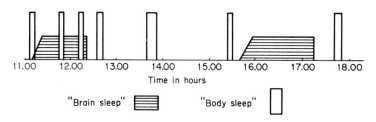

Fig. 2.6. Cataplexic episodes arising in the truncated brain stem do not abolish synchronization in the isolated cerebrum. See periodical, independent repetition of synchronization periods of the *cerveau isolé* ("brain sleep") and paradoxical sleep lapses of decerebrate rigidity ("body sleep"). [From Villablanca, 1966a]

[3] These considerations have been introduced in the final text of this report, following a pertinent remark made by Dr. Purpura in the discussion.

might be tested by comparing the content of noradrenaline and of its precursors in the arterial blood of Villablanca's preparation, during the periods characterized, respectively, by synchronization and desynchronization of the isolated cerebrum. Another control might be represented by an attempt to correlate the EEG patterns of a chronic, high *cerveau isolé*, with the body and pupillary patterns of sleep and wakefulness produced by the cyclic activity arising in the truncated brain stem.

The conclusion of our discussion is that a genuine alternation between wakefulness and synchronized sleep occurs in the chronic *cerveau isolé*. The reappearence of the ability to maintain wakefulness for some time is related to the progress of chronicity, and humoral transmission from the brain stem can hardly account quantitatively for the phenomenon; also there is so far no convincing proof of the existence of denervation hypersensitivity in the isolated cerebrum. Thus the ability to maintain a waking state, and to alternate between sleep and wakefulness, arises within the isolated cerebrum.

The statement that humoral mediation cannot account quantitatively for the existence of a sleep–waking cycle in the isolated cerebrum does not imply that the hypothesis of humoral connections is altogether disproved. We are concerned only with the spontaneous alternation between sleep and wakefulness, and the experiments based on sleep deprivation and of reticular or diencephalic stimulation (see Jouvet, 1972 for the wide literature) will not be discussed. In fact, conditions giving rise to intense arousal might desynchronize the EEG patterns of the isolated cerebrum through humoral mechanisms. Villablanca (1962, 1965) reported occasional desynchronization when the animal was submitted to maneuvers involving strong sensory stimulations. In these conditions adrenaline and noradrenaline discharges might well be elicited reflexly, even when the brain stem is disconnected from the hypothalamus. It is true that the EEG arousal produced by intravenous injections of these hormones (Bonvallet *et al.*, 1954) is related to an increase of blood pressure (Baust *et al.*, 1963), and that the effect should be absent when the cerebrum is disconnected from the brain stem (Bonvallet *et al.*, 1954). However, these experiments were made in acute conditions, and it might be interesting to repeat them after chronic transection of the upper mesencephalon.

V. An Attempt at a Synthesis

Sleep and wakefulness are under the control of ascending systems arising in the brain stem and influencing in several ways the cerebrum. There are several types of neurons characterized by different neurophysiological and neurochemical properties. For simplicity's sake only the two major activating and deactivating systems will be considered. They are tonically active, as shown by experiments of anatomical lesion or of functional inactivation; they are reciprocally organized, even at the level of the brain stem, as shown by the alternation of sleep and waking behavior occurring in the chronic decerebrate preparation.

I believe that most would agree with these conclusions. It is a matter of discussion, and of future experimentation, whether in the normal animal the cycle arises only in the brain stem. If this hypothesis is accepted, the structures of the cerebrum related to sleep and wakefulness would simply register the outcome of a struggle which is decided at the level of the brain stem. They might be regarded as populations of effector neurons, just as the inspiratory or expiratory motoneurons are the effectors for rhythmic signals arising in the respiratory center of the medulla.

I have perhaps oversimplified what seems to me the core of Jouvet's monoaminergic theory of the sleep–waking cycle. In fact, there is little doubt that the cerebrum influences the brain stem, and Jouvet himself pointed out several years ago the importance of this control for synchronized sleep (see Jouvet, 1967a). However, the level where major decisions are taken would be located in the brain stem, according to his interpretation.

Jouvet's hypothesis deserves great attention. I am simply going to offer an alternative explanation, which may have a justification only if it leads to new experiments. It is simply a different way to interpret phenomena which are basically the same.

This is a symposium in which the problem of sleep is attacked from several angles: neurochemistry, neurophysiology, neuropharmacology, clinical neurology. We are all likely to suffer from some kind of professional distortion, and therefore be inclined to think that to maintain sleep and wakefulness is the major task of the central nervous system. This is an important function, of course, but one may be surprised that so many structures of the brain stem are required for the relatively simple task of maintaining a sleep–waking cycle.

The first point I should like to make is that there is perhaps a state of sleep, with an alternation of a synchronized and of a paradoxical phase. *Wakefulness, however, is not a physiological entity*. It is an abstract term to indicate that the "level of activation" must be within given ranges for the usual types of activity to be carried out.

Several experiments have been made by Brunelli *et al.* (1972) on the chronic thalamic pigeon. This preparation provides an ideal background for a simplified study of wakefulness. When the animal is awake, several types of behavior go on, almost without interruption.

There is no such thing as a chronic thalamic pigeon that is merely awake, or if so, this condition is an extremely transient one. The pigeon may spend his waking time preening, pecking, walking around, cooing. All these activities, different as they may appear, have one thing in common, namely that the general activation of the brain is above a critical level. When activation falls below this level the animal is behaviorally asleep and these types of behavior are no longer possible. We all know that an animal must be awake in order to show instinctive behavior.

I realize that in mammals and above all in man the situation is more complex. Even in man, wakefulness may not be dissociated from other activities which involve the central nervous system, such as thinking. However, I prefer to consider the stereotyped and much simpler conditions available in the chronic thalamic pigeon.

No one would question that the ascending reticular system is concerned not only with phasic arousal, or with the maintenance of wakefulness, but also with maintaining a proper level of activity in the central nervous system. These concepts have been developed by Hebb, Lindsley, and several other investigators (see Moruzzi, 1971, for ref.).

The synchronizing or sleep-inducing structures are usually interpreted as being only concerned with interruption of wakefulness. The data which will be presented in later papers will show that every aspect of waking behavior is in fact under the control of these two antagonistically oriented structures of the brain stem. These systems are concerned with the regulation of all the levels of activity of the cerebrum and of course also of the spinal cord, thus controlling every manifestation of waking behavior. The regulation of the sleep–waking cycle is merely one aspect of a broader influence exerted by the ascending systems of the brain stem.

If this view is accepted, it is difficult to think that such a broad influence is controlled simply by cyclic neurochemical changes occurring within the two opposite systems. According to the monoaminergic doctrine, the cause of the sleep–waking cycle is represented by an accumulation of noradrenaline within the brain-stem somata and/or the cerebral endings of the activating reticular system, a phenomenon occurring during sleep; and by a dissipation of the neurotransmitter during wakefulness. According to this interpretation, the 5-hydroxytryptamine should behave in just the opposite way within the sleep-inducing system.

In fact, the same neurochemical changes might also occur as a *consequence* of a prolonged or intense activity of either one or the other of the two antagonistic brain-stem systems responsible for raising (arousal) or lowering (dearousal) the general level of activation. According to our interpretation, opposite ascending influences would simply modulate all kinds of cerebral activities of the waking animal. Obviously any experimental alteration in the metabolism of the monoamines would modify this modulating influence, thus affecting, indirectly, the sleep–waking cycle.

There is of course no crucial proof of either point of view. Brunelli *et al.*

(Chapter 3, this volume) simply suggest an alternative interpretation of the functional significance of the two antagonistic systems of the brain stem.

VI. Summary

The experiments on the chronic decerebrate cat show that neural mechanisms underlying the alternation of sleep and waking behavior are potentially present in the brain stem, after its isolation from the cerebrum.

The experiments on the chronic *cerveau isolé* show that mechanisms underlying the EEG manifestations of synchronized sleep and of wakefulness, and their cyclic alternation, are potentially present when the cerebrum has been isolated from the brain stem by a precollicular section.

A discussion of neurophysiological and neurochemical data leads to the conclusion that two ascending systems arising in the brain stem, the activating reticular system and the deactivating structures of the lower brain stem, modulate cerebral activities which are also reciprocally organized, and able to give rise to a sleep—waking cycle.

CHAPTER THREE

Effects of Pontine Stimulations on
Sleep and Waking Behaviors of the Pigeon

MARCELLO BRUNELLI
FRANCO MAGNI
GIUSEPPE MORUZZI
DANIELA MUSUMECI

This report[1] is concerned with the effects of reticular stimulations on sleep and waking behavior in three experimental conditions: (1) the acute thalamic pigeon, (2) the chronic thalamic pigeon, (3) the male, androgen-treated pigeon, with intact cerebrum.

Our aim was to obtain a constant and predictable background of behavior upon which to study the effects of reticular stimulation. The acute thalamic pigeon provides in fact a background of sleep behavior which may also be observed, although less frequently, in the chronic preparation. The chronic thalamic pigeon and the androgen-treated male, on the other hand, provide several stereotyped background patterns of waking behavior. Our purpose was to compare the effects of electrical stimulations of the *same* area of the pontine reticular formation on sleep posture and on given types of waking behavior.

1. The Sleep–Waking Cycle in the Acute Thalamic Pigeon

The ablation of the cerebral hemispheres provides us with what is called the *acute thalamic pigeon*. In fact, if secondary lesions are avoided, the thalamus

---

[1] Preliminary notes were presented in 1971 at the international Congress of Physiology (München) and at the Accademia dei Lincei. For the full paper see References.

and the hypothalamus are intact. Hence the behavior known as Flourens' syndrome may be generated within the diencephalon and/or the brain stem.

The classical experiments were carried out in the nineteenth century. Ferrier (1876) summarized the results as follows:

> The results of removal of the cerebral hemispheres in pigeons have been described in great detail by Flourens, Longet, Vulpian, and others. A pigeon so mutilated continues able to maintain its equilibrium, and to regain it when disturbed. When placed on its back it succeeds in regaining its feet. When pushed or pinched it marches forward. Should it happen to step over the edge of the table it will flap its wings until it regains a firm basis of support. When thrown in the air it flies with all due precision and co-ordination. Left to itself it seems as if plunged in profound sleep. From this state of repose it is easily awakened by a gentle push or pinch, and looks up and opens its eyes. Occasionally, apparently without any external stimulation, it may look up, yawn, shake itself, dress its feathers with its beak, move a few steps, and then settle down quietly, standing sometimes on one foot and sometimes on both. Should a fly happen to settle on its head it will shake it off. If ammonia be held near its nostrils it will start back. Should the finger be brusquely approximated to its eyes, it will wink and retreat. A light flashed before its eyes will cause the pupils to contract; and if a circular motion be made with the flame, the animal may turn its head and eyes accordingly. It will start suddenly and open its eyes widely if a pistol be discharged close to its head.
>
> After each active manifestation called forth by any of these methods of stimulation, the animal again subsides into its state of repose. It makes no spontaneous movements. Memory and will seem annihilated. When irritated it may show fight both with wings and beak, but it exhibits no fear and makes no attempts at escape. It resists attempts to open its beak for the purpose of introducing nourishment, but should its resistance be overcome, it swallows as usual. If fed artificially it may be kept alive for months, but left to itself will die of starvation, like the frog or fish.

This sleep behavior, however, is not a permanent symptom, as Schrader (1889) was the first to prove, with anatomically well-controlled experiments. It never lasts, in fact, more than 3–4 days and is followed by recovery of waking activities. During the periods of behavioral wakefulness, the animal moves about, its eyes are kept open, and it is obviously able to avoid all obstacles.

The term recovery implies that diencephalic or brain-stem structures are again able to perform functions which had been apparently lost as a consequence of the ablation of the cerebral hemispheres. The point to be discussed is whether the transient sleep behavior is the consequence of the sudden withdrawal of a tonic influence of the cerebral hemispheres. This conclusion would explain the recovery of waking activities on lines similar to those usually accepted for the recovery of reflex activities from spinal shock. This hypothesis may well account for the greater tendency to sleep of the chronic thalamic pigeon.

Brunelli and others (1971a,b) have shown, however, that if the diencephalon is protected during the surgical operation, the recovery of a sleep–waking cycle may begin within 2 hr after the ablation. Without any apparent stimulation, the animal will open its eyes and start to walk around quietly.

Flourens' syndrome is therefore mainly the consequence of diencephalic lesions which may be avoided. The cerebral hemispheres certainly have a great influence on this sleep–waking cycle, as also shown by the fact that the circadian alternation of sleep and wakefulness is lost in the thalamic pigeon. During the first days the tendency to sleep is extreme, as will be shown by the study of the after-effects of nociceptive stimulations. The great tendency of the chronic thalamic pigeon to fall asleep had already been noted by Schrader (1889).

Before presenting the results, a few words on the techniques may be in order. It is easy to implant bipolar electrodes in the pons after ablation of the cerebral hemispheres, by using an appropriate stereotaxic apparatus. The LR and AP parameters may be checked, both anatomically and physiologically. The physiological control is provided by 1/sec stimulation of the nucleus of the fourth nerve (slight synchronous movements of the eyes). The pontine region which has been studied so far lies 1 mm laterally to this nucleus, at the same AP levels. Histological controls show that the tips of the electrodes are localized within the nucleus reticularis pontis oralis.

Two phenomena deserve to be noted in these experimental conditions.
As it might be expected, typical manifestations of arousal may be obtained when reticular stimulation at high rates is applied on a behavioral background of sleep. Rectangular pulses 0.1 msec in duration, at 300/sec will induce opening of the eyes for threshold intensities. These behavioral effects are always accompanied by an increased heart rate (Fig. 3.1A,B); about the same results are observed when arousal occurs spontaneously (Fig. 3.1C) or is produced by noise (Fig. 3.1D).
The arousal is very marked, and phasic in nature, following nociceptive stimulation, e.g., when strong pressure is applied upon the animal's feet. The animal will withdraw and frantically move its wings. Paradoxically, this period of excitation is followed by the reappearance of a typical sleep behavior. This strange phenomenon had been observed by Schrader (1889) following rough handling. An obvious explanation is that any excessive stimulation of the activating system of the brain stem is followed, possibly via feedback channels, by the enhanced activity of antagonistic, sleep-inducing structures, whose existence is supported by experiments to be reported later. On the other hand, sleep is never produced as an aftereffect of nociceptive stimulation in the chronic thalamic pigeon, possibly because in these experimental situations the sleep-inducing structures are overwhelmed by the arousing systems.

The sleep response to nociceptive stimulation recalls the phenomena described by the ethologists as *displacement reactions*. They have been defined by Hinde (1966) as behaviors appearing in conflict situations that are clearly irrelevant to any of the tendencies which are in conflict. It turns out that sleep may appear in the birds as a displacement activity in situations characterized by conflict, frustration, etc., and

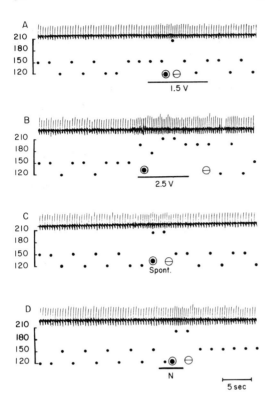

Fig. 3.1 Effect of reticular and acoustic stimulation on the acute thalamic pigeon. Acute thalamic pigeon, 6 days after ablation of the cerebral hemispheres. In each record the upper traces show the EKG, the second traces are the plot of heart rate. The stimulus signal is shown by the black bar; ⊙ and ⊖ indicate opening and closing of the eyes respectively. A and B. Arousal elicited by reticular stimulation (300/sec, 0.1 msec) at 1.5 V and 2.5 V respectively. Note opening of the eyes and increase in heart rate. C. "Spontaneous" arousal. D. Arousal elicited by loud noise (N). Time calibration applies to all records. [From Brunelli *et al.*, 1972]

associated with arousal. Delius (1970) has suggested that this stimulation may lead to a concomitant activation of an arousal inhibiting, and therefore sleep producing system. The functional significance would be to maintain "arousal homeostasis." Apparently these "dearousing systems" are thrown into action by the nociceptive stimulation, and may be strong enough to produce sleep, at least in the acute thalamic preparation.

II. Sleep and Feeding Behavior in the Chronic Thalamic Pigeon

When the ablation of the cerebral hemispheres is made without damaging the diencephalon, periods of behavioral wakefulness—characterized by locomotor activity—appear at a very early stage, even within 2 hr after the operation. In these successful preparations the onset of the usual patterns of waking behavior is also precocious. Self-cleaning activities, particularly preening, may appear within 24 hr. Feeding activities—including pecking movements, seizing and swallowing food, drinking—appear later, within 15–20 days.

Early authors, including Schrader (1889), denied that a thalamic pigeon could become self-sufficient for feeding and drinking. Only in 1938 did Thauer and Peters report that one of their anatomically controlled, thalamic pigeons had started to peck at corn at the 27th day; that it seized and swallowed it 10 days later; finally that after 5 weeks the animal was completely self-sufficient for both feeding and drinking. With improvements in the surgical technique, we have found that this occurs in the great majority of cases. Most of our 58 chronic thalamic pigeons, in fact, became self-sufficient for both feeding and drinking. It is likely that the negative results obtained by earlier investigators were due to surgical damage to the diencephalon.

We should like to point out that the feeding behavior of the thalamic pigeon is not entirely innate; it is likely to be modified, and made specific, by learning processes which occur during the first postsurgical weeks. Hinde (1966, p. 366) recalls that newly hatched domestic chicks and ducklings will peck at any spots which contrast with their background. A narrowing of the range of effective stimuli follows. Chicks will continue to peck at stimuli which subsequently release the action of swallowing, and cease to peck at those which do not. Unspecific pecking can be shown in the thalamic pigeon, since the animal pecks at stationary (small black spots on white paper) and moving stimuli (movement of a pencil), without any feeding significance. Of course, the drive for food will become eventually greater for corn and for other foodstuff, probably because of the reinforcement produced by swallowing and consequent physiological activities.

Pecking movements are easily blocked by pontine stimulations with rectangular pulses at 300/sec, 0.1-msec pulse duration (Fig. 3.2). Control experiments during the implantation showed that for the voltages used (0.9 to 2.2 V), the position of the tip of the bipolar electrodes was critical for about 1 mm. The blockade of pecking is reversible when the pontine stimulation is short lasting. When the stimulation is of long duration, the animal will move, so that the cup containing corn will no longer be within its previous field of vision. The interruption of the pecking movements may then be long lasting.

An interesting observation may be made when trains of rectangular pulses (0.1 msec; 300/sec; lasting 0.2 sec) are applied at a repetition rate of 1/sec. The latency, consisting essentially in a summation time, is then longer by far. At the beginning the interruption of the pecking movements is incomplete. The animal will almost reach the food with its beak, but actual pecking and the reinforcement produced by swallowing the corn will be absent. After a short time pecking behavior will disappear entirely. This is a striking effect and is properly documented on film.

If the same types of pontine stimulation are applied to the same pigeon during the state of sleep, there will be the typical behavioral arousal, characterized by opening of the eyes, occasionally accompanied by extension of

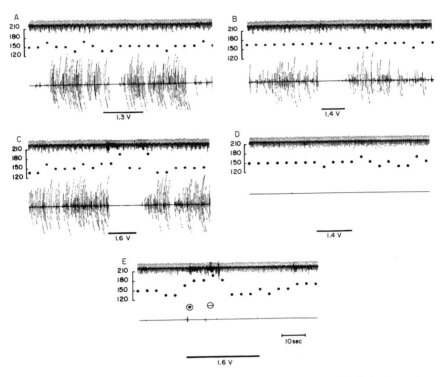

Fig. 3.2. Comparison of the effects of reticular stimulation on pecking behavior and on sleep in the chronic thalamic pigeon. Chronic thalamic pigeon, 8 weeks after ablation of the cerebral hemispheres. Each record shows from top downward: EKG, the plot of the heart rate and microphone record of pecking. Stimulus signal indicated by black bar below each record. A and B. Partial and complete interruption of pecking elicited by reticular stimulation (300/sec, 0.1 msec) at 1.3 and 1.4 V respectively. Note the absence of cardiac acceleration. C. Same as A and B but with stimulus intensity of 1.6 V. Note the increase in heart rate. D and E. Same as B and C, but during an episode of sleep in the same animal. Note the absence of arousal in D and a clear-cut arousal in E, shown by the opening of the eyes (⊙   ⊝) and by the increase in heart rate. Time calibration applies to all records. [From Brunelli *et al.*, 1972]

the neck and exploratory movements of the head. Nevertheless, the arrest of waking activity and the behavioral arousal are elicited at different threshold intensities of stimulation.

The critical voltages for blocking pecking activity in the waking animal (about 1.2 V) are always lower than those required for arousing the same preparation, when it is asleep (about 1.8 V). It might of course be suggested that the same system is likely to have a lower excitability during sleep than during wakefulness. However, a study of the electrocardiographic response suggests that two different anatomical systems are costimulated.

The results of these electrocardiographic controls are shown in Fig. 3.2. During the pecking movements there is no acceleration of heart rate, nor does the frequency of the heart beats substantially change during the blockade of feeding behavior (Fig. 3.2A,B). Arousal of the sleeping pigeon is, on the other hand, always accompanied by an increase in heart rate (Fig. 3.2E). Furthermore, if the intensity of the pontine stimulation is raised in the waking preparation to the levels producing arousal when the animal is asleep, there will be a clear cut increase of heart rate (Fig. 3.2C).

Let us now assume that two antagonistic systems of the brain-stem control not merely the sleep–waking cycle of the thalamic pigeon, but all the aspects of its waking behavior. One system may block pecking movements without influencing heart rate. It is clearly more excitable, at least at the level of the pontine region, so that a selective excitation is possible for the stimulation parameters we used. During sleep, or more simply in the absence of a well-defined waking behavior, the influence of this system cannot be detected, for lack of adequate behavioral background. It will then be missed by the experimenter. By raising the intensity of the stimulation, however, the arousing system will be costimulated. If this type of stimulation is applied during sleep, the arousal phenomenon is observed; it is accompanied by the usual increase of heart rate.

The corollary of this hypothesis is that the system which blocks waking behavior, or at least pecking activities, is stimulated when the electrical pulses are applied to the same pontine region whose stimulation produces arousal on a background of sleep. The effect may be due to direct electrical excitation of ascending fibers or of neurons intermingled with those of the activating reticular system. Deactivating neurons may also be driven transsynaptically, via brain-stem loops, when the ascending activating system is stimulated, thus contributing to arousal homeostasis (see Delius, 1970).

The next step is to determine whether the same electrical parameters which produce reversible arrest of feeding behavior, when applied as a single train of pulses, may eventually lead to sleep behavior, when repetitive trains are used. This working hypothesis has been confirmed by the experiment.

Sleep may in fact be elicited by applying repetitive 0.2-sec trains of rectangular pulses (0.1 msec pulse duration; 300/sec, threshold voltage for arrest of pecking movements). The trains had a repetition rate of 1/sec and lasted for 10 sec, after 10 sec of rest, stimulation was repeated. After four or five applications of these grouped stimulations, in any case always within 2 min, the pigeon fell asleep (Fig. 3.3). This technique recalls Hess's method for producing sleep in the cat, although the time parameters of the stimulations are altogether different. It should be noted, particularly, that the result was obtained very rapidly, after a few trains.

It might of course be objected that the pigeon presented an inherent

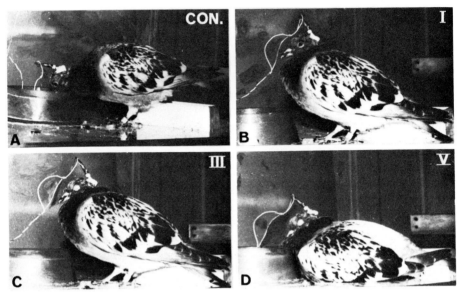

Fig. 3.3. Sleep induced by repetitive train stimulation of the pontine reticular formation in the chronic thalamic pigeon. Chronic thalamic pigeon, 4 weeks after ablation of the cerebral hemispheres. Stimulation of n. reticularis pontis oralis with groups of trains of 60 shocks (300/sec, 0.1 msec pulse duration, 1.5 V) at a repetition rate of 1/sec, for 15 sec, followed by 10 sec of rest. A. Control before stimulation. B, C, and D. After the first, third, and fifth group of trains. [From Brunelli *et al.*, 1972]

tendency toward sleep, one that was counteracted by a strongly motivated feeding behavior. Thus, suppression of feeding activities would be indirect cause of sleep. We have not enough data to permit a statistical evaluation. We may simply note that feeding behavior was abolished by the first group of trains, while at least three groups were required to produce sleep. On the other hand, in several cases it was found that the animal did not resume feeding activity after a single group of trains, possibly because the cup containing the corn had disappeared from the visual field, following a movement. Sleep did not occur as a consequence of this fact. It should be stated, however, that our experiments suggest, but do not prove, that sleep is actively produced by applying repetitive groups of pontine stimulations, for the same parameters which block feeding behavior, when only one train is applied.

So far only one region of the pons has been explored and other regions of the brain stem will be studied during the next year. The effect seems to be rather specific, however, since stimulations of the cerebellar anterior lobe, inhibiting the extensor tone, did not block pecking movements.

III. Sexual Behavior in the Androgen-Treated, Male Thalamic Pigeon

Schrader (1889) had already shown that the chronic thalamic male pigeon may coo and show other sings of premating behavior. He pointed out, however, that this effect was never produced by the sight of the female. We have repeatedly confirmed his observation, which is obviously due to cyclic release of gonadal hormones.

The same result may be obtained, quite easily and in a thoroughly predictable manner, following treatment with androgen. After 15 daily injections of 0.3 mg of testosterone it is easy to provoke the phenomenon designated as *bow-cooing*. The animal bows the head and rotates in the horizontal plane, emitting the typical coo. In confirmation of Schrader's results on the untreated preparation, such an effect is never produced by the sight of the female or of the animal's mirror image, as in the intact pigeon. It is, however, easily and constantly elicited by several types of visual and tactile stimulations, particularly by touching the feathers of the tail. The phenomenon will be designated as *reflex bow-cooing* (Fig. 3.4A,C). It is easily blocked by the usual pontine stimulations, in a fully reversible manner (Fig. 3.4B).

One might be tempted to compare the blockade of either feeding or sexual activities of the chronic thalamic pigeon with the inhibition of the conditioned reflexes occurring during the orienting reaction, Pavlov's external inhibition. The hypothesis may then be advanced that there is a critical level of general activation for each type of waking behavior (see Moruzzi, 1969). Reticular stimulation would simply lead to levels of activation above those of the critical range, thus disrupting the specific behavior.

This hypothesis is disproved by the following observation. The heart rate, which during rest is of the order of 150/sec, may rise to levels up to 500/sec during episodes of vigorous bow-cooing (Fig. 3.4). This striking increase is made possible by the existence—in the resting animal—of a high level of vagal cardio-inhibitory tone, which is strongly reduced by any ergotropic activation. Pontine stimulation will not only block the bow-cooing, but will also reduce the related effects on heart rate (Fig. 3.5). Hence the level of activation, as shown by ergotropic manifestations in the autonomic sphere, is actually reduced by the pontine stimulation.

Here again threshold stimuli producing the blockade of the bow-cooing (Fig. 3.5C) do not activate the arousing system (Fig. 3.5A), which actually increases heart rate (Fig. 3.5B). Thus a selective excitation of the depressing system may be produced for threshold stimulations, when the arrest of waking behavior is taken as an index of the response. Both the deactivating and the arousing systems are likely to be costimulated for intensities producing arousal

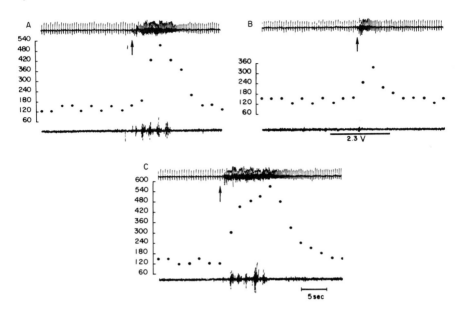

Fig. 3.4. Blockade of "reflex" bow-cooing in the chronic, androgen-treated, male thalamic pigeon. Chronic thalamic pigeon, 12 weeks after ablation of the cerebral hemispheres, treated with 0.3 mg of testosterone daily for 20 days. Each record shows from top downward: EKG, the plot of heart rate, and the microphone record of cooing. A. Reflex bow-cooing, accompanied by a marked increase in heart rate, elicited by tactile stimulation (arrow). B (Continuous with A). Absence of bow-cooing, and moderate increase in heart rate elicited by tactile stimulation (arrow) performed during reticular stimulation (300/sec, 0.1 msec, 2.3 V), indicated by the black bar below the record. Note the lack of cardiac acceleration to reticular stimulation alone. C (continuous with B). "Reflex" bow-cooing with strong increase in heart rate elicited again by tactile stimulation alone. Time calibration applies to all records. [From Brunelli *et al.*, 1972]

on a background of sleep; but of course only the arousing effects may then be detected by looking at the animal's behavior.

Films and tape recordings of cooing behavior provide a convincing demonstration of what appears a striking and consistent effect.

IV. Premating Behavior in the Intact, Androgen-Treated Pigeon

The sight of the female or of its own mirror image evokes vigorous bow-cooing in the intact, androgen-treated male. The level of ergotropic arousal is shown by the striking increase of heart rate, up to 500/min. A reversible blockade of these activities is produced by intensities of stimulation of the same order as those producing an arrest of reflex bow-cooing in the chronic

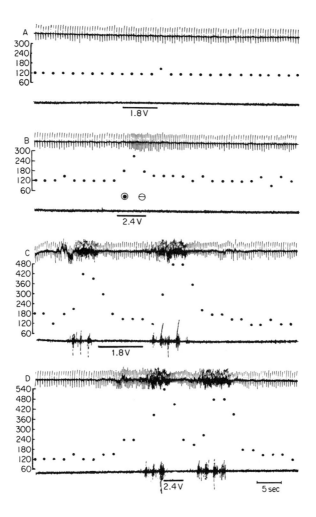

Fig. 3.5. Comparison of the effects of reticular stimulation on sleep and on "reflex" bow-cooing in the chronic, androgen-treated, male thalamic pigeon. Same animal as in Fig. 3.4. Each record shows, from top downward: EKG, the plot of heart rate, and the microphone record of cooing. The stimulus signal is shown by the black bar below each record. A and B. Reticular stimulation (300/sec, 0.1 msec) performed at an intensity of 1.8 V and 2.4 V respectively during sleep episodes. Note lack of arousing effect in A, and the short-lasting arousal (opening of the eyes, ⊙ ⊖, and increase in heart rate) in B, C and D. Same as in A and B, but during bow-cooing elicited by tactile stimulation. Note in both records the reversible blockade of bow-cooing and the decrease of heart rate. The decrease of heart rate is less marked in D (2.4 V) than in C 1.8 V). Time calibration applies to all records. [From Brunelli *et al.*, 1972]

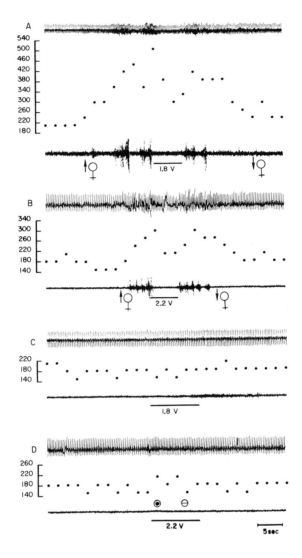

Fig. 3.6. Comparison of the effects of reticular stimulation on bow-cooing and on sleep in the intact, androgen-treated, male pigeon. Intact male pigeon, injected with 0.3 mg of testosterone daily for 15 days. Each records shows, from above downward: EKG, plot of heart rate and microphone record of cooing. The stimulus signal is shown by the black bar below each record. A and B. Bow-cooing elicited by the sight of the female, (between arrows), blocked by reticular stimulation (300/sec, 0.1 msec) at an intensity of 1.8 V and 2.2 V respectively. Note the decrease of heart rate. C and D. The same reticular stimulation as in A and B performed during episodes of sleep. Note lack of arousal reaction in C (1.8 V) and a transient arousal (opening the eyes, ⊙ ⊖) with increase in heart rate in D (2.2 V). Time calibration applies to all records. [From Brunelli *et al.*, 1972]

thalamic pigeon (Fig. 3.6A). Here again the difference of threshold between arrest and arousal responses can be easily demonstrated.

Another premating behavior is referred to by the ethologists as *nest demonstration* or *nest calling*. The bird lies down, almost immobile, repeatedly nodding the head toward the floor and uttering a call, different in type and lower in intensity than during the bow-cooing. The increase of heart rate is clear-cut (Fig. 3.7A,B,C), but by far less pronounced than during the bow-cooing. During

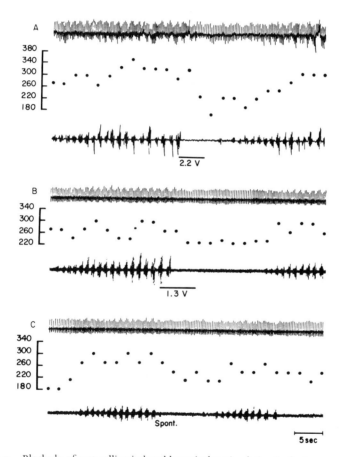

Fig. 3.7. Blockade of nest-calling induced by reticular stimulation in the intact, androgen-treated, male pigeon. Intact male pigeon, injected with 0.3 mg testosterone daily for 15 days. Each record shows from top downward: EKG, plot of heart rate and microphone record of nest-calling. A and B. Blockade of nest-calling by reticular stimulations (300/sec, 0.1 msec) at an intensity of 2.2 V and 1.3 V respectively. (The stimulus signals are indicated by the black bars below the records.) Note decrease in heart rate. C. Spontaneous (spont) arrest of nest-calling. Time calibration applies to all records. [From Brunelli *et al.*, 1972]

the pontine stimulation the nest calling is reversibly suppressed, while heart rate falls to normal levels (Fig. 3.7).

The abolition of the increase of heart rate during the pontine blockade of nest calling disposes of an objection that might have been raised concerning the observations made on heart rhythm during the bow-cooing. It might have been thought that the marked increase in heart rate during bow-cooing could not have been the direct consequence of an arousal; the frantic movements might lead to an increase of heart rate, an effect that would obviously be abolished when the movements disappear as a consequence of the pontine stimulation. Since the same effect on heart is produced during the nest calling, when the animal is immobile, the best explanation of the phenomena is a "dearousing" effect of the pontine stimulation.

V. Conclusions

In 1960 von Holst and von Saint Paul reported that 50-Hz sinewave central stimulation produced several types of behavioral responses in the unanesthetized free-moving chicken, including arrest of pecking, sleep, arousal, and fighting. Of course none of these effects was unknown in the field of mammalian physiology. A cat may stop eating and remain motionless, as though "frozen" in position, when the intralaminar nuclei of the thalamus are stimulated at a rate of 10–30 per sec; this is "the arrest reaction" of Hunter and Jasper (1949). Stimulation of the same region, at a lower rate, may produce sleep, the well-known Hess' phenomena (1927, 1944). Behavioral arousal was elicited by Segundo et al. (1955) by stimulating the reticular formation and several areas of the cerebral cortex in the monkey. Finally, aggressive or fighting behavior was elicited by Hess and several others (see Hess, 1968) by stimulating the hypothalamus. The literature has been fully reviewed by Moruzzi (1972). These phenomena, however, had been observed in the mammals as separate events, probably related to stimulation of different loci of the encephalon. The observations made on chickens by von Holst and von Saint Paul deserve the attention of the neurophysiologist, because the animals presented several of these responses as complex behavioral sequences. For example, the animal may stop eating, look around, and walk, a behavioral response which may be classified as mild arousal; however, it will sometimes start to flutter its eyelids, yawn, fluff its plumage, retract its head and close its eyes, a behavior which may be regarded as sleep.[2] In other cases a rooster was feeding calmly, stopped eating, and fixated a nonexisting object, and finally jumped away fearfully:

---

[2]Similar observations were later reported by Sterman and Clemente (1962b; Fig. 4), following electrical stimulation of the basal forebrain area in the cat.

a sequence of behavior suggesting an arousal of progressively increasing intensity.

Unfortunately von Holst and von Saint Paul (1960, 1967) gave no data on the anatomical localization of the region they stimulated. It was undoubtedly rather extensive, as shown by their schemes, and included (but was certainly not limited to) the brain stem. The authors were mainly interested in the ethological aspects of their findings, but a study of their papers from the physiologist's standpoint might suggest that the arrest of waking behavior was the primary consequence of an arousal. It remained difficult to understand, however, why the initial arousal sometimes progressively increased up to the level of fighting behavior, while sometimes it was followed by sleep behavior, a sign of "dearousal." These results were apparently inconsistent and the final outcome was unpredictable.

When we observed the arrest of pecking following pontine stimulations, our first interpretation went much along the lines of the hypothesis of an excessive level of activation. We thought that the feeding behavior could occur within given ranges of general activation, and that the arousing effects of reticular stimulations simply raised the level above the optimal range.

Of course there was also the alternative possibility that the neural mechanisms underlying waking behavior were simply disrupted by the synchronous excitation of the reticular neurons. In natural conditions the excitation of the activating reticular system is produced by sensory volleys and/or by reverberating circuits with the motivational centers of the hypothalamus. This is likely to be a patterned discharge, one that of course cannot be reproduced by electrical stimulation. This prediction, however, is not confirmed by the experimental results. In fact, one type of behavior, the feeding activity, was replaced by another one, as shown by the fact that the animal which had stopped eating presented some signs of an orienting reaction. We have seen, moreover, that with appropriate patterns of reticular stimulation the animal may initiate feeding behavior several times without reaching its physiological conclusion. This observation in fact gives the impression of a conflict between a specific motivation and a general drive, the gradual increase of the latter finally overwhelming the feeding motivation.

We thus returned to the hypothesis that the electrical pontine stimulation simply produced a general level of activation which was too high with respect to that required by the feeding activities. However, when it turned out that the frantic bow-cooing of the androgen-treated pigeon was just as easily disrupted by the same pontine stimulation, we began to doubt that the arousal hypothesis could be accepted. In fact, the general level of activation of a cooing pigeon is probably much higher than any one which may be produced by mild pontine stimulations. It was at that moment that we decided to take another index of the ergotropic activation occurring during waking behavior or as a consequence of reticular stimulation. We selected heart rate. We have reported in the first part of this paper how we came to the conclusion that there are two antagonistic systems in the brain stem, one leading to arousal and increasing heart rate, another one producing dearousal and eventually leading to sleep, but also abolishing waking behavior when applied as a single train or for a short time. The "dearousal" system might correspond to the EEG synchronizing and sleep-inducing system of the lower brain stem, which has been postulated to account for the results of experiments performed on cats (see Moruzzi, 1972, for ref.).

According to our interpretation, the regulation or, possibly, the modulation of a sleep–waking cycle is simply one aspect of the functional significance of the ascending systems of the brain stem. The significance of the antagonistic systems of the brain stem is in our opinion much wider in its scope. From sleep to strong emotions, most of the neural activities of the waking animal are indirectly controlled by the ascending systems of the brain stem. Sleep would simply be associated with a behavior requiring low but critical levels in the activating influence of the brain stem. There are of course other developments in this way of thinking (Moruzzi, 1969), but they would lead to discussions beyond our present results.

To sum up, in the regulation of any waking behavior during wakefulness two factors should be considered, namely (1) the accumulation of endogenous activity within a specific center (the "motivation") combined with a proper environmental situation and (2) the level of activation (the "general drive"). Only the latter is under the control of the arousing and dearousing structures of the brain stem.

VI. Summary

This report is concerned with the effect of electrical stimulation of the nucleus reticularis pontis oralis on sleep and waking behavior, in both thalamic and intact pigeons. Rectangular pulses (0.1 msec) at the repetition rate of 300/sec were applied through implanted electrodes; films and tape recording of cooing and inkwriter recording were used.

In the *acute thalamic pigeon* sleep behavior is interrupted by short-lasting arousal following pontine stimulation.

In the *chronic thalamic* pigeon the same arousing effect is obtained on a background of sleep, while an arrest of pecking movements is produced during wakefulness.

In the *androgen-treated, chronic thalamic pigeon* arrest of reflex bow-cooing is produced during wakefulness by pontine stimulation, while arousal occurs during sleep.

In the *intact, androgen-treated, male pigeon* the two major premating behaviors, bow-cooing and nest calling, are blocked by pontine stimulations.

Differences of threshold and results of EKG recording suggest that two different systems are responsible for the opposite responses observed during sleep and wakefulness; The activating reticular system is responsible for the arousing effect, while a deactivating system is responsible for the arrest of waking behavior and, eventually, for the onset of sleep.

Discussion

Bremer: I have had some experience with acute thalamic pigeons. Among the things that struck me in your demonstration is the fact that the acute thalamic pigeon falls into sleep as a result of nociceptive stimulation. It would be interesting to test the spinal reflexes at that moment. A simulated death syndrome (the so-called Richet inhibition), with abolition of spinal reflexes, is produced in the frog by nociceptive stimulation. It has been shown by Gerebtzoff (1948) in my laboratory that the syndrome results from the activity of a bulbar inhibitory center. Its destruction or paralysis is immediately followed by the reappearance of the spinal reflexes.

Moruzzi: We have not tested the spinal reflexes in our acute thalamic pigeons. The sleep-inducing effect of a nociceptive stimulation is observed only during the period of wakefulness in the acute preparation, where the tendency to sleep is extreme. This paradoxical response is no longer observed in the chronic preparation, possibly because the sleep-inducing structures are then overwhelmed by the arousing system.

Bremer: What is the flying ability of the chronic thalamic pigeon?

Moruzzi: The thalamic pigeon does not fly spontaneously during the first weeks after ablation of the cerebral hemispheres. However, when thrown in the air the pigeon flies and lands with precision, as shown by Ferrier and others in the past century. Spontaneous flying appears only in the chronic stage, when the animal has become self-supporting for feeding and drinking.

Andersen: What criteria did you use to determine that the bird is actually asleep? I am asking this question because perhaps it is in a different state.

Moruzzi: After ablation of the cerebral hemispheres, we may only say that the animal is behaviorally asleep, as shown by closure of the eyes, neck and leg posture etc. The acute preparation may be awakened for a short time, and only with strong sensory stimulation; then it soon subsides into the sleep-like state. The acute behavioral syndrome is in fact one of lethargy rather than of true physiological sleep.

CHAPTER FOUR

Role of the Thalamus in Sleep Control: Sleep–Wakefulness Studies in Chronic Diencephalic and Athalamic Cats[1]

JAIME VILLABLANCA

The participation of the thalamus in the physiology of sleep and wakefulness is a controversial subject. In the past several years, the general tendency has been to assign to the thalamus, and in fact to the whole rostral brain, a secondary role in the control of these processes (see review by Jouvet, 1967a). The main factor responsible for this trend has been the impressive data collected in support of the caudal brain stem in the basic regulation of sleep and wakefulness. These data include: the demonstration by the Magoun school of the ascending activating influences of the reticular formation (see review by Magoun, 1958); the discovery of sleep-inducing structures in the caudal brain stem (see review by Magnes et al., 1961b); and the more recent discovery that rapid eye movement sleep (REMs) can exist almost unchanged in the decerebrate preparation (Jouvet, 1962b; Villablanca, 1966a). This last finding, together

[1]This paper was written at the Mental Retardation Center of the Neuropsychiatric Institute, University of California at Los Angeles, aided by USPHS Grants HDO5953, HDO4612 and MHO7097. The experiments on the diencephalic and athalamic cats were performed at the Departamento de Medicina Experimental, Escuela de Medicina, Universidad de Chile, Santiago, aided by Grant G68–429 from Foundations Fund for Research in Psychiatry, New Haven, Connecticut, U.S.A.

with supporting evidence, most of which has come from Jouvet's laboratory, indicates that REM sleep is independently and entirely controlled by the brain stem. All the above studies followed Bremer's classical experiments (Bremer, 1935–1936). Bremer's observation of a "permanent sleep syndrome" in the acute *cerveau isolé* was interpreted as being the result of a specific deafferentation with the neocortex being deprived of the steady flow of excitatory impulses which are essential for the maintenance of the waking state (Bremer, 1960).

Following the above discoveries, it would almost seem a lost cause to consider the contribution of the rostral brain in the control of sleep and wakefulness. Yet, there are investigators who maintain that the forebrain has an important role in this regard. Probably the one investigator expressing the latter viewpoint the strongest has been W. P. Koella. His arguments will not be mentioned here, but readers are referred to his review (1967). Koella has cleverly assembled the evidence for the diencephalic participation in sleep control; he has borrowed Sherringtonian terminology to call the thalamus " the head ganglion of sleep," a concept which conceives of the diencephalon as being a super-center coordinating the many units which participate in "the sleep controlling apparatus."

More recently, there have been further investigations the results of which do not support the view of Koella (Naquet *et al.*, 1965; Angeleri *et al.*, 1969); these findings will be discussed later. At this point, I shall only quote what I consider to be the major conclusion from Angeleri's study. (1969, p. 661):

> The absence in the present experiments of changes in sleep after thalamic lesions places the observations of Naquet *et al.* on a firmer basis, eliminates the doubts left by earlier descriptions of animals with chronic thalamic lesions, and renders even more problematical the interpretation of the effects of low frequency electrical stimulation of the massa intermedia of the thalamus.

The last-mentioned stimulation experiments are precisely those performed by Hess (1944), Monnier (1950), Akert *et al.* (1952), Hess *et al.* (1953), Akimoto *et al.* (1956), and Monnier and Tissot (1958), all of which give supporting evidence for an important thalamic participation in sleep regulation. Angeleri *et al.* (1969, p. 662) concluded with: "This is equivalent, nevertheless, to an admission that the thalamus is not a centre that plays a primary and essential role in the regulation of sleep."

Our interest in the participation of the rostral brain structures in sleep–wakefulness regulation began with our experiments in the chronic *cerveau isolé* of the cat (Villablanca, 1962, 1965, 1966b). Since Moruzzi has reviewed these studies in another chapter, it is unnecessary to summarize the results here. According to those studies, it seemed obvious to us that if the rostral brain is able to display alternation in sleep-wakefulness, exhibiting both EEG and behavioral components independently from the brain stem and from the remaining visual and olfactory afferents, it follows that some structures in the rostral brain should be responsible. Our interest was focused on the diencephalon when we found that in acute cats the EEG spindle bursts persisted in the thalamus after complete removal of all structures above the diencephalon (Villablanca and Schlag, 1968). It seemed worthwhile, therefore, to examine the behavioral correlates of the EEG spindle bursts in the chronic animal as well as to study their changes with time.

In a series of experiments performed during the past 2 years, we have centered our attention in studying chronic cats in which the entire neocortex, the striatum, and most of the rhinencephalon were removed; in this context, these animals are called "diencephalic" cats. The EEG and behavior of these animals were compared with those of a preparation which we call "athalamic" because the thalamus had been totally ablated.

At this point, it should be emphasized that this was not a search for a "sleep center." We think that sleep–wakefulness, as any of the other complex central nervous system functions, e.g., movement and sensibility, is the result of a complex integrative process in which there is a specialization of nervous structures acting to perform certain aspects of this function. However, I do not think that we will ever be able to designate any particular area of the brain as having the main responsibility for the whole phenomenon. According to this concept, we are more concerned with what the thalamus contributes to sleep physiology, than with whether or not it is the main "sleep center." (See Chapter 15.)

I. Methods

The data were collected from eight "diencephalic" and seven "athalamic" cats; three cats in each group were kept alive for more than 6 months, after which they were sacrificed. Three cats in each group lived for less than 1 month (diencephalic) or less than 2 months (athalamic), either because they were hyperactive and inflicted irreparable damage to their heads or cranial electrode pedestal (diencephalic), or because postural abnormalities made it impossible to keep them for a longer period (athalamic).

The diencephalic cats were first implanted bilaterally (three animals) with tripolar electrodes in the thalamus on the left (A8.5, L4, H + 2) and right (A10, L3.5, H + 2) side respectively or unilaterally (five cats) (A7.5, L3, H + 2 and A10, L3, H + 2), and in the pontine reticular formation (P5, L2, H-6), using the stereotaxic atlas of Snider and Niemer (1961). A bipolar electrode was implanted in the neck muscles. In a second operation 15–20 days later, the left cerebral hemisphere was removed and the right hemisphere was either removed (two cats) or disconnected from the brain stem at the level of the internal capsule (six cats) by aspiration according to previously described techniques (Villablanca, 1966c). In the latter animals, bipolar electrodes were also implanted in the frontal, parietal, and occipital areas in order to monitor the EEG of the "isolated" hemisphere.

The thalamus was removed by aspiration through the midline using a transcallosal approach in order to minimize direct cortical damage. At the same time, bipolar electrodes were implanted bilaterally in the frontal, parietal, and occipital cortices and in the nuchal muscles. A tripolar electrode was implanted in the pontine reticular formation (P5, L2, H-6).

Diencephalic and athalamic cats were submitted to 24-hr observation–recording sessions; these were conducted on 10 to 12 different dates, 10–20 days apart, for as long as 6 months in six cats. Overt behavior was the main criteria used to define the sleep–wakefulness continuum. Numerous polygraph recordings were performed during the observation sessions; during the first postoperative month they represented about 10% and thereafter about 30% of each 24-hr observation period.

The reasons for relying mainly on behavioral criteria to monitor sleep–wakefulness were as follows: First, in the beginning, it was impossible to restrict the animals for long recording periods. Two to 3 days following surgery the animals became extremely hyperactive; the diencephalic cats, in particular, walked persistently (obstinate progression) for hours (a maximum of 17 hr continuous walking was recorded in one cat). Activity was not as marked in the athalamic as in the diencephalic cats, yet they also manifested obstinate progression or walked with their heads hyperextended and tried to climb any obstacle in their path; invariably, they would fall backward and hit their heads. Therefore, their confinement in a cage was contraindicated. We found that it was best to keep them in a circular corral with smooth walls and a foam mattress floor. After the first postoperative month, the cats were much less active, except for three athalamic cats which manifested exaggerated postural abnormalities. Second, the EEG correlates of sleep in diencephalic and athalamic cats were not known at the initiation of this study, except for the well-established relationship between the pontine reticular formation EEG and REMs which persist even in decerebrate animals (Jouvet, 1962b; Villablanca, 1966a). Third the oculopupillary behavior, which was used as the main behavioral index of sleep–wakefulness, has been demonstrated both in intact (Berlucchi *et al.*, 1964b) and in brain-lesioned cats (Villablanca, 1966a,b) to be a sensitive and reliable correlate of the sleep–wakefulness state; a similar sensitivity of the pupils' size to fluctuations of vigilance appears to occur also in man (Eckhard *et al.*, 1964).

At the beginning of each session, a plastic hollow cylinder was fitted in one of the cat's eyes in order to prevent eye closure, the contralateral eye being used to monitor eyelid position. In the diencephalic cats illumination was kept constant, moderate, and indirect, in order to reduce the effect of the light reflex upon pupil size; the pupils were nonreactive to light in athalamic cats and remained fully dilated while the animals were awake.

The results of the 24-hr sessions were plotted every 5 min or at shorter intervals if changes were evident. The time spent by each animal in each sleep–wakefulness stage was expressed as a percentage of the 24-hr period; an average of these percentages, including the values for all the animals observed at each given postoperative day, was then calculated. In the case of the diencephalic cats the percentages were no different when sleep-wakefulness was evaluated by behavioral criteria alone or when both behavioral and polygraphic criteria were used. Athalamic cats, instead, often exhibited an EEG-behavioral dissociation which will be described later on in this paper; in these cases the behavioral criteria were used to define sleep–wakefulness. The controls were taken from 37 recording–behavioral sessions of 6–24 hr duration, carried on in similar laboratory conditions in normal cats employed in other sleep–wakefulness experiments (Villablanca, 1966a), as well as in nine of the cats reported here.

Drug studies were performed in five diencephalic and in six athalamic cats. Preliminary trials were conducted in both intact and operated animals to determine the dose of Pentothal which, when given intraperitoneally, would produce a subanesthetic, quiescent state. This effect was obtained with 38.6, 14.7, and 8.3 mg/kg in intact, athalamic, and diencephalic cats respectively. Pentothal was given to an operated animal immediately after a 24-hr sleep–wakefulness observation session and simultaneously to an intact control cat; the observations were continued for approximately 4 hr. Sleep and wakefulness were evaluated in the same manner as described above with the exception that longer polygraphic recordings were performed in these animals (about 40% of the 4-hr additional time).

II. Results and Discussion

All brains were macroscopically and histologically inspected. With regard to the neuroanatomical findings, only a few comments will be made since this is not intended to be a neuroanatomical study. First, in the diencephalic cats, the thalamus was left essentially intact (Fig. 4.1) as was the hypothalamus, subthalamus, and caudal brain stem; bilaterally, the piriform cortex, basal forebrain area, and anterior perforate substance were the only parts constantly found to be connected to the diencephalon. Other remnants were small and probably nonfunctional. Second, in all athalamic cats most of the thalamus was removed (Fig. 4.2); however, the lateral geniculate body (in at least three cats) was spared unilaterally, and in one case the rostral thalamus was only partially

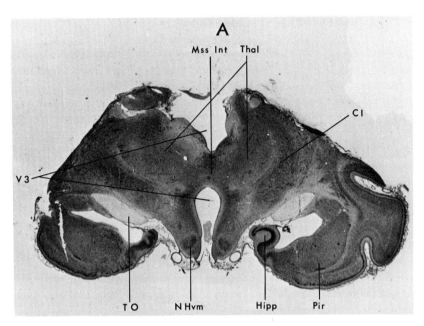

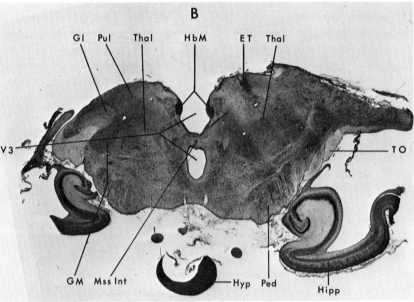

Fig. 4.1. Cresyl violet-stained frontal sections of a diencephalic cat brain at: (A) approximately A10 (Snider and Niemer's Atlas); (B) approximately A7. The animal was sacrificed 187 days after complete removal of the neocortex and striatum. CI, capsula interna; EL, electrode tract; GL, corpus geniculatum laterale; GM, corpus geniculatum medials; HbM, nucleus habenularis medialis; Hipp, formatio hippocampalis ventralis; Hyp, hypophysis; Mss Int, massa intermedia thalami (note atrophy); Pir, lobus piriformis; Pul, pulvinar; Thal, thalamus; T O, tractus opticus; V 3, ventriculus tertius (note enlargement); III, third nerve. [From Villablanca and Marcus, 1972]

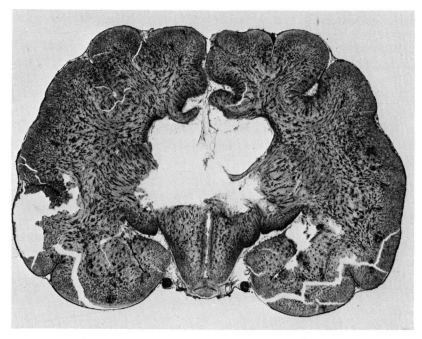

Fig. 4.2. Golgi-Cox impregnated frontal section at approximately A9 (Snider and Niemer's Atlas) of an athalamic cat brain. The animal was sacrificed 185 days after removal of the thalamus. [From Villablanca and Salinas-Zeballos, 1972]

removed. Additional damage was done to the fornix and the internal capsule in some animals. Third, we are aware that in chronic-lesioned animals, morphological changes may occur in structures not directly touched by the surgery. On the one hand, it has been demonstrated (Bard and Rioch, 1937; Carreras et al., 1966; Emmers et al., 1965; Murray, 1966; Walker, 1938) that a severe degeneration of the thalamus occurs after extensive cortical removal although a part of the cell population remains (Carreras et al., 1966; Walker, 1938), particularly in the midline. On the other hand, we have been unable to find any information in the literature concerning indirect anatomical effects of massive thalamic lesions; a cursory examination of the Golgi-Cox impregnated brain sections of our athalamic cats did not reveal any striking cortical neuronal changes.[2]

Because of the nature of this paper, each set of results will be discussed immediately after its presentation in relation to the pertinent available evidence from the literature and, if possible, a conclusion will be drawn.

---

[2]We thank Dr. A. Globus—University of California at Irvine–for kindly assisting us in inspecting our Golgi-Cox impregnated histology slides.

A. Sleep–Wakefulness Patterns (Diencephalic and Athalamic Cats)

1. Quantity of Sleep

Four stages were identified in the sleep–wakefulness continuum of both the diencephalic and athalamic animals. The cat was considered to be awake when it either stood, walked, or engaged in any other activity (e.g., licking or mewing), or when it was quiet, but kept its eyelids open, nictitating membranes retracted, eyeballs centered in the orbit, and its pupils dilated. The animal was considered to be drowsy when it sat quietly or crouched with eyelids half closed, nictitating membranes protruding variably and the pupils reduced and fluctuating in size (although no smaller than 5 mm in width) with the eyeballs exhibiting slow, often dissociated movements. The cat was considered to be in nonrapid eye movement sleep (NREMs) when it lay down in a random or curled-up position with eyelids closed, nictitating membranes protruding and eyeballs tending to rotate inward and downward, with the pupils smaller than 5 mm in width and exhibiting less fluctuations. Finally, the animal occasionally lapsed into typical episodes of REM sleep with all the behavioral and ocular features described for this stage of sleep in intact (Berluchi *et al.*, 1964b) and chronically decerebrate cats (Villablanca, 1966a).

The average percentage of the time spent by the animals in each sleep–wakefulness stage during each 24-hr observation period is shown graphically for diencephalic cats in Fig. 4.3 and for athalamic cats in Fig. 4.4. The outstanding finding of this study was the impressive reduction of both NREMs and REMs in both athalamic and diencephalic animals, the reduction being more marked and more regular in the diencephalic than in the athalamic cats. In both groups of animals, the sleeplessness lasted as long as they survived; it tended to increase in the diencephalic cats after the first postoperative month. The cumulative sleeping time averages for all the observation periods of control and brain-lesioned cats are shown in Fig. 4.5. It can be seen that the insomnia in diencephalic cats was such that during their 6 months of survival they remained in NREMs only 6.3% of the observation time compared to 38.2% for the control cats, and in REMs 0.8% of the observation time compared to 13.8% for the controls. For the athalamic cats, the figures were 11.8% and 2.5% for NREMs and REMs respectively. As far as we know, this is the first time that such a marked and permanent suppression of both NREMs and REMs has been demonstrated as a consequence of a lesion in the rostral brain.

Although there have been many studies in decorticate animals, several factors limit their comparability to the present results. In most cases, the authors were only secondarily interested in sleep; moreover, REM sleep was not known as a separate entity at the time most of the experiments were performed. Finally, although the extent of the decortication was not always clearly stated, it appears that usually only a neodecortication was done.

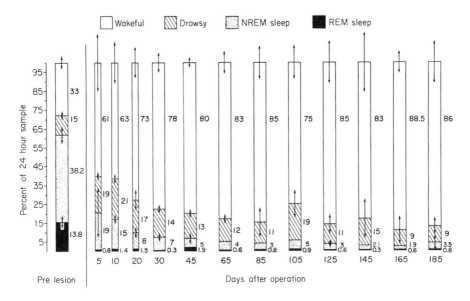

Fig. 4.3. Percentages of sleep–wakefulness stages during 24-hr sessions following the complete removal of the neocortex and striatum (diencephalic cat). Numbers beside the bars indicate the average percentages of each sleep–wakefulness pattern for five cats up to the 45th postoperative day and for three cats thereafter. The standard deviations are indicated, except when smaller than 1, by arrows. [From Villablanca and Marcus, 1972]

Hyperactivity has been a common finding in decorticate dogs (Goltz, 1892; Kleitman and Camille, 1932). Kleitman and Camille (1932) reported a predominance of locomotor activity in decorticate dogs, yet they did not provide any figures concerning the actual sleeping time of their animals. Hyperactivity after decortication has been likewise described for cats (Wang and Akert, 1962) and in a more sleep-oriented study (Rioch, 1954), it was found that decorticate cats slept approximately 12 hr, whereas intact cats slept for 18–20 hr. Rioch's observations, however, were made intermittently with a photographic camera.

There appears to be only one previous study (Jouvet, 1962b) concerning both REMs and NREMs in decorticate animals. In that study, NREM sleep was reported to be almost entirely absent, whereas REM sleep was found to be within the normal range (15–20% of the observation time). Those experiments were performed in cats with the limbic system and the striatum essentially intact; this anatomical difference may explain the contrasting REMs results between Jouvet's study and the present report. According to studies in which motor activity of neodecorticate cats and rats was compared to that of diencephalic cats (Wang and Akert, 1962) and rats (Sorenson and Ellison, 1970), it appears that the presence of striatum and/or rhinencephalon is important

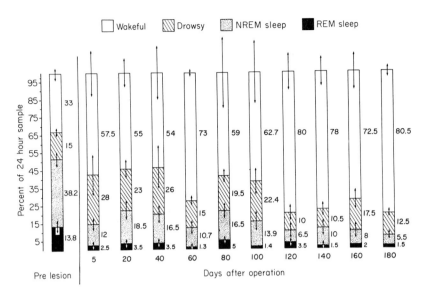

Fig. 4.4. Percentages of sleep–wakefulness stages during 24-hr sessions following the complete removal of the thalamus (athalamic cat). Numbers beside the bars indicate the average percentages of each sleep–wakefulness pattern for five cats up to the 60th postoperative day and for three cats thereafter. The standard deviations are indicated, except when smaller than 1, by arrows. [From Villablanca and Salinas-Zeballos, 1972]

for a normal quantity of sleep and wakefulness. Those studies reported permanent behavioral activity in diencephalic cats and rats versus inactivity in the striatal cats and only moderate activity in striatal rats.

There are fewer studies in athalamic than in diencephalic animals. To our knowledge, the study of Naquet *et al.* (1965) is the only one dealing with completely thalamectomized animals. Unfortunately, no quantitative information concerning sleep and wakefulness could be obtained from their report. However, their description (1965, p. 123) that "during the first days after the operation the phases of wakefulness and the phases of slow waves were predominant," and that "the phase of sleep with fast activity was very short and may not exist at all," suggests a decrease in REMs in these athalamic cats. Other authors have studied animals with more restricted thalamic lesions. Bach-y-Rita *et al.* (1966) reported a decrease in both NREMs and REMs in two of their cats which had the thalamus removed unilaterally. Angeleri *et al.* (1969) found a significant, persistent reduction of REMs (down to 5% of the observation time) in their cats which had unilateral lesions of specific nuclei. A similar observation, although less well documented, was made earlier by Lena and Parmeggiani (1964) after lesioning the midline thalamic nuclei in cats. Finally, there

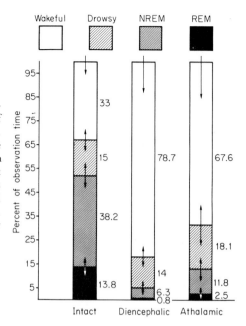

Fig. 4.5. Comparison between percentages of sleep–wakefulness stages of intact, diencephalic, and athalamic cats. Numbers besides the bars represent the average cumulative percentages of each sleep–wakefulness pattern for intact (control) cats and for all the 24-hr sessions represented in Fig. 4.3 (diencephalic) and Fig. 4.4 (athalamic). The standard deviations are indicated, except when smaller than 1, by arrows.

is a single human surgical case in which a period of 96 hr of total insomnia was reported (Bricolo, 1967) after bilateral thalamic lesions of both specific and nonspecific nuclei. NREMs recovered partially, yet REMs remained absent for an unspecified period. In summary, the literature appears to support our finding of an insomnia in both diencephalic and athalamic cats.

We postulate that the sleep reduction after a lesion in the rostral brain is due to an imbalance which occurs between opposing rostral brain influences which favor sleep on the one hand and oppose sleep on the other. Accordingly, we propose that rostral brain mechanisms modulate caudal brain-stem structures that participate in sleep regulation, particularly REMs.

Since chronic cats with high complete mesencephalic transection do not manifest a decrease in either REMs (Jouvet, 1962b; Villablanca, 1966a) or NREMs (Villablanca, 1966a), it suggests that rostral structures do not exert much control over caudal brain-stem sleep mechanisms. However, the present findings in diencephalic and athalamic animals necessitate a revision of this interpretation. Accordingly, we postulate that, in the intact animal, *both enhancing and suppressing rostral brain influences impinge upon the caudal brain sleep mechanisms and modulate their function in a balanced manner.* Consequently, mesencephalic transection, by completely removing both types of influences, would not induce a large disturbance in the balance. On the other hand, an imbalance might occur when only some areas of the rostral brain are removed, as in neodecortication or thalamectomy, since in both of these conditions rostral brain influences would be only partially removed.

More specifically, to explain the sleeplessness of diencephalic and athalamic cats, we postulate that in these cases there has been a net withdrawal of sleep-enhancing influences; these influences descend upon the brain stem either from the neocortex, striatum, rhinencephalon or thalamus, or from all these areas, since their complete removal or partial damage created the insomnia. The tendency to a more pronounced sleeplessness in diencephalic than in athalamic animals (Fig. 4.5) can probably be accounted for on the basis of the more extensive removal of sleep-enhancing influences in the diencephalic cats. The progressive nature of the retrograde thalamic degeneration (Carreras *et al.*, 1966) could explain the further reduction in sleep after the first month in the diencephalic animals.

The sleep-suppressing effect may hypothetically be ascribed to the hypothalamus and subthalamus. There is evidence that these structures possess arousal properties (Ranson, 1939; Nauta, 1946; Ingram *et al.*, 1951; Hess, 1954; Koella and Gellhorn, 1954; Collins, 1954; Naquet *et al.*, 1965; Bach-y-Rita and Baurand, 1966), and both structures were undisturbed by surgery in our experiments. The hypothalamus has been demonstrated to remain functional after its complete isolation (Woods *et al.*, 1966). It is possible that the hypothalamic influence may favor wakefulness rather than suppress sleep, yet this does not change our basic hypothesis of an imbalance among elements of a descending rostral brain control.

The experiments just reported, as well as some of the supporting evidence cited, bear on the physiology of sleep and wakefulness in general inasmuch as they strongly suggest an important participation of the rostral brain in the control of sleep and wakefulness alternation. The thalamus appears to be particularly essential for an adequate balance in this control. That this is the case is indicated by the fact that its entire removal markedly alters such a descending control.[3]

2. *Effects of Pentothal*

If there is a dynamic interplay between enhancing and suppressing rostral brain structures which control the sleep mechanisms of the caudal brain stem, then it follows that under conditions of imbalance (such as those prevailing in diencephalic and athalamic cats), the remaining dominating influence could be blocked, thereby tending to reestablish a balance. By administering Pento-

---

[3]An alternative explanation for the effect of thalamectomy would be that it destroys fibers passing through the thalamus but originating in other forebrain sleep-wakefulness controlling structures.

thal to our operated cats, observations were made which supported such an hypothesis.

The results presented in Fig. 4.6 were obtained from 13 experiments. Essentially, a large sleep "rebound," particularly for REMs, was the outstanding

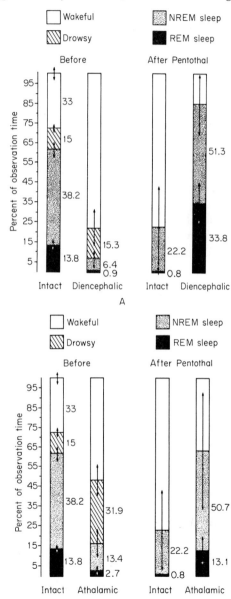

Fig. 4.6. The effects of intraperitoneally administered, subanesthetic doses of Pentothal on the percentages of sleep–wakefulness stages of: (A) intact (38.6 mg/kg) and diencephalic (8.3 mg/kg) cats; and (B) intact and athalamic (14.7 mg/kg) cats. The numbers beside the bars represent the average cumulative percentages for 13 experiments. See text for details.

effect of Pentothal in both the diencephalic and athalamic cats; these effects contrasted with the marked REMs suppressing effect of the drug in intact animals. The effect was more marked and regular in the diencephalic cat (Fig. 4.6A) in which there was a 37-fold increase in REMs with respect to the predrug condition and more than a twofold increase in relation to NREMs value in predrug, intact cats. Jouvet (1962b) reported periodic occurrence of REMs in neodecorticate cats treated with 15 to 20 mg/kg of Nembutal, whereas no REMs was observed with larger doses (30 mg/kg). Several barbiturates have been found to reduce REMs both in intact cats and in man (see Hartmann, 1967).

We interpret this data in the following way: first, in the diencephalic and athalamic animals, the caudal brain stem REMs mechanism had not been destroyed by surgery, but only functionally blocked by the sleep-suppressing mechanism; second, the activity of the blocking structure itself (supposedly, the hypothalamus or the subthalamus) was cancelled by the barbiturate, thereby eliminating the only remaining suppressive rostral influence upon caudal brain mechanisms. Therefore, with no influence descending from the rostral brain, a "neutral" point was reestablished which allowed for the sleep "rebound." In other words, under the action of the barbiturate, diencephalic and athalamic cats are comparable, with regard to sleep–wakefulness control, to cats with complete high mesencephalic transection, in that in all three conditions the caudal brain-stem mechanisms appear to operate free from rostral influences.

3. Sleep Postures

In the diencephalic cat, all the sleeping postures of the intact animal were seen at one time or another, and some cats exhibited them at all times. On the other hand, we never observed any of the normal somnic or presomnic postures in athalamic cats, i.e., they did not curl or roll up in the typical sleeping position of cats—and only fragments of the crouching posture were seen—nor did they stretch with the back arched and yawn, which are characteristic of the intact cat upon awakening. Gate ataxia and postural alterations were conspicuous motor disturbances in the athalamic cats, particularly in the early postoperative period.

Our findings in diencephalic cats are in agreement with observations in chronic decorticate cats (Rioch, 1954) and dogs (Kleitman and Camille, 1932), although, in contrast to our cats, the striatum was apparently left intact in those preparations. The observation that electrical stimulation of the diencephalon evokes the typical sleep postures (Hess, 1944; Akert et al., 1952) more easily and naturally than stimulation elsewhere (see Koella, 1967) is also in line with the present finding. We are not aware of any other sleep studies conducted in chronic cats with the thalamus totally removed. Naquet et al. (1965) did not describe the sleeping postures in their athalamic cats which lived for a maximum of 12 days.

Chronic cats with mesencephalic transection (Villablanca, 1966a) sleep in random positions. Since the hypothalamus was intact in both our diencephalic and athalamic animals, this structure cannot be implicated in causing any of the postural defects. Therefore, it seems safe to conclude that the thalamus itself is necessary for a full display of the normal postural patterns that are concomitant with sleep in the intact animal.

B. EEG—BEHAVIORAL OBSERVATIONS

1. Diencephalic Cats

a. EEG spindle bursts. In all diencephalic cats, the electrothalamogram (EThG) in the acute postoperative state was different from that in the chronic condition. During the first 3–5 postoperative days, rhythmic waves, occurring at the frequency (8–12 Hz) of cortical spindles and exhibiting a characteristic waxing and waning, were recorded from the thalamic leads (Fig. 4.7A). Their amplitude (15–50 μV) was about one-third the amplitude of the spindle waves recorded from the same leads in the intact cat. These spindle bursts were present when the cat was behaviorally drowsy or in NREMs, and they lasted until the animal shifted to REMs or awakened. Often they appeared as soon as the animal stopped its ongoing activity and at this time, they exhibited a relatively large voltage and a frequent rate of occurrence. During the following few moments, both voltage and rate of occurrence declined and attained a steady state. A decrease in neck muscle tone and ocular signs of drowsiness coincided with the abrupt onset of the spindle bursts. When the animal lapsed into REMs episodes, the EMG activity decreased markedly and almost simultaneously, bursts of spikes appeared at the pontine level (Fig. 4.8). After a delay of 15–30 sec, the spindles disappeared from the EThG. Likewise, at the end of the REMs period, if the animal continued sleeping, the spindles reappeared earlier than the EMG activity or the cessation of the pontine spikes.

On the third to the sixth postoperative days, the characteristics of the spindle waves changed in that they were lower in voltage, decreased in occurrence and altered in wave frequency (Fig. 4.7B). Usually, by the fifth postoperative day, no single distinctive feature of the spindle bursts could be observed. Similarly, whereas Pentothal induced profuse spindling during the first 3–5 postoperative days, it was ineffective in doing so thereafter.

Morison and Basset (1945) reported rhythmic spindle waves in the thalamus of neodecorticate cats and yet, doubts were cast upon this observation after the findings that spindle waves were absent in the thalamus of decorticate rabbits (Sergio and Longo, 1959) and cats (Jouvet, 1962b). However, in recent years,

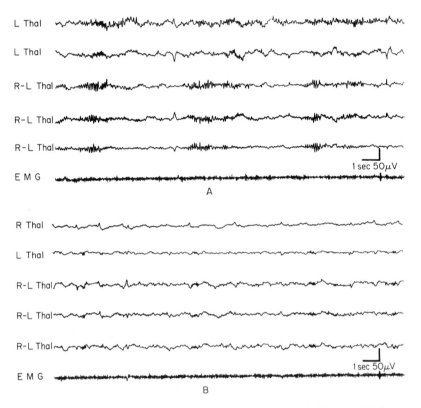

Fig. 4.7. Electrothalamogram of a behaviorally drowsy diencephalic cat on: (A) the second postoperative day showing the presence of spindle bursts; and (B) the fourth postoperative day showing the fading spindle activity. R Thal, right thalamus; L Thal, left thalamus; R-L Thal, right-left thalamus; EMG, electromyogram. R-L recordings are bipolar combinations between different leads of tripolar bilateral electrodes. All recordings are bipolar. [From Villablanca and Marcus, 1972]

the original Morison and Basset results have been repeatedly confirmed in diencephalic (Kellaway *et al.*, 1966; Villablanca and Schlag, 1968) and neodecorticate animals (Andersson and Manson, 1971). Whereas all the above experiments, except Jouvet's, were performed in acute or anesthetized cats, the present studies were performed in freely moving chronic diencephalic animals. In the latter condition, during the first to the fifth postoperative days, there is a positive correlation between the EThG spindling activity and the animal's behavior, i.e., the spindle waves are associated with drowsiness and with NREM behavioral sleep as occurs in the intact animal. This eliminates the suggestion (Jouvet, 1962b) that they could be related to irritation or diaschisis secondary to surgery in the acute preparation.

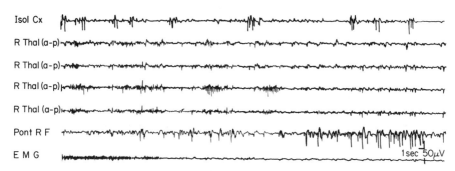

Fig. 4.8. EEG of a diencephalic cat on the third postoperative day showing the arrest of spindle burst activity about 35 sec after the onset of behavioral REMs. Isol Cx, isolated cortex; recording from frontal-parietal cortices of the isolated hemisphere. Note the absence of electrocortical changes with the onset of REMs. R Thal (a-p), right thalamus (anterior-posterior) indicates bipolar recordings between different leads of two tripolar electrodes—one located about 2 mm in front of the other—in the right thalamus; Pont R F, pontine reticular formation; EMG, electromyogram.

One wonders why the rhythmic thalamic EEG activity disappeared in diencephalic cats 3–4 days following surgery. It is possible that this is related to the retrograde degenerative cell changes which occur in the thalamus after surgery. More specifically, it suggests that the presence of spindles is linked to the integrity of the larger thalamic cells, since these are the first to degenerate (Carreras *et al.*, 1966). The finding of an early deterioration of the rhythmic activity fits well with Andersen's concept (Andersen and Andersson, 1968) that the recurrent axon collaterals of thalamic cortical projection cells are involved in the generation of the spindle burst; indeed, the axons of these larger cells and their collaterals should degenerate the earliest after cortical excision.

b. EEG synchronization. Although the spindle bursts disappeared, the EThG of the chronic diencephalic animal was not uniform thereafter. Changes related to sleep–wakefulness in our preparations were observed by visual inspection of the record or by employing the Drohocky Voltage Integrator (Goldstein and Beck, 1965). When the cat was awake, there were very low voltage waves (usually under 25 μV) of irregular frequencies, but having abundant components of frequencies over 10 Hz. (Fig. 4.9A). This EThG activity was similar to that recorded during the waking state from the thalamus of the same animal before surgery. As the level of vigilance decreased, there was a progressive increase in voltage and decrease in frequency of the EThG waves (Fig. 4.9B). When the animal was in behavioral NREMs, the background EThG voltage had at least doubled the voltage which prevailed during the waking state; this was further substantiated by counting the output of the integrator

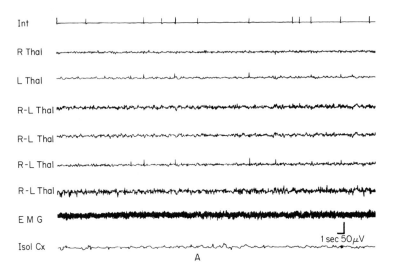

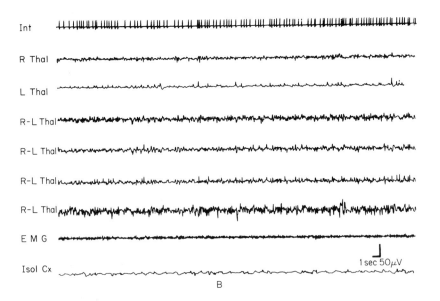

Fig. 4.9. EEG of a diencephalic cat on the 87th postoperative day showing the difference between the electrothalamographic activity during (A) wakefulness and (B) behavioral NREMs. Int, integrator; output of the Drohocky Integrator displaying pulses of voltage-integrated activity from the right thalamic lead. Note the marked increase in the number of pulses during NREMs. Other abbreviations as in Figs. 4.7 and 4.8. [From Villablanca and Marcus, 1972]

(Figs. 4.9 and 4.10) during behavioral sleep and wakefulness. In addition, during NREMs the frequency of the waves was slower but irregular. These EEG patterns ceased immediately when the animal awakened (Fig. 4.10) or went into REMs. From these data, there appears to be an analogy between the EThG of the diencephalic animal and the electrocorticogram of the intact cat, i.e., the EThG of diencephalic cats appears to be "synchronized" during NREMs and "desynchronized" during wakefulness.

The persistence of a slower, higher voltage EThG pattern during NREMs in chronic diencephalic cats may indicate a thalamic participation in the generation of slow wave EEG activity other than spindle bursts. We are aware however, that the present observation must be confirmed inasmuch as it has been reported (Jouvet, 1962b) that no signs of synchronization are observed in the thalamus of chronic decorticate cats.

c. EEG-behavioral coupling. Olfactory (sardine) and auditory (clicks, or noises familiar to the cat) stimuli were employed to assess the effects of external stimulation on the EEG and behavior. The diencephalic cats were highly reactive to smell and especially to sound. Subtle noises triggered brisk body movements with ocular arousal and orientation of the head toward the source of noise. Stronger, sudden sounds, e.g., handclaps, produced startle reactions with hissing and growling and even escape reactions characterized by sudden, fast, slinky running movements.

In all diencephalic cats, the EThG was closely correlated with behavior,

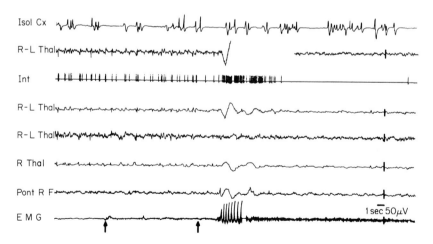

Fig. 4.10. EEG of a diencephalic cat on the 21st postoperative day showing electrothalamographic activity during sudden arousal by olfactory stimulation presented between arrows (see text for description of EEG-behavioral coupling). Abbreviations as in Figs. 4.7 and 4.8. [From Villablanca and Marcus, 1972]

i.e., a "synchronized" EThG recorded from a behaviorally sleeping cat reverted to a "desynchronized" pattern as soon as the animal awakened either spontaneously or by stimulation (Fig. 4.10). Furthermore, olfactory or acoustic stimuli of just enough intensity to produce a weak ocular arousal simultaneously changed the EThG "synchronized" activity to a less synchronized one.

2. *Athalamic Cats*

a. Cortical desynchronization and synchronization. During the first 10 postoperative days, irregular high voltage slow waves prevailed in the electrocorticogram (Fig. 4.11) of the athalamic cats with a dominant frequency of 2–4 Hz and an amplitude over 100 μV; this pattern resembled the EEG of NREMs in intact cats. With behavioral arousal this synchronization either did not change or the occurrence of the slow waves, as well as their voltage, tended to decrease.

With the passage of time following thalamectomy, EEG patterns which progressively resembled the desynchronized EEG of waking in intact cats were seen during the waking state. However, it was not until the 15th to 25th post-

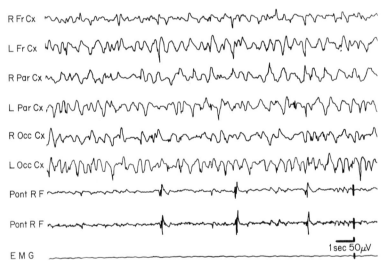

Fig. 4.11. EEG of an athalamic cat during behavioral REMs on the 6th postoperative day showing (1) the synchronized electrocorticographic pattern prevailing during the early postoperative period and (2) the dissociation between the pontine and EMG activity and the electrocorticogram. R. Fr Cx, right frontal cortex; L Fr Cx, left frontal cortex; R Par Cx, right parietal cortex; L Par Cx, left parietal cortex; R. Occ Cx, right occipital cortex; L Occ Cx, left occipital cortex; Pont R F, pontine reticular formation; EMG. electromyogram. The two pontine recordings are from two different leads of a tripolar electrode. All recordings are bipolar. [From Villablanca and Salinas-Zeballos, 1972]

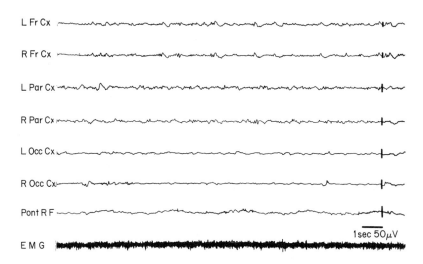

L Fr Cx

R Fr Cx

L Par Cx

R Par Cx

L Occ Cx

R Occ Cx

Pont R F

1 sec 50μV

E M G

Fig. 4.12. EEG of an athalamic cat during wakefulness on the 94th postoperative day showing electrocortical desynchronization. Abbreviations as in Fig. 4.11. [From Villablanca and Salinas-Zeballos, 1972]

operative day that a rather typical desynchronized EEG was observable (Fig. 4.12).

The EEG during REMs showed several unusual features. During the first 10 postoperative days, typical episodes of REMs, could occur without any change in the synchronized EEG pattern which prevailed at this stage (Fig. 4.11). However, at this time REM episodes often tended to be associated with EEG desynchrony; this association, like that seen during behavioral arousal, increased with the passage of time. The degree of desynchrony during REMs was directly proportional to the density of EEG pontine spikes, i.e., the slow waves disappeared from the EEG when there were frequent and dense bursts of pontine spikes (Fig. 4.13). Furthermore, more phasic EEG events had to occur to maintain a relatively desynchronized EEG during REMs in the acute than in the chronic state. At any rate, good cortical desynchrony was seen earlier after thalamectomy during REMs (15 postoperative days) than during behavioral wakefulness (15–25 postoperative days). Finally, the initiation of cortical desynchrony never coincided with the behavioral onset of REMs which constantly started in advance. In the acute animal there was a lag of up to several minutes between both events; this delay shortened and was never longer than 60 sec after 1–2 months.

The 8–12 Hz rhythmic spindlelike bursts were completely absent in the cortex from the very beginning in all athalamic cats; the absence persisted for as long as the animal survived and the rhythmic waves could not be induced

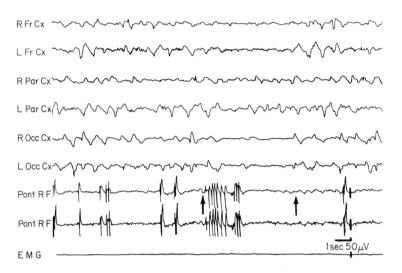

Fig. 4.13. EEG of an athalamic cat during behavioral REMs on the 6th postoperative day showing (1) the partial dissociation between the electrocorticogram and the pontine and EMG activity and (2) the tendency for cortical desynchrony (between arrows) to occur with dense bursts of pontine spikes. Abbreviations as in Fig. 4.11. [From Villablanca and Salinas-Zeballos, 1972]

by administration of Pentothal. Behavioral drowsiness in the chronic athalamic cat was heralded by the appearance of intermittent slow waves starting mainly in the frontal leads (Fig. 4.14) but spreading quickly to the rest of the cortex. Their occurrence and amplitude increased gradually if the cat continued to sleep and reached a fully developed pattern of EEG synchrony consisting of almost continuous irregular high voltage slow waves (Fig. 4.15).

The effect of visual, acoustic, and olfactory stimulation on the behavioral and EEG manifestation of sleep was studied in all cats. It was found that olfactory stimulation was the most effective in waking the animal; the acoustic and visual modalities followed in efficacy in the same order.

b. EEG-behavioral coupling. During approximately the first 10 postoperative days, the level of behavioral arousal of the athalamic cats could not be predicted by just looking at the animal's electrocorticogram; therefore, there existed a clear EEG-behavioral dissociation at this stage which decreased progressively with time. As a rule, however, in the chronic animal there was an EEG and behavioral coupling except during transitional periods (sleep to wakefulness, NREMs to REMs, or vice versa). An example of this transitional dissociation is shown in Fig. 4.16. Although the cat behaviorally awoke, as evidenced by ocular, EMG, and postural signs, the EEG remained synchronized; if the behavioral wakefulness persisted, the EEG desynchronized slowly.

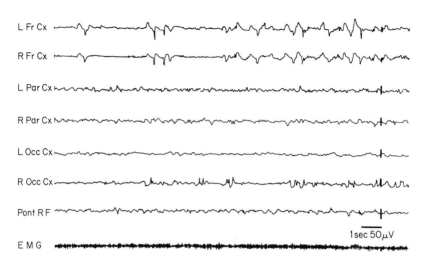

Fig. 4.14. EEG of an athalamic cat during the onset of drowsiness on the 94th post-operative day showing (1) the absence of electrocortical spindle bursts and (2) the initiation of slow wave activity occurring mainly in the frontal cortex. Abbreviations as in Fig. 4.11.

The longer the survival of the animal, the shorter was the delay of desynchronization with arousal, reaching a minimum delay of 10–20 sec after 3 months.

Several of our observations in athalamic cats have been previously reported. Kennard (1943) found a slower frequency in the skull EEG of monkeys after ablation of the massa intermedia or unilateral thalamic lesions. Knott et al. (1955) observed a marked reduction in the frequency of the EEG of cats—which persisted for a few days—with lesions predominately of the intralaminar nuclei. When the lesions encroached upon the region of the anterior thalamic nuclei, the EEG slowing lasted longer. In addition to reporting the occurrence of lasting high voltage slow waves after rostral thalamic lesions, Chow et al. (1959) found that with total destruction of the rostral thalamus there was a dissociation between EEG and behavioral arousal during the first postoperative days. Furthermore, they observed that in the long-term, chronic animal, the EEG spindle bursts were abolished and recovered only partially. Bach-y-Rita et al. (1966) reported homolateral absence of ECoG spindle bursts in their chronic cats with a massive unilateral thalamic lesion. In the experiments of Angeleri et al. (1969), unilateral destruction of the specific nuclei of the thalamus produced a homolateral increase in 2–5 Hz EEG activity which was more marked in the acute condition as well as in the cases in which the specific nuclei involvement was more extensive. Apparently the fast EEG activity recovered only in those cases in which the lesion affected only a few of the specific nuclei. The spindle bursts were affected, although not completely

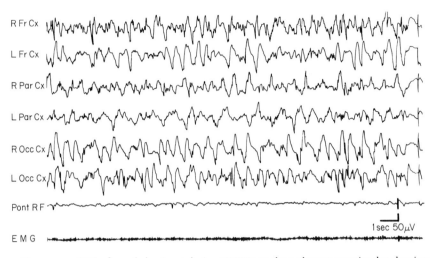

Fig. 4.15. EEG of an athalamic cat during NREMs on the 14th postoperative day showing (1) slow wave electrocortical activity and (2) absence of electrocortical spindle bursts. Abbreviations as in Fig. 4.11.

abolished, when the nonspecific nuclei were lesioned or when there was destruction of many specific nuclei. In the totally thalamectomized cats of Naquet *et al.* (1965), the spindle waves no longer were observed in the electrocorticogram.

The evidence presently available indicates that the rhythmic spindle waves have a thalamic origin. Two of the main sources of data justifying this assertion have been dealt with in this paper. They include the demonstration of the persistence of the spindle bursts during the first postoperative days in the thalamus of the diencephalic cat, and the absence of the spindle bursts after thalamic lesions. A third line of evidence stems from electrophysiological experiments which have been covered by Anderssen's lecture (see page 127 of this volume) and by the monograph of Anderssen and Anderson (1968). Furthermore, it appears that the diencephalon is the only structure from which the spindles can spontaneously originate. On the one hand, it has been demonstrated that spindle waves are present in the diencephalon disconnected from supradiencephalic and lower brain-stem areas (Kellaway *et al.*, 1966; Villablanca and Schlag, 1968; Anderson and Manson, 1971). On the other hand, it is known that spindles do not occur spontaneously either in a cerebral hemisphere disconnected from the diencephalon (Kellaway *et al.* 1966; Villablanca, 1966c), or in the brain stem separated from the rostral brain (Jouvet, 1962b; Villablanca, 1966a).

The desynchronizing role of the thalamus on the cortical EEG is supported by data collected in stimulation experiments. Several authors have demon-

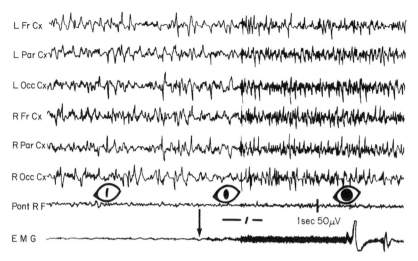

Fig. 4.16. EEG of an athalamic cat on the 34th postoperative day showing the dissociation between the electrocorticogram and behavior during the transition from behavioral NREMs to wakefulness. At the arrow, the cat aroused according to EMG and behavioral criteria; however, the electrocorticogram did not desynchronize until about 40 sec later when the cat stood. Note change in paper speed. Abbreviations as in Fig. 4.11. [From Villablanca and Salinas-Zeballos, 1972]

strated that desynchronization of the EEG can be induced by high frequency stimulation of the so-called nonspecific thalamic system (Jasper, 1949; Jasper *et al.*, 1948; Moruzzi and Magoun, 1949; Starzl *et al.* 1951; Jasper and Ajmone-Marsan, 1952; Akimoto *et al.* 1956). Concomitant with the EEG effects, behavioral manifestations of phasic arousal have been observed (Jasper, 1960; Hösli and Monnier, 1962). Using the stimulation technique, Nakamura and Ohye (1964) studied the individual role of thalamic nuclei in the thalamically induced desynchronization of the ECoG in acute cats. They concluded that the corticopetal impulses arising in the thalamic relay nuclei are involved in suppressing the 2–4 Hz delta waves, whereas the nonspecific thalamic areas appear to be involved in suppressing the neocortical 8–12 Hz spindle bursts.

Schlag and Chaillet (1963) reported that a partial interruption of the mesencephalon at the level of mesodiencephalic junction—sparing the tegmental reticular system—prevented the EEG arousal induced by high frequency stimulation of the intralaminar and midline nuclei. This suggests that the desynchronizing effect of thalamic stimulation is mediated by the caudal brain-stem reticular formation. It should be pointed out, however, that the latter experiments were performed in acute animals and hence, the possibility remains that in a chronic preparation such stimulation may be effective in desynchronizing the cortex. In other words, it is suggested that the thalamus might exert its influence upon the cortex by means of both cortical and subcortical connections.

When the thalamus is no longer a source of desynchronization for the neocortex, the only remaining desynchronizing structure is probably the reticular activating system. It is well known that there are extrathalamic pathways for the ascending desynchronizing effect of the brain-stem reticular formation (Starlz *et al.*, 1951; Nauta and Kuypers, 1958; Tissot and Monnier, 1959). The other two areas with known potentiality for producing cortical desynchronization, namely the hypothalamus (Ranson, 1939; Ingram *et al.* 1951; Hess, 1954; Koella and Gellhorn, 1954; Collins, 1954) and the subthalamus (Naquet *et al.*, 1965; Bach-y-Rita and Baurand, 1966), apparently influence the neocortex mainly via the thalamus (see Crosby *et al.*, 1962) and their action would thus be greatly impaired in the athalamic cat.

The finding that in the athalamic cat cortical desynchronization accompanying REMs reappears earlier postoperatively than that observed during wakefulness, indicates that either the desynchrony during REMs is stronger than that of wakefulness in the intact cat or that the extrathalamic route is more efficient in conducting the caudal brain-stem desynchronizing influences arising during REMs than those originating during wakefulness. We do not know of any data supporting either possibility.

The EEG-behavioral dissociation is another intriguing problem. It has been shown that complete dissociation between electrocorticographic events and the behavior of the animal's body occurs after mesencephalic transection (Villablanca, 1966a). This finding has been interpreted as an experimental separation of rostral structures controlling sleep–wakefulness from those areas having a similar function but located behind the transection (Villablanca, 1966a; see Moruzzi's chapter in this book). The EEG-behavioral dissociation probably results from the interruption of ascending and descending pathways interrelating both rostral and caudal sets of controlling mechanisms in the intact animal. Partial dissociation has been reported to occur in animals with either incomplete mesencephalic transections or incomplete reticular formation lesions (Hubel and Nauta, 1960; Feldman and Waller, 1962; Hobson, 1965). These findings may be explained as a partial disruption of the pathways normally coupling rostral and caudal sleep–wakefulness controlling mechanisms. Similarly, this may explain the dissociation occurring in athalamic cats, since it is known that influences ascending from the caudal brain stem pass through the thalamus (Nauta and Kuypers, 1958; Scheibel and Scheibel, 1958; Cowan *et al.*, 1964; Bowsher, 1967).

An alternative hypothesis is that the thalamus has EEG-behavioral coupling properties of its own. There are at least two arguments in support of this postulate: first, in the chronic *cerveau isolé* cat with a transection just behind the third nerve nuclei (Villablanca, 1966b) there is an adequate coupling between the ECoG and the oculopupillary behavior which suggests that an independent rostral brain mechanism (probably thalamic) is responsible; second, as stated above, in diencephalic cats there is an adequate EEG-behavioral coupling.

III. Conclusions

From the foregoing, it is apparent that sleep and wakefulness can still continue after lesions obliterating most of the thalamus. Are we to conclude that the thalamus has no important role in sleep–wakefulness physiology? Although it is well known that movements can continue after removal of the motor cortex, ablation of the striatum, section of the pyramids, and, as a matter of fact, after the removal of the whole forebrain, no physiologist would maintain that the cerebrum does not have an important role in the physiology of movement.

According to our results, we propose that the sleep–wakefulness which remains after thalamic destruction is severely altered, both from a quantitative as well as from a qualitative standpoint. What remains is sleep-wakefulness with marked traits of "dissolution," to borrow Jacksonian terminology.

To be more specific and in an attempt to conclude with an answer to our initial question as to what the thalamus contributes to sleep–wakefulness physiology, let me summarize the main conclusions stemming from the present experiments and the supporting evidence presented in this paper. The thalamus appears to be:

1. Essential for an adequate balance between enhancing and suppressing influences of the rostral brain impinging upon caudal brain-stem sleep-wakefulness controlling structures. A permanent, pronounced reduction of both NREMs and REMs is created after inflicting direct or indirect damage to the thalamus

2. Essential for the performance of most of the postural manifestations concomitant with sleep. Most of the somnic and postsomnic sleep postures disappear after thalamectomy, whereas they are present in the diencephalic cat

3. Essential for the generation of EEG rhythmic spindle waves. It has been shown that the spindle waves persist in an isolated thalamus and disappear when the thalamus degenerates or is surgically removed

4. Important as a cortical desynchronizing mechanism. The EEG desynchronization during wakefulness and during REMs is markedly impaired after thalamectomy and recovers slowly in the chronic condition.

5. Important for the normal coupling of rostral brain and caudal brain stem sleep–wakefulness controlling mechanisms and hence for an adequate EEG-behavioral coupling. A striking EEG-behavioral dis-

sociation is produced by large thalamic lesions and this dissociation decreases with long-standing chronicity.

Finally, we do not maintain that the thalamus is "the head ganglion of sleep"; however, we suggest emphatically that the thalamus is important for the normal display of the sleep–wakefulness cycle.

ACKNOWLEDGMENT

I wish to express my gratitude to A. L. Fierro and A. D. Hermosilla for their technical assistance, Drs. R. Marcus and M. E. Salinas-Zeballos for their participation in some stages of the research, and A. F. Koithan and G. M. Ruiz de Pereda for the histological work. I am indebted to R. J. Marcus (Department of Psychiatry, UCLA) for kindly assisting me in reviewing and editing the English version of this manuscript.

Discussion

Jouvet: I do not think that you can demonstrate a quantitative change in paradoxical sleep just by looking at the behavior of ten cats; in order to do this, you must perform EEG recordings from leads placed in adequate structures. We have found that two convenient locations are the hippocampus and the pontine reticular formation (Jouvet, 1962b). Using these techniques in decorticate cats we have demonstrated that during the first 2–3 postoperative days paradoxical sleep stays within normal levels (Jouvet, 1962b). After the first week we found that paradoxical sleep represents 10% of the observation time. We do not think that this is a significant decrease in paradoxical sleep because we find the same percentage in sham-operated animals.

Villablanca: First, let me reiterate that we performed many 2–24-hr duration polygraphic recording sessions in our cats (76 in the diencephalic and 53 in the athalamic) and that the results were included in Figs. 4.3 and 4.4. During the first postoperative month they represented about 10% of observation periods inasmuch as the operated cats, particularly the diencephalic cats, could not be restrained for long recording periods (which in itself indicates that they were not in REMs) and that at that early stage of the research we did not know at all whether we were going to find any constant EEG-behavioral correlation in these animals (in fact we found that in the athalamic animals there was an almost total dissociation between the electrocortico-gram and the behavior and an abnormal onset of EEG and behavioral signs of REMs). After the first month the polygraphic recordings were increased to encompass about one-third of the total observation time. At this time it was clear that there was a correlation between the thalamic EEG and NREMs in the diencephalic cats and at the same time the dissociation between the EEG and behavior was reduced considerably in the athalamic animals. The EEG recording thus became more meaningful. In fact, after the first postoperative month the percentages of the sleep–wakefulness patterns were not significantly different when the states were evaluated by behavioral criteria alone or when both behavioral and polygraphic criteria were used. Furthermore, our experience indicates (Villablanca, 1965, 1966b) that pupillary and ocular behavior are highly reliable indices of the different stages of sleep and of wakefulness in animals with extensive CNS lesions, as is the case in intact cats (Berlucchi et al., 1964b).

Concerning the comparison between the results in decorticate cats reported in your 1962 paper (Jouvet, 1962b) and the present results, we should first recognize that they are in agreement in that NREMs is drastically reduced. The results concerning REMs are totally different since you reported that REMs represented 15 to 20% of the total observation time in your decorticate cats. I would suggest that this is because we are dealing with two different experimental animals; in your 1962 paper your animals are described as only neo-decorticated and hence I assume that the striatum was intact as well as the ventral and dorsal hippocampus (as stated in Fig. 11 of that paper); in contrast our cats were essentially diencephalic animals since *both* the striatum and limbic system were ablated or extensively lesioned. I have quoted experimental data (see text) suggesting that the presence of the striatum and limbic system might influence sleep and wakefulness in decorticate animals. You have now added some new information and stated that, indeed, your chronic decorticate cats spent 10% of their time in REMs and so do sham-operated animals. I think that this figure represents in fact about a 33% decrease in REMs. However, I do not understand why sham-operated animals also show such a decrease.

Jouvet: If we were to accept that the striatum facilitates PS, we would still be left with an important problem; this is, how could we explain the finding that PS is not reduced significantly in mesencephalic and pontine cats. This is a point in which both your experiments and ours show similar results.

Villablanca: This would be a difficult problem if we were to conceive of the striatum as the *only* rostral brain structure influencing the caudal brain-stem mechanisms involved in REMs. Instead, what we are proposing is a *dual* control whereby both enhancing and suppressing influences impinge upon caudal brain-stem mechanisms and modulate their function in a balanced manner. Both types of influences are removed in the mesencephalic and pontine cats and hence the basic REMs mechanisms, which are situated caudal to the brain-stem transection, can operate freely and in an almost automatic manner as you yourself have demonstrated (Jouvet, 1965b). A *partial* forebrain lesion instead would then create an imbalance in the descending control, resulting in a dominance by one of the influences, i.e., sleep suppressing or wakefulness enhancing, as postulated for the present experiments. A similar model has been proposed for other CNS functions as for example the descending forebrain control of caudal brain-stem mechanisms related to the tonus of the postural muscles; an imbalance in this descending control can cause an exaggeration (hypertonus) or a decrease (hypotonus) in postural tonus.

Jouvet: From my standpoint when attempting to decide which brain areas are the most closely related to sleep control, it is important to define the location of the smallest brain lesion which can induce the longest total insomnia. At the present time I think that the only lesion fulfilling these requirements is the one destroying the raphe nuclei of the brain stem. I am still waiting for someone to demonstrate such an insomnia after destruction of another similarly small brain area.

Villablanca: I am not disputing the fact that the brain stem contains the basic mechanisms for sleep and wakefulness, as it does contain the basic mechanism for many other CNS functions. What I am trying to demonstrate is that these mechanisms are not autonomous but that they are under important controls descending from the rostral brain. In other words, that the destruction of the raphe nuclei produces insomnia does not mean that they are the only structures concerned with sleep regulation. This would imply a return to the concept of a "sleep center" which I think is untenable in view of our present knowledge. Furthermore, it does not mean that they are the most important structures in this control either because they may subserve a very primitive, unsophisticated "sleep" function. Discrete lesions of the brain-stem nuclei and pathways related to motor control can have devastating effects in the performance of movements and yet no one would maintain that the forebrain has no importance in such a control.

Albe-Fessard: I would like to recall that Drs. Naquet, Denavit, Lanoir and myself (1965) have also studied cats without a thalamus. The survival period of the animals was only 12 days and the EEG recording periods were 2 to 4 hr every 24 hr. The main finding in these cats was the absence of EEG spindle bursts. An important question concerning all these preparations is, in my thinking, the state of the cerebral cortex after 12 days of thalamectomy. Another group of cats in our experiments received only a medial thalamectomy, the ventrobasal complex and lateral geniculate being preserved. Spindle bursts persisted on the posterior cortical areas in these cases.

Koella: The surgical bilateral thalamectomy and the long survival of the animals in Dr. Villablanca's work are certainly an accomplishment; I wish he would tell us a little more about the technique.

Villablanca: The operation was performed through a midline craneotomy. The sagittal sinus was sectioned between two ligatures and the underlying falx was cut at this level. After gently retracting the cerebral hemispheres, the corpus callosum was aspirated in the midline, exposing the third ventricle and the dorsal thalamus. The thalamus was removed by aspiration. Natural landmarks were used as references to delimit the thalamus (thalamostriate junction, outer edge of the fornix, columna fornicis, anterior and posterior commissures) except for the ventral and lateral boundaries. To delimit the lateral thalamic boundary, a needle was stereotaxically placed slightly medial to the lateral limit of the thalamic mass (and removed after the ablation); the tip of the two lateral needles and the level of the anterior commissure were used as references for the ventral limit of the suction. At the end, the bone defect was covered with a prosthesis of cranioplastic material.

Koella: Concerning the interesting discussion which this work has promoted, I would like to suggest an integrative viewpoint. I am sure that both Drs. Villablanca and Jouvet are correct concerning the participation of the cerebral cortex and the raphe nuclei in the control of sleep; but Drs. Clemente and Sterman (Sterman and Clemente, 1962a) and Dr. Parmeggiani (Parmeggiani and Zanoco, 1963) were probably also correct when they suggested a participation of the basal forebrain area and the hippocampus respectively. Now, sleep is not a simple thing. There are a number of factors which play on the "input-side" of the "system," e.g., an internal clock, a "need" or "pressure" for sleep, probably biochemical in nature, neurohumoral influences, external and internal neuronal factors. Furthermore, some of these may be involved in the form of negative as well as positive feedback loops. Also, on the output side we have the numerous sleep signs, manifestations of functional changes taking place with the onset of sleep, and of particular sleep states. All these multiple inputs and outputs make it necessary that many structures participate in the organization of sleep.

What we would like to propose here, as we have done in a previous publication (Koella, 1967), is that the activity of all these areas must in some way be interrelated or integrated to achieve a smooth, coordinated control of sleep.

CHAPTER FIVE

Forebrain Mechanisms for the Onset of Sleep

MAURICE B. STERMAN
CARMINE D. CLEMENTE

With few exceptions the two basic patterns of slow wave sleep (SWS) and rapid eye movement sleep (REM) are present with remarkably similar characteristics from marsupials (Van Twyver and Allison, 1970) to man (Williams *et al.*, 1964). Because of this similarity and the consistent sequential appearance of these two patterns during sleep, it has been concluded generally that their neural substrates appeared simultaneously in evolution (Snyder, 1966) and represent separate but integrated components of a fundamental sleep mechanism organized in the brain stem (Jouvet, 1967a). This assumption has directed the strategies which most investigators have developed in seeking the neural substrate for a sleep mechanism in the mammalian brain. Several observations, however, are in discord with these conclusions. Studies of electroencephalographic and other physiological patterns in several reptiles (Klein *et al.*, 1964; Tauber *et al.*, 1968) and in the echidna, a primitive mammal (Allison and Goff, 1968b), indicated the presence of SWS with no clear manifestations of REM. Conversely, studies of the human fetus (Sterman and Hoppenbrouwers, 1971) and newborn infants (Parmelee and Stern, 1972) indicate that periodic REM may be present in the absence of an integrated SWS. Additionally, experiments carried out in brain-transected cats have shown that the two patterns can clearly be dissociated, with SWS appearing in the isolated forebrain (Bremer, 1935;

83

Villablanca, 1966a,b; Slosarska and Zernicki, 1969) and REM in the isolated brain stem (Jouvet, 1961, 1962, 1965a,b; Matsuzaki *et al.*, 1964). These findings suggest that alternate conclusions and strategies are possible.

In a recent electrophysiological and behavioral study of the salamander (*Ambystoma tigrinum*), Lucas *et al.* (1969) found none of the characteristic mammalian polygraphic manifestations of sleep and waking states, thus confirming the previous observations of Hobson (1967) and Hobson *et al.* (1968) in several amphibians. Yet, the salamander exhibited periods of behavioral activity (elevated head, locomotion, feeding, and withdrawal from stimuli) alternating in a regular manner with periods of quiescence (lowered head, inactivity, and regular respiration). From a behavioral standpoint, the resulting picture is one of periodic activity and quiescence (Fig. 5.1). Perhaps this relatively simple dichotomy in behavior is a phylogenetic antecedent to the more clearly expressed central and peripheral patterns of sleep and wakefulness which appear with higher levels of encephalization.

Kleitman (1963, 1967), however, drew attention long ago to another periodic alternation in state, that occurring during sleep between the SWS and REM patterns. He felt that this periodicity reflected a "basic rest–activity cycle" which could modulate brain activity during wakefulness also. He attributed this to a neural integration *more primitive* than the sleep–waking processes. There is now substantial evidence that a shorter and more basic periodicity of this type does exist both in man as an approximately 90-min cycle (Globus, 1970; Kripke *et al.*, 1971; Othmer *et al.*, 1969; Friedman and Fisher, 1967; Sterman, 1972), and in the cat as a 20-min cycle (Sterman *et al.*, 1972). As was mentioned previously, the pontine cat is capable of expressing, simul-

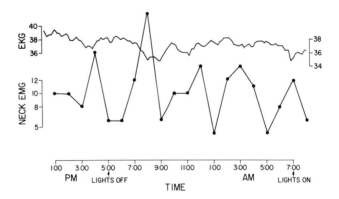

Fig. 5.1. Modulation of motor behavior over a 24-hr period in the tiger salamander. Note that periodic increases in neck EMG, reflecting head position and general somatic activity, describe a rest–activity cycle of 3–4 hr in this poikilothermic animal.

taneously, SWS and REM in recordings obtained from the separated forebrain and brain stem, respectively. In several of our investigations (McGinty *et al.*, 1971; Sterman, 1972), we have observed this same dissociation of states. Moreover, we have noted that the periodic occurrence of REM in the isolated brain stem of the cat can show a strong similarity in period to that determined in the normal animal, although classification of the states of sleep and wakefulness becomes arbitrary at best. These findings confirm the conclusion of Jouvet 1965b, 1967a,b, 1969a,b) that the neural substrate of the REM state is organized within the pontine level of the brain stem. However, together with the other considerations noted above, these facts could be interpreted as indicating that this mechanism is, in fact, independent of sleep and represents a neural integration functionally more basic and phylogenetically antecedent to the mammalian sleep–waking rhythm.

It is indeed possible, therefore, that the intrinsic physiological integration of the salamander limits this animal to a "basic rest–activity cycle" whose 3–4 hr period reflects the characteristically low metabolic activity in this poikilothermic animal. Several investigators have demonstrated a relationship between REM periodicity and basal metabolic rate (Weiss and Roldan, 1964; Jouvet, 1967a; McGinty *et al.*, 1971). From this point of view, subsequent adaptations in the highly successful mammalian series could be attributed to the development of brain mechanisms which provided for sustained periods of activity followed by sustained periods of quiescence. Within these states, however, the rest–activity cycle continued to be manifest, perhaps serving as the temporal unit from which wakefulness and sleep were knit (Kleitman, 1967). We propose that the capacity for maintenance of the waking state was attendant upon the functional evolution of a nonspecific mesodiencephalic reticular formation (Magoun, 1952; Rossi and Zanchetti, 1957) and that for sleep upon the parallel development of forebrain mechanisms antagonistic to this activating system. If, indeed, advantage did accrue to organisms developing mechanisms for sustained wakefulness and sustained sleep, evolution would have made several attempts at maximizing one or the other before arriving at the more or less balanced arrangement seen in most mammals. Consistent with this possibility are the findings that the shrew, an insectivore, shows little if any sleep in laboratory observations (Van Twyver and Allison, 1969) while the primitive opossum consistently sleeps 75–85% of the time under similar conditions (Snyder, 1966; Van Twyver and Allison, 1970).

Our concern over the past decade has been with the elucidation of what was to us a requisite forebrain involvement in the process of sleep. The findings of Hess (1943), Nauta (1946), and Kaada (1951), in particular, focused our attention in this regard to basal forebrain structures. In a continuing series of investigations we have established that (1) electrical stimulation, at both high (300 Hz) and low (5–7 Hz) frequencies, of the preoptic area of the hypothalamus and adjacent basal telencephalic structures (collectively termed the "basal forebrain region") elicits EEG slow waves (Sterman and Clemente, 1962a) and behavioral sleep (Sterman and Clemente, 1962b). In other studies, stimulation of this area slowed runway performance through an apparent inhibitory influence upon mesencephalic reticular formation (Sterman and Fairchild, 1966) and produced postsynaptic inhibition (hyperpolarization) of brain stem (Nakamura *et al.*, 1967) and spinal cord (Sauerland *et al.*, 1967) motor reflex discharge. (2) These induced EEG and behavioral patterns can be associated with a previously neutral environmental event (i.e., a tone) which in turn acquires the capacity to elicit sleep conditionally (Clemente *et al.*, 1963). (3) Bilateral destruction of this area results in a marked suppression of all sleep patterns and a corresponding increase in wakefulness with associated hyperactivity (Sterman *et al.*, 1964; McGinty and Sterman, 1968). (4) Projections from this area connect it functionally with orbital cortex, hippocampus, amygdala, midline thalamus, and mesencephalic reticular formation (Clemente and Sterman, 1963, 1967; Mizuno *et al.*, 1969). Many of these findings subsequently were confirmed in other laboratories (Kaneko *et al.*, 1962; Hernandez-Peon, 1962; Nielson and Davis, 1966; Nauta, 1964; Scheibel and Scheibel, 1967; Morgane, 1969; Roberts and Robinson, 1969; Taylor and Branch, 1971; Madoz and Reinoso-Suarez, 1968; Bremer, 1970a).

We have attempted to understand the mechanism whereby activation of elements within this basal forebrain region can influence ongoing behavior and initiate sleep. Several explanations can be considered. One that has been forwarded recently is that the effects of electrical stimulation, the procedure employed in our early studies, are not functionally significant, but merely another reflection of the proclivity for the EEG to be synchronized by almost any kind of regular, low frequency central or peripheral stimulus (Jouvet, 1967a,b, 1969a,b). This explanation is, unfortunately, a gross over-simplification which does not consider the important procedural and physiological discrepancies among the many investigations which have employed electrical stimulation. This point was elaborated recently by Doty (1969), who stressed the unique capacity for high frequency basal forebrain stimulation to induce sleep rapidly in a normal behaving cat, unlike stimulation of other structures, such as caudate, thalamus, and brain stem, where low frequencies and long delays were required (high frequencies produce arousal). Electrical stimulation of the basal forebrain region produced EEG synchronization which was often preceded by both gross and specific behavioral adjustments antecedent to sleep (finding a corner, lying down, and assuming a characteristic sleep posture). Moreover, these responses became rapidly associated with contingent environmental circumstances which, in turn, were capable of eliciting the same sequence of behavioral and physiological changes without application of electrical stimulation.

A more reasonable explanation for the sleep influences of basal forebrain manipulations could derive from the proximity of this region to important regulatory mechanisms in the adjacent hypothalamus. Taylor and Branch (1971) reported that EEG synchronization induced by basal forebrain stimulation was accompanied by an inhibition of pituitary-adrenal function, as indicated by a corresponding phasic depression of adrenal steroid secretion (Fig. 5.2). What is known about state-specific variations in plasma corticosteroids indicates that their levels in both cat and man are lowest at the onset of peak sleep periods (Krieger, 1970; Weitzman et al., 1966). However, the depression of plasma corticosteroid levels in the Taylor and Branch study could not be directly responsible for sleep onset, since the time course of humoral changes lagged significantly behind induced EEG synchronization. It is likely that the delayed suppression of ACTH secretion following basal forebrain stimulation was secondary to other more direct changes in neural

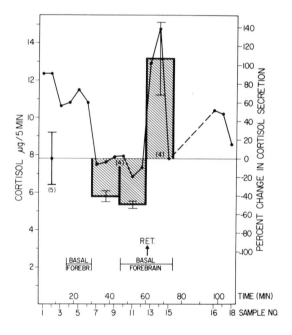

Fig. 5.2. Effects of basal forebrain and reticular formation stimulation on cortisol secretion in the cat. Solid and dashed lines indicate typical response patterns in one animal, while vertical bar (control base line) and cross-hatched columns show mean percentage changes in a group of five cats. Thirty sec of low-frequency basal forebrain stimulation were delivered every minute for 15 and 30 min, respectively, as indicated by horizontal bars at bottom. A single 10-sec stimulus applied to reticular formation is indicated by arrow during the second basal forebrain stimulation period. Note delayed tonic inhibitory effect of forebrain stimulation on pituitary-adrenal activity and phasic reversal resulting from brief brain-stem stimulation. [From Taylor and Branch, 1971]

integration resulting from this stimulation. Since the neural mechanisms of the stress-induced and circadian ACTH secretions have been found to be different (Hodges, 1970), the phasic changes in corticosteroid levels noted above may have resulted from a reduction in stress consequent to stimulation of the basal forebrain area in these surgical preparations and reflected by the occurrence of generalized EEG synchronization.

The preoptic-anterior hypothalamic region in general has been associated with thermoregulatory mechanisms in the mammalian brain. Roberts and Robinson (1969) showed convincingly that thermal stimulation of an area overlapping with the basal forebrain region produced behavioral and EEG sleep patterns in the cat. They concluded from this observation that thermo-receptors in this region were an important source of input to the sleep-regulating influences represented there. Comparable experiments were more recently reported by DeArmond and Fusco (1971). It is conceivable that local heating resulting from electrical stimulation of this region activates the first line of thermal–regulatory defense against hyperthermia in the mammalian system, namely behavioral quiescence. That this is not the sole function of this area, however, is indicated by some differences in electrically and thermally induced sleep patterns. In the former, the induced behavioral response frequently, but not always, included the heat-retaining postural response of curling up and burying the head into the midsection, as is usually the case under natural sleep conditions in the domestic cat. Thermal stimulation resulted in behavioral quiescence characterized by a stretching out of the body and, at higher inten-sities, panting. The feature common to both types of stimulation is a suppres-sion of ongoing behavior, a consistent result of basal forebrain stimulation. We have seen this also in relation to aggressive behavior (Sterman and Clemente, 1962b), and feeding (Sterman et al., 1969). Moreover, stimulation of the basal forebrain produced a suppression of motor reflex responses (Clemente and Sterman, 1967) and reticular formation evoked potentials (Bremer, 1970a), both of which are consistent, neurophysiologically, with these behavioral observations. The termination of ongoing behavior can serve many aspects of physiological regulation, including heat loss, and is also an essential pre-requisite for sleep. Specifically organized regulatory processes within the hypothalamus and adjacent limbic structures may utilize a common basal fore-brain mechanism for behavior suppression to their respective ends, all of which can ultimately involve sleep.

Because of the current interest in neurochemical mediation of sleep, as indicated clearly in this text, and the delay in sleep disturbances which we described in our earlier studies of lesions placed in the basal forebrain area (3–7 days), it has been suggested that the influences induced by stimulation in this region be viewed within the context of neurochemical mechanisms. We have carried out a number of subsequent investigations, directed at two pertinent questions in this regard: (1) What is the time course of events relating basal forebrain influences to behavior? (2) What relationships exist between the basal forebrain sleep mechanism and the raphe nuclei serotonergic system of the brain stem described by Jouvet (1967a,b, 1969a,b).

Two experiments relate to the first question. In previous studies of basal forebrain lesion effects, we had not examined behavior immediately following tissue destruction for a number of technical reasons. In a recent study of the temporal organization of sleep and waking states in the cat (Lucas and Sterman, 1972), the basal forebrain area was damaged bilaterally *in unanesthetized animals* with the delivery of current between focal electrode tips placed in the preoptic region with a generalized indifferent lead in neck muscle tissue. The animals showed no adverse response to this procedure. Long-term, continuous poly-graphic recordings were obtained immediately before the placement of lesions and on days 1, 3, 7, 14, and 26 afterward. Bilateral lesions of this area, but not of posterior thalamus or dorsal midbrain, often produced an immediate and profound suppression of sleep. These animals became acutely hyperactive, circled the chamber incessantly, but showed no lasting disruption of temperature regulation or feeding (Fig. 5.3). In fact, animals trained to perform an operant response for food continued to do so during prolonged periods of wakefulness such that it was possible to conclude that more or less normal periodicity in alimentary behavior was preserved. The disruption of sleep patterns persisted for several weeks and showed a gradual, and sometimes only partial, recovery by 26 days (Fig. 5.4). The rather regular ultradian sleep-

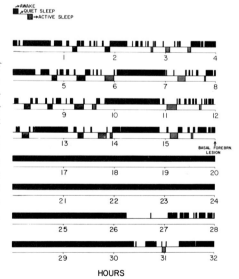

Fig. 5.3. Schematic representation of physiological state patterns in a cat over a continuous 32-hr period at midpoint of which the basal forebrain region was damaged bilaterally (arrow). Lesions were produced without anesthesia or other disturbances of the animal. Note the regular alternation of waking and sleep periods (sleep–waking cycle) prior to placement of lesions. The sleep–waking cycle is replaced by continuous wakefulness for at least 10 hr following the lesion and remains disrupted for periods in excess of several months.

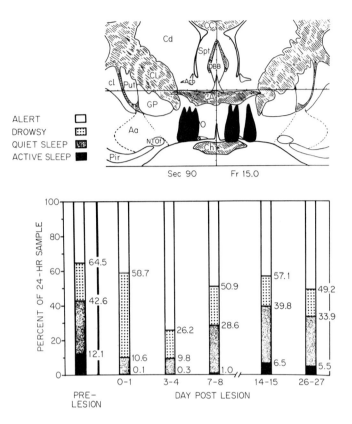

Fig. 5.4. Diagrammatic representation of bilateral basal forebrain lesions in a cat, together with resulting alterations in 24-hr percentage values for four basic physiological patterns on test days following destruction of this tissue. The first postlesion 24-hr sample was obtained immediately after placement of the lesions. Numbers indicate pattern percentages on sample days. [From Lucas and Sterman, 1972]

waking cycle of the cat (see, for example, first 16 hr of Fig. 5.3) was badly fragmented, while the rest–activity cycle (determined by performance episodes in waking and by the eventual reappearance of recurrent REM during sleep) remained comparable in period to prelesion data. Thus, the disturbances produced by basal forebrain lesions were both immediate and progressive and involved primarily a disruption of the sleep pattern and sleep–waking cycle and not the shorter, 20-min, rest–activity cycle reflected by recurrent performance and REM episodes.

Some indication of temporal events involving the basal forebrain region directly with sleep may be provided by recent studies from our laboratory of the spontaneous activity of preoptic cells in behaving cats. Recording of extracellular unit activity during normal transitions between wakefulness and sleep

has been made possible by the development of fine wire microelectrode techniques (Harper and McGinty, 1973). Most cells in the brain change their rate
or pattern of discharge as the animal moves from wakefulness through the two
basic patterns in sleep. Harper has found that many preoptic cells, however,
show a rather distinctive alteration in discharge specifically with the onset of
sleep. These elements, whose discharge during waking behavior is irregular and
rather low in rate, showed a marked increase in discharge rate and an intense
bursting pattern in direct correspondence to the assumption of a quiet posture
and the onset of EEG slow wave activity (Fig. 5.5). Once a true sleep state is
achieved, as indicated by spindle burst and slow wave activity in the EEG, these
units returned to their presleep pattern and rate of discharge. It is conceivable
that such elements give rise to a diffuse descending pathway whose projections
into midbrain tegmentum act to terminate or inhibit ongoing behavior, elicit
resting postures and reduce corticopetal discharge, such that a changed central
integration can be achieved which results in sleep behavior.

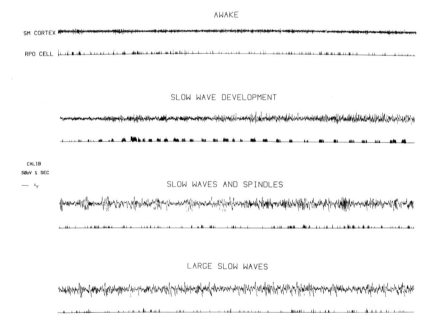

Fig. 5.5. Comparison of sensorimotor cortex EEG activity and basal forebrain (right preoptic)
are a single-cell spike discharge during wakefulness, sleep onset, early slow wave sleep, and late
slow wave sleep in the same cat. Note the distinctive increase in firing rate and bursting discharge
pattern during the transition to slow wave sleep. The cell responded with this characteristic
pattern on each of many occasions when the animal initiated sleep during a prolonged recording
period.

The basal forebrain region was found previously to receive inputs from frontal cortex and thalamus, to be involved in a number of limbic system feedback pathways, and to respond to thermal and neurochemical influences. Efferent projections from this region include medial and midline thalamus, epithalamus, and mescencephalic tegmentum. More recently we have found physiological evidence for a direct projection to the more rostral midline raphe nuclei, providing a possible integration with brain-stem serotonergic elements felt by Jouvet (1969a,b) to be involved in the sleep process. Electrical stimulation of the basal forebrain area in cats elicited evoked neuroelectric potentials and altered unit activity within the rostral raphe nuclei. Additionally, stimulation of the diffusely projecting dorsal raphe nucleus resulted in a subtle alteration of discharge pattern in basal forebrain units. Thus, a reciprocal organization might exist between the rostral raphe nuclei and basal forebrain region such that a feed-back modulation of serotonin release is directed by descending elements of the latter. Some of the possible pathways and neurochemical mediators involved in such reciprocal organisation have been reviewed recently by Morgane and Stern (1972).

In summary, then, what can we presume to know about the role of the basal forebrain region in sleep? We can conclude that it is not involved in the brain-stem mechanism responsible for REM sleep, which we consider to reflect a more primitive neural periodicity, endorsing Kleitman's concept of a basic rest–activity cycle. Electrical, chemical, and thermal stimulation of the basal forebrain region elicits slow wave sleep, while its destruction suppresses this pattern, produces hyperactivity, and disrupts the normal temporal organization of sleep and waking behavior. Basal forebrain cells become specifically active concurrent with this transition to sleep. It is clear that elements originating in this region exert some fundamental influence upon other brain structures, thereby providing for the onset and regulation of normal sleep patterns. We propose that projections to the thalamus and the midbrain reticular formation could block afferent input volleys and initiate EEG synchronization through the suppression of sensory and motor functions. The relationship of the basal forebrain region to the brain stem raphe nuclei suggests a means of influencing the production and release of serotonin, which would also tend to mediate this integrative function.

Like most of our knowledge of functional brain mechanisms underlying complex behaviors, concepts about sleep remain diffuse and depend more upon theoretical advocates than unequivocal scientific evidence. Future investigation might well find today's concepts both naive and narrow. Sleep is most likely modulated by a number of functional influences, as are other integrative processes. For example, most control systems in the brain have been found to be regulated by both tonic and phasic mechanisms. Thus, sleep may serve basic regulatory needs of the organism by virtue of its systematic alternation with wakefulness. On the other hand, acute adjustments directed by neocortical (cognitive) or hypothalamic (homeostatic) influences allow the central nervous system to utilize this process to advantage in its more phasic activities. It is likely that the basal forebrain region, by virtue of its numerous projections, participates in both of these manifestations of the sleep process.

Discussion

Steriade: I was impressed by the increase of spontaneous firing you showed in preoptic neurons at the beginning of sleep. This is quite opposite to what we have observed in principal (relay type) thalamic VL cells at the very onset of slow sleep, where there was a sudden silence in the spontaneous discharges which preceded the EEG signs by a few seconds (Steriade *et al.*, 1971b). We ascribed this silence to a disfacilitation resulting from abrupt withdrawal of tonic excitatory impingement from the waking reticular formation on VL cells. Now, I think it can be inferred that the intense firing in preoptic neurons at the onset of sleep may inhibit the mesencephalic reticular neurons, as suggested by recent data of Bremer (1970a) and consequently account for the striking supression of discharges we observed in VL neurons.

Jouvet: What are these same preoptic neurons doing at the beginning of paradoxical sleep? Do they stop firing?

Sterman: No, firing rates are generally increased, but the pattern of discharge remains irregular and bursting is rare. The increased rates do not approach those seen at sleep onset and lack the regularity and bursting characteristics of that period.

Dement: One of the most important points of your presentation is that the same behavioral effects can be obtained by either fast or slow stimulation of that basal forebrain region. This has to be studied because it is quite different from other structures such as the thalamus.

Schlag: When you talk of the basal forebrain region, what is your feeling? Do you think of it as a cellular population situated there or do you attribute the effects of stimulation or lesion to passing fibers of cortical origin?

Sterman: In studies of reflex excitability during sleep we have observed that an inhibitory influence from the preoptic region can persist for several days after neocortex and adjacent limbic structures have been removed. This suggests that there are neurons in this area which retain an autonomous inhibitory function, at least temporarily, after higher level inputs have been withdrawn. But I prefer not to conceptualize this as a center; I do not believe in centers.

Villablanca: What happens if you make very large lesions of the pre-optic area?

Sterman: With large lesions, parts of the adjacent hypothalamus are destroyed, with consequent alterations of other basic functions. Neverthe-less, Dr. McGinty and I (1968) found that large bilateral lesions at the caudal preoptic level produced disruptions of sleep patterns which per-sisted after transient temperature and feeding irregularities had passed. If the lesions produced a transection of the basal forebrain at this level, the hyperactivity and suppression of sleep became progressively worse until, by 7–10 days postlesion, sleep was totally abolished. These animals literally collapsed from exhaustion, showed marked extensor rigidity, and died. The behavior and consequences were similar to those described years ago by Nauta (1946) after anterior hypothalamic transections in the rat.

Dement: Why did the animals die?

Sterman: Superficial autopsies showed no obvious pathology; however, it is likely that some metabolic failure ultimately was responsible. I would like to think that these animals died of a pathologically sustained suppression of sleep, but it is very possible that other regulatory complications resulting from the lesions were the primary cause of death.

Jouvet: How much percentage of reduction in sleep did you reach with moderate lesions?

Sterman: That varied with the size and location of the lesions. With well-placed lesions, 3–4 mm square, REM was often minimal or totally abolished for over a week and slow wave sleep reduced by 75% or more (see, for example, Fig. 5.4). Sleep pattern percentages often returned to normal ranges by 4–6 weeks, but Dr. Lucas and I (1972) found that the temporal organization of these patterns (sleep–waking rhythm) remained disrupted for over 6 months.

Moruzzi: Dr. Bremer, would you like to comment on the relations of this basal forebrain area with the brain-stem reticular formation?

Bremer: I tried to verify the hypothesis that a cerebral hypnogenic area—I chose the preoptic one for technical facilities—owes, at least in part, its sleep-inducing property to an active inhibition of the ascending reticular system. The experiments, which are still in progress, have been performed in the *encéphale isolé* cat, after it had been verified that the diffuse cortical synchroniza-tion, which Sterman and Clemente (1962a) had shown to be induced by a low frequency preoptic stimulation, could be similarly obtained in this prepar-ation, provided it was in an optimal functional state. This condition is impor-tant, for I could confirm and extend the observation which Sterman and Clemente (1962a) had already made that all the effects of the preoptic activation are suppressed by even the slightest depression of the brain. The observations involved the recording, by macro- and microelectrodes, of the field potential evoked in the mesencephalic reticular tegmentum and in nonspecific thalamic nuclei by weak electrical pulses applied on the preoptic area. The response is a positive potential of 20 to 60 msec duration, eventually preceded by a brief negative wave or by a burst of multiunit spikes and often followed by a slow reboundlike negative wave. The field potential is increased, sometimes markedly, by temporal summation (optimal interval: 3 msec) and by the recruiting build-up, resulting from a low frequency stimulation. It is resistant to strychnine and picrotoxin. The designation of the P wave as the extracellular counter part of a postsynaptic inhibition of the neuron population explored is indicated by the concomitant depression of single or multiunit discharges of reticular neurons and of their responses to a sensory stimulus. Particularly demonstrative of the inhibitory power of the preoptic stimulus was the suppressive effect it exerted on the excitatory response (negative field potential) of the center median to a testing mesencephalic reticular shock within an 80-msec interval of the two stimuli. Their succession in a reverse order (reticular shock preceding) resulted in a striking increase of the center median positive field potential evoked by a testing preoptic shock. I have tentatively interpreted this effect as the manifestation of a negative feedback relation between the arousal system and the hypnogenic one, tending to a stabilization of the vigilance level, as Bonvallet and Allen (1963) had already suggested for the relation between the bulbar hypnogenic "center" and the ascending reticular formation.

Sterman: Our earlier experiments with brain stimulation in a runway situation attempted to test this reciprocal antagonism hypothesis behaviorally. The basal forebrain and the reticular formation were stimulated simultaneously or in succession. I have shown you the results. The idea of a balance between basal forebrain and tegmental systems may seem simplistic, but it works. There is also good evidence for a direct projection to the thalamic nonspecific systems from basal forebrain, which may provide for another point of interaction between opposing neural influences.

Purpura: If this is the place to make suggestions, I think that a high priority should be given to experiments where the effects of stimulation in the basal forebrain and in the region of the tractus solitarius should be tested by intracellular recordings from thalamic neurons. Some years ago, when Clemente and Sterman's data appeared, we tried to do these experiments using basal forebrain stimulations, but we never obtained clear synchronized activities over the cortex in *encéphale isolé* preparations. They were never as reliable as the 8 to 12/sec rhythms elicited by medial thalamic shocks.

Sterman: I do not know whether these were acute or chronic preparations, but if the animals were not completely recovered from the physiological aftereffects of transection, I would not be surprised by the difficulty which you encountered. The normal functioning of sleep mechanisms appears to require a stabilized internal and external milieu, since high resolution analysis indicates that sleep is rather fragile. Concerning the relationship of this region to the thalamus, Clemente and I (1963) tried very early to record thalamic responses to stimulation of the preoptic region. We found moderate responses in ventralis medialis and reuniens and larger ones in center median and the intralaminar nuclei. Degeneration studies subsequently showed strong projections to these nuclei, ascending with the inferior thalamic peduncle.

Purpura: Is the medial thalamic system necessary for these effects of basal forebrain stimulation? I am asking that because you also postulate a direct downstream projection.

Sterman: Thalamic interactions may mediate the EEG synchronizing influence only. In my opinion, a critical experiment remains to be done. This would involve placement of bilateral preoptic lesions in a *cerveau isolé* preparation showing sustained EEG synchronization as well as other signs of sleep.

Schlag: Villablanca and I (Villablanca and Schlag, 1968) did that. Our lesions were a little more dorsal: just rostroventral to the anterior pole of the thalamus where you expect the projections to arrive. In acute *cerveaux isolés*, all EEG activities in the frequency range of spindles were immediately wiped out. These were curious preparations because fast rhythms were prevented by the midcollicular transection and spindles were prevented by the lesion rostral to the thalamus. Only irregular waves around 3/sec persisted although almost all thalamocortical projections were still intact. We were very surprised by this result because it showed that desynchronizing action was not necessary to abolish spindles.

Andersen: Where is this prethalamic lesion? Does it cut the ansa lenticularis?

Schlag: Yes, it does in most cases, but up to now we have been unable to ascribe the effects to any particular structure or path. There are many functionally different pathways in this region.

I do not think that thalamic connections with the orbitofrontal cortex are crucial though. With Mme Petre-Quadens, we have tried to see whether it would be possible to block the spindles by a transection some millimeters more rostrally. Such a transection has to be quite extensive. Theoretically, it should be equivalent to a prethalamic lesion if the effect is due to the interruption of thalamocortical projections. But there was no consistent effect on the EEG. Therefore, we believe that a disconnection of the thalamus from the basal forebrain area is a more likely hypothesis than a disconnection from the orbitofrontal cortex to explain the disappearance of spindles.

Bremer: Let us remind ourselves that diffuse nonconvulsant electrocortical synchronization does not necessarily mean sleep. When Dr. Sterman stimulates the preoptic area with repetitive small current pulses, the EEG "synchronization" does not appear immediately. It develops after a delay, sometimes a long one, in the form of sleep spindles. We are faced with the fact that the two well-documented hypnogenic areas possess in common the capacity, when stimulated at a low frequency, of driving directly the thalamo-cortical electrogenesis at this frequency. But this synchronization is not always accompanied by behavioral sleep and the electrocortical driving opposes the appearance of the sleep spindles when the frequency of these waves is higher than the stimulation one. The functional significance of this property of the hypnogenic structure and, more precisely, its relation with the sleep determinism remains to be found.

CHAPTER SIX

Intracellular Studies of Thalamic Synaptic Mechanisms in Evoked Synchronization and Desynchronization of Electrocortical Activity[1]

DOMINICK P. PURPURA

Transitions from one to another sleep state or from sleep to wakefulness and vice versa are associated with complex alterations in electrocortical activities as well as variations in neuronal discharge patterns at many neuraxial sites. The neurophysiologist interested in defining the basic synaptic mechanisms underlying these dynamic alterations in brain function is faced with a task of enormous proportions. Perhaps the most difficult involves the choice of operational approach that will permit analysis of mechanism with a minimum of physiological distortion.

Leaving aside any consideration of the anatomical substrate responsible for triggering one or another sleep–wakefulness state, one useful experimental approach is to examine the intimate behavior of single neurons at different sites over long periods of time and attempt to relate change in state with alterations in neuronal activity. Were it possible to utilize the intracellular recording technique in such chronic experiments, information would be forthcoming that would bear directly on the issue of synaptic processes. Unfortunately such an experimental approach is not feasible in the freely moving animal with

[1] Supported in part by National Institutes of Health Grant NS-07512.

99

currently available techniques of intracellular registration. Thus the decision must be made whether to settle for chronic extracellular unit data and forego analysis of synaptic mechanism or opt for an approach that may permit definition of synaptic mechanism in concomitants of sleep–wakefulness behavior in the absence of the behavior itself. Both approaches may not be entirely satisfactory but neither are they without redeeming value, if the data obtained in one are correlated with the findings derived from the other. Such correlative approaches are urgently needed lest the vast amount of data obtained in chronic extracellular recordings in behaving animals exceed the capacity for "adequate interpretation." The assumption here is that intracellular data obtained in experimental preparations that mimic physiological processes subserving sleep–wakefulness activities should provide the basis for an "adequate interpretation." This is more than an article of faith in the resolving power of the intracellular approach to the study of complex processes. It is an assertion that synaptic mechanisms underlying events that have their counterpart in behavioral activities are not likely to be irrelevant to the genesis of these behaviors. Specifically, in the case of sleep–wakefulness activities, change of state is generally accompanied by alterations in the amplitude and frequency of electrocortical potentials. Similar, if not identical alterations in electrocortical activities can be replicated in experimental situations that permit analysis of synaptic processes but provide no information on their relationship to behavioral state. Nevertheless, it would be surprising indeed if the processes disclosed in the "model situation" were fundamentally different from those underlying the alterations in electrocortical potentials accompanying sleep-wakefulness activities in the behaving animal.

For the past decade we have sought to apply the foregoing philosophical approach to intracellular studies of the elementary thalamic synaptic mechanisms involved in two types of evoked electrocortical activities in locally anesthetized-paralyzed *encéphale isolé* cats. The first type of activity provides a model system for the pattern of *electrocortical synchronization* observed in the behaving animal during the transition from quiet wakefulness to drowsiness or light sleep. This pattern, typified by the 6–12/sec recruiting response, is readily elicited by low-frequency (6–12/sec) stimulation of medial and intralaminar nonspecific thalamic nuclei (Dempsey and Morison, 1942a; Morison and Dempsey, 1942).

The second type of electrocortical activity provides a model system for the pattern of electrocortical desynchronization that occurs in transitions from sleep to wakefulness in response to spontaneous or evoked arousal stimuli in the behaving animal. This pattern may be induced by high frequency (50–200/sec) stimulation of thalamic nonspecific nuclei (Dempsey and Morison, 1942a; Jasper, 1949) or ascending components of the brain-stem reticular activating system (Moruzzi and Magoun, 1949).

Utilization of these two model systems for studying induced EEG synchronization and desynchronization has provided information concerning the subcortical as well as the cortical stages of these operations and processes (Purpura, 1970). The following survey focuses on the intrathalamic synaptic events underlying synchronization and desynchronization of thalamocortical neuronal activity, and considers the consequences of thalamic internuclear operations as they relate to transmission of specific activity in some thalamic relay nuclei. It will be shown that the synaptic mechanisms disclosed in these intracellular studies are sufficient to account for a wide range of alterations in the functional activity of neurons at different neuraxial sites during events which have their counterpart in changes in sleep–wakefulness states. The reader is referred to a recent review for references to many of the intracellular studies of neurons in the mammalian brain carried out by other workers (Purpura, 1971). The following survey is limited to examination of selected aspects of work from the author's laboratory on problems relevant to the subject matter of this volume.

I. Synaptic Mechanisms in Generalized Thalamocortical Synchronization

Typical long-latency recruiting responses recorded from the pericruciate cortex of *encéphale isolé* cats rarely exhibit a significant component in response to the first stimulus of a low-frequency train of stimuli delivered to medial thalamic (MTh) nuclei (Fig. 6.1A). However, this initial stimulus has dramatic effects on ongoing discharges of neurons in widespread parts of the rostral thalamus (Purpura and Cohen, 1962). The pattern of extracellular unit discharges is abruptly interrupted by this stimulus and may be replaced by a rhythmic burst of spikes superimposed upon early and late focally recorded negativities (Fig. 6.1B). The unit is silenced during a prominent extracellularly recorded positivity. Even higher frequency injury discharges of extracellularly recorded units are silenced during this positivity (Fig. 6.1C). Although there may be variations in latency and amplitude of the focal positivity recorded from different thalamic nuclei, the relationship of the positive potential to cessation of unit discharge is basically similar (Fig. 6.1D–J).

The intracellular synaptic events underlying the extracellular field potentials shown in Fig. 6.1 are summarized in Fig. 6.2 (Purpura and Shofer, 1963). Again it can be seen that the first stimulus of the recruiting train which evokes very little response at the level of the cortex is effective in altering the pattern of ongoing activity of thalamic neurons. For the most part this initial "command" stimulus elicits a prominent and prolonged inhibitory postsynaptic potential

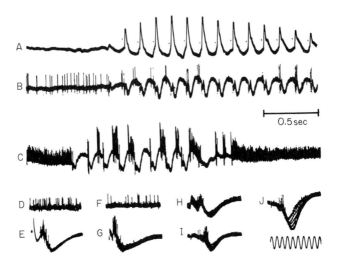

Fig. 6.1. Examples from different experiments of long-latency "recruiting" positivities recorded with extracellularly located micropipettes in different regions of the thalamus during medial thalamic-induced recruiting responses. A. Cortical surface-negative recruiting response (pericruciate cortex). B. Simultaneously recorded recruiting positivity in ventral anterior thalamus. Spontaneous unit discharges are abolished during the focal positivity but are grouped on the succeeding negativities. C. Coarse movement of a relatively large micropipette initiates high frequency injury discharges of units in rostral VL. Injury discharges are suppressed during the 7/sec evoked focal positivity. D and F. Spontaneous activity of units in VL and VA, respectively. E and G. Suppression of unit activity in these locations during recruiting positivity. Note different patterns of early focal negativity and associated multiunit discharges. Examples of extracellular recordings in Ret. (H) and VL (I and J) illustrate the various relationships of unit discharges and slow waves observed in different nuclear groups during recruiting responses. Superposed traces in D, E, F, G, H, I, and J. Calibration for D, E, F, G, H, I, and J are shown in J, 100 Hz, 0.3 mV. [From Purpura and Cohen, 1962]

(IPSP) which is synchronized in many cells. Additional stimuli of the low frequency MTh-repetitive train evoke short-latency excitatory postsynaptic potentials (EPSPs) which may give rise to a variable number of spike discharges. EPSP–IPSP sequences may occur without alteration (Fig. 6.2B and 6.2D) or there may be IPSP alternation (Fig. 6.2C). In some neurons of the intralaminar nuclei high frequency spike bursts terminated by IPSPs may be observed (Fig. 6.2E). The development of the EPSP–IPSP sequence is noteworthy since this may evolve from a background of increased membrane polarization (Figs. 6.2B and Fig. 6.3). Additionally, the early EPSP may not be prominent with the first stimulus but it is generally markedly potentiated with the second and subsequent stimuli (Fig. 6.2).

Although neurons in the same and different thalamic nuclei may exhibit

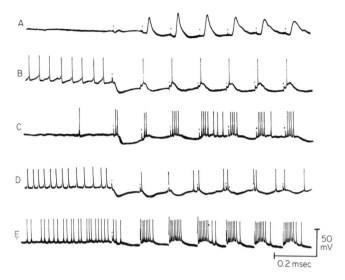

Fig. 6.2. Patterns of intracellularly recorded activities of thalamic neurons during cortical recruiting responses evoked by 7/sec medial thalamic stimulation. A. Characteristics of surface-negative recruiting responses (motor cortex) elicited throughout the experiment from which the intracellular records (B–E) were obtained. B. Neuron in ventral anterior region of thalamus exhibiting prolonged IPSP following first stimulus then EPSP–IPSP sequences with successive stimuli. C. Relatively quiescent ventrolateral neuron develops double discharge with first stimulus. The ensuing IPSP is succeeded by another evoked EPSP and cell discharge. Note alternation of IPSP. D. Neuron with discharge characteristics similar to that shown in B. E. Neuron in intralaminar region exhibiting an initial prolonged IPSP that interrupts spontaneous discharges. The second and all successive stimuli evoked prolonged EPSPs with repetitive discharges that are terminated by IPSPs. [From Purpura and Shofer, 1963]

different patterns of EPSP–IPSP sequences, under favorable conditions a remarkable degree of synchronization is detectable in intracellular recordings from thalamic neurons located in different parts of the thalamus (Fig. 6.3). It is evident from this that while the interneuronal networks responsible for eliciting temporal patterns of EPSP–IPSP sequences must be complex indeed to affect elements in different nuclear groups, their overt actions are relatively simple as seen in the prolonged IPSPs interrupted by shorter duration EPSPs. One consequence of this EPSP–IPSP sychronization in many thalamic neurons is to produce membrane oscillations which account for the extracellular recorded "spindle waves" of the thalamus (Purpura and Cohen, 1962). Of course such data support the hypothesis that PSPs are largely responsible for brain waves in general (cf. Purpura, 1959). A second consequence is to limit discharges of thalamic neurons to the phases between prolonged IPSPs. In essence the prolonged IPSP is the basic synaptic event in the generalized synchronizing process at the thalamic level (Purpura and Cohen, 1962).

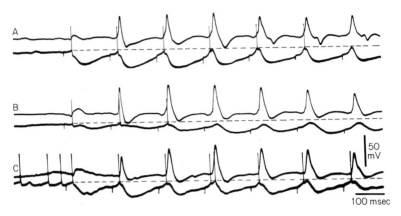

Fig. 6.3. Temporal relations of EPSP–IPSP sequences in neurons situated in different thalamic regions during motor-cortex recruiting responses (upper channel records) evoked by 7/sec stimulation of medial-thalamic, nonspecific nuclei. The three unidentified neurons were impaled at different depths from the dorsolateral surface of the exposed thalamus during a single penetration of the microelectrode. Depths as follows: A, 2.0 mm; B, 4.5 mm; C, 6.5 mm. Timing of the first three spike discharges elicited by EPSPs is synchronized in the three elements. IPSP latencies and duration are similar except during late phases in B. Note IPSP summation leading to progressive hyperpolarizing shift of membrane potential during continued stimulation. Dashed lines are drawn through "firing levels" determined by first synaptically evoked response of each series. [From Purpura *et al.*, 1966a]

It is a point of considerable importance that IPSPs may summate sufficiently to prevent EPSPs from attaining firing level (Fig. 6.3B). Thus it is not necessary for spike discharge to occur on the recovery phase of the IPSP or in relation to the EPSP for repetition of the EPSP–IPSP sequence. Nor is the total cessation of discharges frequently observed during the period of MTh stimulation referable to some obscure effects of cellular impalement since the same can be observed in extracellular recordings of "giant spikes" (Fig. 6.4). These data contradict the view that postanodal exaltation following the IPSP of thalamic neurons is an important feature of the thalamic synchronization mechanism as emphasized by Andersen and Andersson (1968). Suffice it to say that reconsideration of this problem has led Andersson and Manson (1971) to reject the postanodal exaltation hypothesis (cf. Purpura, 1969 for further discussion of this issue) in favor of the view of the present author that rhythmical activity is maintained by alternating EPSP–IPSP sequences.

Stimuli to medial and intralaminar thalamic nuclei are not only effective in inducing recruiting responses but in triggering "spindle bursts" with a variable latency after the last stimulus in an initiating train (Morison and Dempsey, 1942). Figure 6.5 illustrates a series of such spindle waves at the cortical level and the intracellular synaptic events accompanying these in

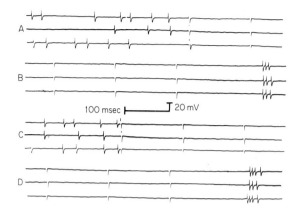

Fig. 6.4. Inhibiting effects of low-frequency medial thalamic stimulation on extracellularly recorded "giant spikes" of a neuron located in the ventro-anterior thalamus. Three series of stimuli are shown from continuous recordings of several minutes' duration. The last stimuli in B and D are followed by a long latency spontaneous burst whose occurrence is remarkably precise.

recordings from a thalamic neuron. The prominent increase in membrane polarization produced by the summation of IPSPs and the interruption of these by EPSPs with and without spike discharge are noteworthy (Purpura et al., 1966a).

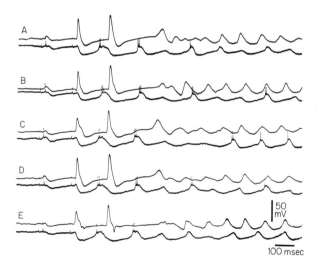

Fig. 6.5. Relationship between electrocortical activity and intracellularly recorded EPSP–IPSP sequences elicited in a thalamic neuron by three stimuli delivered to medial thalamus. A–E. Five series of responses evoked after an interval of several seconds between stimuli. Note the remarkable regularity of the PSP pattern in relation to the spindle waves triggered by the three stimuli that evoke abortive recruiting responses. [From Purpura et al., 1966a]

In view of the central importance of prolonged IPSPs in the process of thalamocortical synchronization, attention has been focused on the nature of the synaptic mechanism underlying the IPSP. The question that has been examined is whether the prolonged suppression of neuronal discharge seen in association with an increase in membrane polarization is entirely due to a conductance-increase mechanism or another event, i.e., disfacilitation or a nonconductance increase type of IPSP. The question has been answered unequivocally with the demonstration of a marked increase in membrane conductance, as tested by injected current pulses, throughout the entire period of discharge suppression associated with the prolonged summating IPSPs (Fig. 6.6) (Feldman and Purpura, 1970). This indicates a transmitter-induced activation of inhibitory receptor sites on thalamic neurons for periods lasting as long as seconds during prolonged phases of thalamocortical synchroniza-

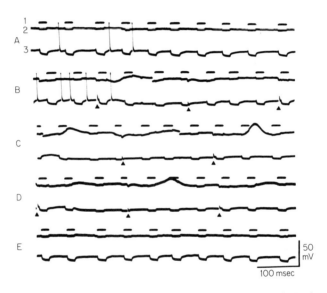

Fig. 6.6. Relative membrane resistance changes in a thalamic neuron during low frequency (5-Hz) stimulation of medial thalamus (MTh). Neuron located in VA-VL regions of the thalamus. *1*, marker channel indicating time and duration of transmembrane current injection; *2*, cortical surface recording of evoked recruiting responses; *3*, intracellular record showing membrane potential changes produced by 25-Hz, 20-msec duration, 2-nA inward current pulses. A. Control. Neuron exhibits several 50 mV spontaneous spike discharges followed by a quiescent phase. B. MTh stimulation is initiated at first arrowhead (▲) during a burst of spontaneous spikes. Increase in membrane polarization begins 30–40 msec after the stimulus and exhibits variations in relation to subsequent stimuli (▲) in C and D. Recruiting responses exhibit "alternation" characteristics (C_2, D_2). Membrane resistance changes follow the time course of the evoked membrane potential increase. E. Several seconds after cessation of stimulation. [From Feldman and Purpura, 1970]

tion. The implication here is that transmitter operations subserving complex and prolonged transformations in neuronal activity in cortico-diencephalic organizations may have a different time course than at other junctions. Whether such prolonged transmitter effects are referable to the activity of repetitively discharging inhibitory interneurons or differences in kinetics of transmitter-receptor activation and inactivation has not been clarified.

A closely related problem concerns the identity and location of the inhibitory interneurons responsible for generating the prolonged and synchronized IPSPs in thalamic neurons. The Scheibels (1966, 1967) have implicated neurons of the thalamic nucleus reticularis in the generation of diffusely distributed IPSPs (of the type shown in Figs. 6.2 and 6.3) because these neurons project axons to virtually all parts of the thalamus. Physiological studies have supported this hypothesis in showing that various inputs to reticularis neurons initiate prolonged high frequency discharges in these cells (Schlag and Waszak, 1971). Obviously the identification of such elements as inhibitory neurons is valid only to the extent that prolonged IPSPs are of necessity generated by high frequency discharges of inhibitory neurons. If such is the case, then candidate inhibitory neurons must be diffusely distributed in the thalamus as originally proposed by Purpura and Cohen (1962) (Fig. 6.7). It remains an open question whether the prolonged summating IPSPs are related to the discharge of reticularis neurons whereas the more phasic IPSPs examined by Andersen and Eccles (1962) and Andersen and Andersson (1968) are referable to the activity of locally distributed inhibitory interneurons in a recurrent pathway (see Andersen, Chapter 7 in this volume). For present purposes it is sufficient to emphasize the operation of powerful inhibitory synaptic pathways within

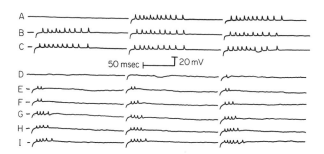

Fig. 6.7. Two patterns of extracellularly recorded unit activities of thalamic neurons during 7/sec medial thalamic stimulation. A, B, and C. Continuous record of a "VA unit" silent prior to stimulation. The first stimulus evokes 12 discharges, the second 11, and all subsequent stimuli, 10 each. D, E, F, G, and I. Unit probably in n. reticularis exhibiting progressive increase in number of discharges during prolonged medial thalamic stimulation. [From Purpura and Cohen, 1962]

the thalamus whose activation is capable of synchronizing the discharges of neurons in widespread parts of the thalamus.

Activation of the *generalized* synchronization process by low frequency stimulation of medial and intralaminar thalamic nuclei does more than influence the discharge characteristics of thalamic neurons (*vide infra*) and neocortical elements (Purpura and Shofer, 1964; Purpura *et al.*, 1964). For if this were the case there would be little reason to implicate the rostral (thalamic) component of the generalized projection system in the modulation of a variety of forebrain and brain-stem neuronal organizations. On the contrary, it has been established in intracellular studies that activation of the thalamic generalized projection system is capable of synaptically influencing neurons of the corpus striatum (Purpura and Malliani, 1967; Malliani and Purpura, 1967) mesencephalic reticular formation (Maekawa and Purpura, 1967c) and amygdaloid complex (Santini and Purpura, 1969). As is evident from examination of typical patterns of intracellularly recorded events from neurons in these different locations (Fig. 6.8), the effects of medial thalamic stimulation are dependent upon the synaptic organization of elements that comprise the local neuronal population as well as the biophysical properties of these elements (cf. Purpura, 1971).

The synaptic effects observed in different cortical basal ganglia and brain-stem organizations following stimulation of the generalized thalamic projection system are indicative of important parallel processing operations of this system (Purpura, 1970). Indeed, it is unlikely that another projection system of the brain will be found to have so widespread an influence upon different neuronal organizations as that described here in connection with the mechanisms of generalized thalamocortical synchronization. The implications of these intracellular data for the genesis of alterations in discharge characteristics observed during sleep–wakefulness activities in many neuraxial sites are self-evident.

II. Thalamic Synaptic Mechanisms during Reticulocortical Activation

It has long been established that high frequency stimulation of thalamic or brain-stem components of the ascending reticular activating system induces electrocortical flattening or desynchronization under appropriate experimental conditions (Dempsey and Morison, 1942a; Hunter and Jasper, 1949; Jasper, 1949; Moruzzi and Magoun, 1949). The effect produced by high frequency (25–200/sec) stimulation of medial thalamic nuclei thus differs markedly from that produced by low frequency (6–12/sec) stimulation. The preceding section has considered the intrathalamic synaptic events observed

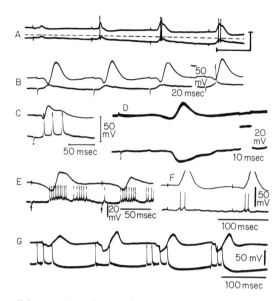

Fig. 6.8. Parallel processing of unspecific thalamic output in synaptically related neuronal subsystems. Upper channel records, obtained from motor cortex, display the characteristics of recruiting responses elicited in different preparations during medial-thalamic stimulation. A. Typical responsiveness of a pyramidal-tract neuron in motor cortex. Dashed line drawn through firing level. Nonspecific thalamic stimulation elicits a progressively incrementing EPSP with a slow rise time and a prolonged decay phase. Calibrations: 50 mV, 100 msec. [From Purpura *et al.*, 1964] B. Intracellular synaptic events recorded in a caudate neuron during nonspecific thalamic stimulation. Note remarkable similarity in EPSP characteristics in the caudate and PT neuron. [From Purpura and Malliani, 1967] C. Pattern of EPSP and spike discharges generally observed in putamen neurons. D. Long-latency IPSP detectable in a neuron of the nucleus entopeduncularis during medial-thalamic stimulation. [C and D from Malliani and Purpura, 1967] E and F. Characteristics of discharge patterns of neurons in mesencephalic reticular formation during medial thalamic stimulation. [From Maekawa and Purpura, unpublished] G. Responsiveness of a neuron in the amygdaloid complex during stimulation of intralaminar nuclei of the nonspecific projection system. [From Santini and Purpura, unpublished]

during low frequency stimulation and has emphasized the prominent involvement of prolonged IPSPs and EPSP–IPSP sequences in the evoked EEG synchronization. The problem examined now concerns the nature of the alterations in these synaptic events accompanying reticulocortical activation.

In the first approach to this problem, intracellular recordings were obtained from rostral and ventral tier neurons of the dorsal thalamus during low and high frequency stimulation of the medial thalamic nonspecific nuclei (Purpura and Shofer, 1963). The results of this study are summarized in the experiment illustrated in Fig. 6.9. In this experiment low frequency medial thalamic (MTh) stimulation elicited typical EPSP–IPSP sequences in a

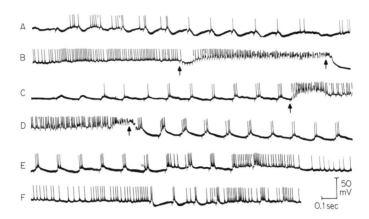

Fig. 6.9. Effects of repeated high frequency medial thalamic stimulation on a ventromedial neuron exhibiting preactivation recruiting pattern characterized by short-latency EPSPs and prolonged prominent IPSPs. A–E. Continuous record. A. 7/sec medial thalamic stimulation succeeded by a phase of hyperexcitability (B). At first arrow in B, a prolonged IPSP is initiated by the first stimulus of the high frequency (60/sec) repetitive train. Successive stimuli after the IPSP evoke summating EPSPs associated with high frequency spike attenuation. D. Second period of 7/sec medial thalamic stimulation after repolarization initiates only prolonged slowly augmenting EPSPs. Changes in stimulus frequency between arrows, in C and D, induce high frequency repetitive discharges superimposed on depolarization whose magnitude is related to stimulus frequency. F. Several seconds later. Note reappearance of IPSPs during 7/sec medial thalamic stimulation. [From Purpura and Shofer, 1963]

ventromedial thalamic neuron (Fig. 6.9A). The first of a high frequency train of MTh stimuli initiated an IPSP but all subsequent stimuli resulted in a profound synaptically induced soma depolarization with superimposed partial spikes (Fig. 6.9B). Resumption of the low frequency MTh stimulus now resulted in EPSPs without obvious IPSPs (Fig. 6.9C). Under these conditions a second period of high frequency MTh stimulation elicited a rapid soma depolarization with continued postactivation enhancement of excitatory drives (Figs. 6.9D and 6.9E), Partial recovery of the EPSP–IPSP sequence during low frequency MTh stimulation is seen in Fig. 6.9F.

These and other data (Purpura and Shofer, 1963) indicate that the major synaptic events observed in thalamic neurons during the transition from evoked EEG synchronization to MTh-induced desynchronization is a "blockade" of the synchronizing IPSP and augmentation of excitatory synaptic drives in a large proportion of thalamic neurons. Inasmuch as stimulation of the same region of the thalamus at two different frequencies produces fundamentally different synaptic events in thalamic neurons (which are associated with different overt electrocortical activities), it follows that the interneuronal organizations responsible for these events must be selectively responsive to different input frequencies. Since the chief effect of the high frequency stimulation is to attenuate or block the development of prolonged IPSPs, this suggests that high frequency stimulation activates a second high threshold inhibitory system which is inhibitory to the interneurons generating prolonged IPSPs (Purpura and Shofer, 1963). Alternatively it might be argued that the prolonged IPSPs are not eliminated but masked by the development of powerful excitatory synaptic activities.

Further exploration of this problem has been made possible by utilizing the experimental paradigm of Moruzzi and Magoun (1949). The latter workers showed that if electrocortical synchronization (recruiting responses) was elicited by low frequency stimulation of medial thalamic nuclei, concomitant high frequency stimulation of the ascending brain-stem reticular activating system of the pontomesencephalic tegmentum would effectively block the evoked synchronization. Results obtained in two different experiments in which combined low frequency MTh stimulation and high frequency brain-stem reticular formation (BSRF) stimulation was carried out during intracellular recording from thalamic neurons are shown in Fig. 6.10 (Purpura *et al.*, 1966a,b).

In both experiments of Fig. 6.10 low frequency MTh stimulation elicited

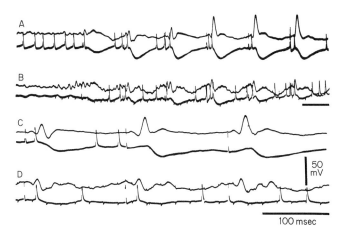

Fig. 6.10.   Intrathalamic synaptic events associated with suppressing effect of high frequency (50/sec) BSRF stimulation on thalamocortical recruiting responses. A. Unidentified ventrolateral thalamic neuron exhibits characteristic EPSP–IPSP sequences during evoked recruiting responses to 7/sec MTh stimulation. B. Prior BSRF stimulation blocks recruiting response at the cortex and markedly attenuates synchronizing IPSPs. C and D. From another unidentified thalamic neuron. C. 7/sec MTh stimulation alone. D. Simultaneous low frequency MTh and high frequency BSRF stimulation. Note marked attenuation of prolonged IPSPs and variable increase in cell discharges. Time bar in (B), 100 msec. [From Purpura *et al.*, 1966a,b]

typical EPSP–IPSP sequences in thalamic neurons in association with long-latency recruiting responses (Figs. 6.10A and C). Combined low frequency MTh stimulation and high frequency BSRF stimulation resulted in attenuation or blockade of the prolonged IPSP component of the EPSP–IPSP sequence induced by MTh stimulation (Figs. 6.10B and D). Additionally, BSRF stimulation increased the discharge frequency of the thalamic neurons by attenuating the IPSP and increasing excitatory synaptic drives. A close correlation was noted between the time course of the reticulocortical activation following BSRF stimulation and the suppression of synchronizing IPSPs in thalamic neurons (Purpura *et al.*, 1966a,b).

It is not to be inferred from the results shown in Fig. 6.10 that high frequency BSRF stimulation is effective in blocking only the IPSPs evoked in thalamic neurons by MTh stimulation. On the contrary, BSRF stimulation is equally effective in attenuating IPSPs generated in thalamic relay cells by stimulation of their afferent projection pathways (Fig. 6.11). Moreover, such blockade of IPSPs may persist for many seconds following cessation of BSRF stimulation.

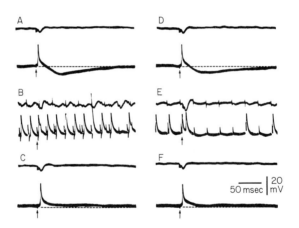

Fig. 6.11. Effects of high frequency brain-stem reticular formation (BSRF) and medial thalamic (MTh) stimulation on responses of a VL relay cell to brachium conjunctivum (BC) stimulation. Upper traces are monopolar recordings from motor cortex, negativity upward. A. Control BC stimulation (at arrows) evokes a cell discharge which arises from a small EPSP. The spike potential is succeeded by a prominent depolarizing afterpotential and a prolonged IPSP. Despite the low amplitude of the spike potential in this cell, stable responses were recorded for many minutes. B. Increase in VL cell discharge during 60/sec BSRF stimulation. The degree of induced depolarization in this element may be appreciated by comparison of the separation between traces in these records and those in A. BSRF stimulation also evokes responses in motor cortex which are similar to those elicited by BC stimulation. C. Several seconds after BSRF stimulation, BC-evoked IPSP is eliminated and the depolarizing potential succeeding the spike is prolonged. D. Recovery of IPSP 30 sec after C. E. 50/sec MTh stimulation. Note facilitation of cortical surface-evoked responses and intermittent discharges. F. Several seconds after cessation of MTh stimulation BC-evoked IPSP is eliminated. [From Purpura *et al.*, 1966b]

The conclusion to be drawn from intracellular studies of the interaction between medial thalamic and BSRF stimulation is that thalamic neurons participating in the mechanism of evoked EEG synchronization also participate in the mechanism of EEG desynchronization. Basic differences in discharge characteristics of thalamic neurons during these two modes of activation are entirely referable to differences in the patterns of their synaptic inputs. What particularly characterizes these differences is the presence or absence of prolonged IPSPs. IPSPs that are prominently displayed during evoked EEG synchronization or during the operation of recurrent inhibitory pathways are attenuated or inhibited during BSRF stimulation. Viewed in this fashion *inhibition of inhibition* at the thalamic level must be considered a major factor in the development of reticulocortical activation. This, in association with a demonstrable augmentation of excitatory synaptic inputs, satisfactorily accounts for the overt alternations in thalamic neuronal activity observed during the transition from EEG synchronization to EEG desynchronization (Purpura and Shofer, 1963).

III. Thalamic Internuclear Interactions during Synchronizing and Desynchronizing Activities

The fact that the evoked EEG synchronization induced by low frequency stimulation of thalamic nonspecific nuclei is accompanied by a prolonged period of inhibition of a large proportion of thalamic neurons has important implications for the analysis of factors modulating input-output functions in thalamic relay nuclei. This is well illustrated in the case of the cerebellothalamocortical projection pathway (Cohen *et al.*, 1962; Purpura, 1970; Purpura *et al.*, 1965). Both relay and nonrelay elements of the nucleus ventralis lateralis (VL) are profoundly influenced by synaptic pathways arising in medial and intralaminar thalamic nuclei. This is evident in the large proportion of VL cells that exhibit EPSP–IPSP sequences during low frequency MTh stimulation. Indeed, VL cells may display prominent and prolonged IPSPs for 70–80% of the time during which evoked EEG synchronization is induced. It is clear that during this time VL relay activity will be strongly inhibited (Fig. 6.12). Thus if relay activity elicited by brachium conjunctivum stimulation is timed to occur at any phase of the prolonged summating IPSP evoked by low frequency MTh stimulation, the monosynaptic EPSP generated by the brachium input is both attenuated and removed from the firing level of the VL neuron. Only when the relay activity occurs in relation to the EPSP component of the EPSP–IPSP sequence evoked by MTh stimulation is VL transmission facilitated (Purpura *et al.*, 1966b). Such a nonspecific–specific internuclear interaction serves as an effective "gating" mechanism for modulating as well as limiting output in response to a high frequency cerebellothalamic afferent

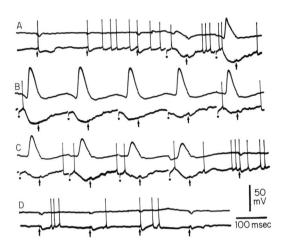

Fig. 6.12. Inhibition of VL cell discharges evoked by 7/sec brachium conjunctivum (BC) stimulation (at arrows) during concomitant 7/sec medial thalamic stimulation (indicated by dots under shock artefacts). Medial thalamic stimulation precedes BC stimulation by 70 msec during the interaction. A–D. Continuous record. Medial thalamic stimulation elicits a typical long-latency surface-negative recruiting response in motor cortex. A sequence of small EPSPs and more prominent prolonged IPSPs are observed in the VL cell. A–C. Inhibition of BC-evoked discharges is secured during the thalamocortical recruitment. D. Cessation of medial thalamic stimulation reveals persisting but variable inhibition of BC-evoked discharges. [From Purpura *et al.*, 1965]

input (Purpura *et al.*, 1966a). One consequence of this interaction will be seen in a relative inhibition of VL relay activity during EEG synchronization.

Unlike VL relay cells, neurons of the thalamic ventrobasal complex that receive monosynaptic excitatory input from medial lemniscus afferents (Maekawa and Purpura, 1967a) are weakly influenced by low frequency MTh stimulation (Maekawa and Purpura, 1967b). In contrast, medial thalamic stimulation has a significant synaptic effect on VB interneurons that exhibit long-latency PSPs in response to lemniscal stimulation (Fig. 6.13). The differences in the potency of internuclear interaction between medial thalamic and VL organizations on the one hand, and between medial thalamic and VB organizations on the other, suggests a significant "bias" of the internuclear system toward thalamic nuclei with projections to motor and premotor cortex. Alternatively, such differences may reflect operational failures to activate components of the nonspecific thalamic system that have internuclear relations with VB. In this context it should be noted that the spontaneous development of rhythmic 8–12/sec waves in somatosensory cortex is frequently associated with rhythmic EPSP–IPSP sequences in VB relay cells (Fig. 6.14) (Maekawa and Purpura, 1967b). Under these conditions VB relay neurons may exhibit

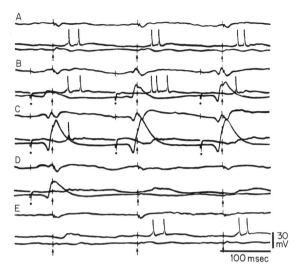

Fig. 6.13. Effects of MTh stimulation on VB neuron exhibiting long latency EPSPs and repetitive discharges to medial lemniscus (ML) stimulation. The third beam record in this figure represents simultaneously evoked recruiting response from anterior sigmoid gyrus. Note differences in the characteristics of recruiting responses in anterior sigmoid gyrus and in posterior sigmoid gyrus (upper channel records). A–E. Continuous record. A. Prior to MTh stimulation, ML stimulation elicits long latency EPSP and associated spikes. Build-up of recruiting responses in B and C results in development of long latency IPSPs in VB neuron which suppresses spike discharges. Depressant aftereffects of MTh stimulation are shown in D and recovery of control responsiveness to ML stimulation in E. [From Maekawa and Purpura, 1967b]

prolonged IPSPs which effectively block transmission of lemniscal afferent input. Evidently the spontaneously occurring rhythmical waves in the VB-somatosensory projection system are generated by activity in thalamic organizations which are not influenced by MTh stimulation. The converse of this may also be seen, especially in the VL-motor cortex projection system. Figure 6.15 illustrates examples of simultaneous recordings from a VL relay neuron and the motor cortex projection area during a spontaneous spindle burst and during evoked recruiting responses. The spindle burst was not associated with synaptic events in the VL relay neuron whereas MTh stimulation elicited prominent EPSP–IPSP sequences. These data bear on the problem of the variable relationship of different varieties of synchronized electrocortical activity in specific cortical areas to synaptic events in relay cells reciprocally linked to these areas.

The reciprocal relations between specific relay nuclei and cortical projection areas provide a means whereby synchronized discharges in relay elements may be facilitated or inhibited by corticepetal activities. As noted above, the effects of nonspecific thalamic stimulation on specific relay activity during evoked

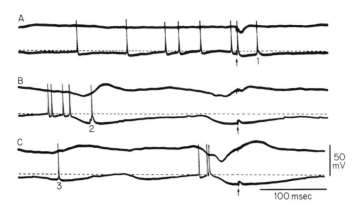

Fig. 6.14. Membrane potential changes in an identified VB relay cell during spontaneously developing cortical spindle waves. Horizontal dashed lines are drawn through base line membrane potential levels to emphasize magnitude and duration of membrane hyperpolarizations during different phases of electrocortical waves. A–C. From a continuous record in which segments have been removed to permit alignment of monosynaptic responses to medial lemniscus (ML) stimulation (at arrows). During spontaneous IPSPs relay discharges are blocked, revealing the ML-evoked EPSPs in isolation. Spontaneous spike discharges are modulated in frequency during IPSPs. Some of these spikes arise from a level of increased membrane polarization (1 and 3), and one exhibiting multiple brief depolarizations (cf. Maekawa and Purpura, 1967a) is shown in B (2). [From Maekawa and Purpura, unpublished]

EEG synchronization signify the operation of equally potent control mechanisms regulating transmission in afferent projection systems. Until recently, little consideration was given to the effects observed in nonspecific thalamic neurons following stimulation of specific thalamic nuclei. It is now established that specific and nonspecific nuclei are reciprocally related by internuclear pathways (Desiraju and Purpura, 1970).

The demonstration of internuclear synaptic pathways arising in VA-VL nuclei and distributing to medial and intralaminar (nonspecific) thalamic nuclei has been accomplished by intracellular registration from medial thalamic neurons during low frequency stimulation of VA-VL regions. The most commonly encountered synaptic events in such studies are illustrated in Figs. 6.16 and 6.17. In many instances the first of a repetitive train of VA-VL stimuli elicited a very short latency, prolonged IPSP in medial thalamic neurons (Fig. 6.16A). This inhibition of nonspecific neuronal activity occurred in association with the development of typical primary cortical responses. The second and subsequent stimuli which gave rise to augmenting responses were accompanied by temporal changes in IPSPs of medial thalamic neurons (Figs. 6.16B and C).

A second pattern of synaptic activity observed in medial thalamic neurons during VA-VL stimulation is shown in Fig. 6.17. In this pattern the initial

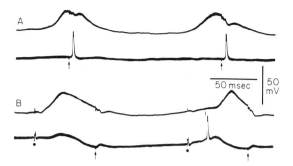

Fig. 6.15. Comparison of different relationships between electrocortical waves in motor cortex (upper channel) and intracellular synaptic events in an identified VL-relay neuron. Brachium conjunctivum (BC) stimulation (at arrows) evokes a VL-relay discharge and a prominent specific response of motor cortex. A. No effect is observed in the VL neuron during the spontaneous spindle waves of motor cortex. B. During medial thalamic stimulation (dots below shock artefacts) prominent EPSP–IPSP sequences are observed in association with surface-negative recruiting responses. VL-relay discharges are inhibited during the IPSPs. [From Purpura, McMurtry, and Maekawa, unpublished]

VL stimulus evoked a long latency prolonged IPSP upon which powerful EPSPs were superimposed with successive stimuli. Medial thalamic cells exhibiting this pattern of synaptic activity in response to VL stimulation were also influenced by corticepetal volleys (Fig. 6.18). As in the case of ventral tier specific projection neurons, elements of the thalamic nonspecific projection nuclei may be powerfully influenced by activity arising in the cerebral cortex. Thus, the evidence from intracellular recordings in neurons located in specific (VL) and nonspecific nuclei clearly indicates that activity generated in nonspecific thalamic nuclei and cerebral cortex may modulate transmission in VL. At the same time VL stimulation can profoundly inhibit or activate nonspecific neurons and the latter may also be strongly influenced by corticothalamic projections. While each of these interacting synaptic systems can be functionally dissected one from the other, it must be borne in mind that in the intact animal they are operated in concert. It follows from this that the interneuronal machinery of the thalamus must be continuously modulated by a variety of inputs which have one feature in common: their capacity to operate reciprocally related interneuronal pathways that elicit synchronizing EPSP–IPSP sequences in specific *and* nonspecific neurons.

The final problem to be considered in this section on basic synaptic mechanisms regulating thalamic relay transmission is concerned with the manner in which reticulocortical activation alters input–output functions in specific thalamocortical projection systems. It was shown above that during evoked EEG synchronization VL relay transmission is markedly depressed by virtue of

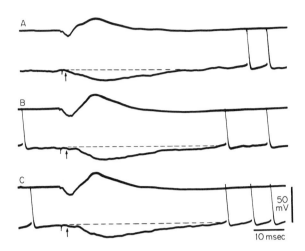

Fig. 6.16. Alterations in characteristics of IPSPs elicited in a neuron of the medial thalamus (MTh) during repetitive stimulation (6 Hz) of n. ventralis lateralis (VL). Upper channel records are surface-evoked responses (negativity upward) recorded from motor cortex. A–C. First three responses to VL stimulation at 6 Hz. A. First stimulus elicits a typical positive-negative primary response in motor cortex. Intracellular recording from a MTh neuron located at a depth of 4.5 mm from the surface of the thalamus reveals a 1. 5–2.0 msec latency IPSP (at arrow). B. The second stimulus occurring 140 msec after the first produces an "augmented" surface-evoked response. This is associated with a 2 msec increase in latency of the IPSP which may have been interrupted by a small EPSP. The IPSP is increased in duration and is succeeded by a more prominent EPSP that elicits a spike potential. C. The third stimulus evokes essentially similar cortical surface and intracellular synaptic events as the second stimulus. Base line membrane potential is indicated by the dashed lines. [From Desiraju and Purpura, 1970]

the prolonged IPSPs elicited in VL cells subsequent to low frequency MTh stimulation (Fig. 6.12). Since one of the prominent effects of brain-stem reticular formation (BSRF) stimulation on synchronizing EPSP–IPSP sequences in VL cells is to attenuate or block the IPSPs, it can be expected that BSRF stimulation superimposed on low frequency MTh stimulation will counteract the inhibition of relay transmission observed during the evoked EEG synchronization. This has been confirmed in intracellular studies which are summarized in Fig. 6.19 (Purpura *et al.*, 1966b).

Identification of a VL neuron monosynaptically excited by brachium conjunctivum stimulation is shown in Fig. 6.19A. During low frequency MTh stimulation the IPSP elicited in the VL cell blocked the relay discharge, revealing the monosynaptic EPSP in isolation (Fig. 6.19B). It is important to note that high frequency BSRF stimulation *alone* increased the discharge frequency of the VL neuron (Fig. 6.19C), thereby indicating a powerful facilitatory influence of reticular activation on VL relay transmission, as originally shown in extracellular studies (Frigyesi and Purpura, 1964). When BSRF stimulation is initiated during low frequency MTh stimulation, the IPSP produced by the latter stimulation is greatly attenuated along with restoration of relay transmission (Fig. 6.19D). However, it should be pointed out that the balance of countervailing synaptic effects elicited during the two modes of stimulation may at one time favor BSRF stimulation and at other times favor MTh stimulation, at least in respect to the increase in discharge frequency initiated by reticulocortical activation. In the example of Fig. 6.19D, BSRF stimulation effectively suppressed electrocortical recruiting responses (compare Fig. 6.19B and 6.19D) but the BSRF-induced augmentation of VL discharge was eliminated by the MTh stimulation despite the fact that relay transmission was restored. The data emphasize the variable effects of different inputs with different degrees of synaptic security as regards their capacity to activate VL relay cells.

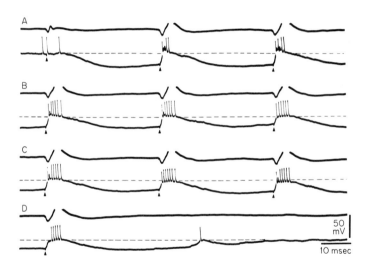

Fig. 6.17. Dramatic enhancement of short-latency prolonged EPSPs superimposed on long-duration IPSPs in an MTh neuron (depth, 5.5 mm) during 5 Hz VA–VL stimulation. Arrow heads indicate stimulus artefacts. A. The first stimulus elicits a spike discharge on a short-latency EPSP that is not well illustrated. A prolonged IPSP with a latency of 30–40 msec follows the initial synaptic events. The second and subsequent stimuli delivered during the residual membrane hyperpolarization of the prolonged IPSP evokes a polysynaptic "giant" EPSP, with superimposed high frequency spikes and partial spikes. A–C. Continuous recording. Two-sec strip of record removed between C and D. In D, the last stimulus of the repetitive train elicits a smaller EPSP with delayed discharges. The terminal IPSP exhibits a superimposed spontaneous EPSP and spike discharge before return to base line membrane potential level as indicated throughout by the horizontal dashed lines. [From Desiraju and Purpura, 1970]

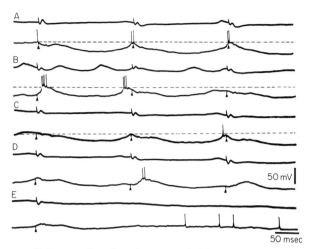

Fig. 6.18. Intracellular recordings from the same medial thalamic neuron studied in Fig. 6.17. A–E. Continuous record during low frequency stimulations of the corona radiata of pericruciate cortex (at arrow heads). Note that the first stimulus triggers a repetitive series of EPSP–IPSP sequences which resemble the PSP patterns evoked by VA–VL stimulation in Fig. 6.17. Dashed lines indicate membrane potential base line level in the absence of stimulation. [From Desiraju and Purpura, unpublished]

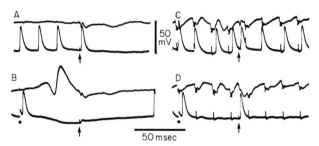

Fig. 6.19. Alterations in PSPs of a VL relay cell during combined low frequency MTh stimulation and high frequency (60/sec) BSRF stimulation. In this figure sample records were taken from continuous film strips during 7/sec BC stimulation or combined 7/sec MTh and BC stimulation. A. Spontaneous activity of the VL cell is interrupted after an evoked response to BC stimulation. Note low level IPSP succeeding the evoked discharge. B. Conditioning 7/sec MTh stimulation (indicated by black dot) elicits a long latency recruiting response in motor cortex and an EPSP–IPSP sequence in the VL cell. The prolonged synchronizing IPSP blocks cell discharges and reveals the underlying low-amplitude specific EPSP evoked by testing 7/sec BC stimulation. C. During 60/sec BSRF stimulation VL cell discharge frequency is increased by small short latency reticulo-VL EPSPs. D. BC responses are conditioned by 7/sec MTh stimulation during high frequency BSRF stimulation. Comparison of D and B reveals that BSRF stimulation attenuates the synchronizing IPSP, thus permitting restoration of BC-evoked discharges. Note small superposed reticulo-VL EPSPs on residual synchronizing IPSP. Complete suppression of cortical surface recruiting response during BSRF stimulation is shown in D. Short latency cortical-evoked responses were prominent in this experiment during BSRF stimulation. [From Purpura et al., 1966b]

IV. Comment and Conclusion

The argument has been advanced in this brief survey of intracellular studies that the synaptic mechanisms observed in thalamic neurons during evoked EEG synchronization (recruiting responses, spindle waves) and EEG desynchronization (reticulocortical activation) are likely to be set into operation when similar electrocortical alterations are found in association with changes in sleep–wakefulness activities in the behaving animal. It is important to point out that these intracellular studies were carried out in locally anesthetized paralyzed *encéphale isolé* cats in order to avoid the complicating effects of barbiturate anesthesia. Despite this, it may be argued that electrical stimulation of medial thalamic and brain-stem reticular regions can hardly serve as an appropriate model for reproducing the electrocortical events observed in the freely moving and behaving animal. However, since publication of most of these intracellular studies, investigations in which extracellular recordings have been obtained in chronic preparations exhibiting sleep–wakefulness behavior have been interpretable largely on the basis of the synaptic mechanisms described here (Steriade *et al.*, 1969a; cf. Steriade and others in this volume). There is thus good reason to believe that the intracellular synaptic events disclosed in these studies constitute the basis for the alterations in spontaneous discharge characteristics observed in a number of thalamic neuronal organizations during transitions from sleep to wakefulness and vice versa (Baker, 1971; Hubel, 1960). In accordance with this view, it can be inferred that the appearance in neurons of synchronized rhythmical bursts of discharges succeeded by long silent periods is largely due to EPSP–IPSP sequences and that attenuation of IPSPs and increase in excitatory synaptic drives characterize the intracellular events in neurons exhibiting desynchronized firing patterns.

Differences should be noted in respect to the ease with which transmission is influenced in two fundamentally different specific thalamic projection pathways during evoked EEG synchronization. Whereas powerful modulatory effects have been observed in VL by stimulation of nonspecific-specific internuclear pathways, this has not been observed in VB relay cells. Recent findings in behaving cats with chronically implanted VB electrodes have indicated that the response characteristics of VB cells to afferent input are not significantly influenced by alterations in sleep–wakefulness behavior (Baker, 1971). On the other hand, the latter investigations have disclosed consistent changes in spontaneous activity of VB neurons during sleep and wakefulness. Evidently different types of control systems must be capable of influencing the activities of neurons in the same and different thalamic nuclei. This suggests the need for caution in attempts to extrapolate the results obtained in one type of experimental situation to another. A case in point is the remarkably different activity of VB cells in the barbiturate anesthetized animal (Andersen *et al.*, 1964b) and in the unanesthetized (Mountcastle *et al.*, 1963) and behaving animal (Baker, 1971). There can be no question but that such differences reflect the operation of different input systems that modify relay transmission in VB neurons under the different experimental situations.

No apology is necessary for the failure of the author to provide a simple diagrammatic representation of the possible neuronal circuitry underlying the synaptic effects observed in thalamic neurons during evoked EEG synchronization and EEG desynchronization. Most likely these would only serve to satisfy the casual reader rather than the data. It is more important to stress the primary conclusion drawn from the data that the different synaptic events observed during the different types of electrocortical activity are attributable to interactions in *interneuronal networks* with different input characteristics. The inference in this is that "switching" of pathways within such networks may occur in response to changes in input frequency or by activation of new inputs. This is evident in the "inhibition of inhibition" that characterizes the blocking action of reticular stimulation on the thalamic synchronization process, as noted above. For present purposes and until much more is known about thalamic interneuronal organizations and their efferent and afferent relations, such an explanation seems the most parsimonious. Alternatives to this which require recurrent pathways, special properties of thalamic neurons including postanodal exaltation phenomena (cf. Andersen, Chapter 7 and discussion in Purpura, 1969) may also play a role in the synaptic events described here. But it is doubtful if these can be as important in the production of different patterns of synaptic activities during neuronal synchronization and desynchronization as interactions in interneuronal networks. If it is possible to discern any pattern in the evolution of comparative morphophysiological studies of "nervous systems," it is in attempts to define the interneuronal interactions in these structures. This is equally applicable to vertebrate spinal cord and invertebrate ganglia. Doubtless the same approach applied to brainstem and forebrain structures will further clarify the interneuronal transactions revealed in the present studies in connection with synaptic events that have their counterpart in complex sleep–wakefulness behaviors.

Discussion

Steriade: Dr. Purpura's intracellular findings in paralyzed cats are well corroborated by our observations on fluctuations in VL focal responses during the sleep–wakefulness continuum in chronically implanted, behaving preparations (Steriade *et al.*, 1969b). The presynaptic component of the VL response evoked by cerebellothalamic stimulation (reflecting the action potentials in the afferent pathway) did not change in amplitude during various stages of sleep and waking. In spite of the constancy of this input, the monosynaptically relayed VL response virtually disappeared during drowsiness with EEG spindles, was reduced during sleep with slow wave as compared to waking, and showed a dramatic increase during paradoxical sleep (see Fig. 8.2B of Chapter 8).

Purpura: I think that it is an important point because it shows that there is never a necessity to involve a presynaptic inhibitory mechanism to explain these changes in the VL nucleus.

Steriade: Now, I have a point concerning your hypothesis on the dis-inhibition induced by brain-stem reticular stimulation. When we recorded neurons from the cat's pre-cruciate gyrus or monkey's precentral cortex and observed a significant reduction in duration of the tested (afferent or recurrent) inhibition during waking as compared with slow sleep, some neurons were also seen to increase their mean discharge rates during waking, but other ones did not significantly alter their spontaneous firing (Steriade *et al.*, 1971; see also Chapter 8 in this book). In the latter case, when reduction in the evoked inhibition during waking is apparently independent of an increase in the excitatory drive (compare stages W and D in Fig. 8.26 of Chapter 8 in this book), we may infer an inhibition of inhibitory interneurons. On the other hand, the reduction of the antidromically elicited inhibition of VL neurons during reticular arousal was always associated with a considerable increase in their spontaneous firing (Steriade *et al.*, 1971a). Furthermore, we could drive VL neurons at short latencies and without failure by fast reticular pulses, thus indicating a high-security monosynaptic excitatory projection from the mesencephalic tegmentum to the VL. I wonder whether excitation—a strong one as the evidence indicates—may overwhelm inhibition and, thus, be solely responsible for the reduced inhibition during waking in the VL?

Purpura: I believe that this problem has a general interest for our audience to understand what happens to cerebral mechanisms during sleep. It is not just a continuous dialogue between specialists.

The answer to the question of whether excitation is responsible for all the effects one sees in the VL nucleus is probably not a definite "no." We also have observed excitatory drives in the VL with stimulation of the reticular formation. But, first, bear in mind that natural arousal does not necessarily produce as much excitation as an electrical stimulation. Second, it seems that the best way to determine the responsible mechanism is to study membrane resistance changes accompanying potential variations in these thalamic neurons. We did this study to see whether or not the IPSPs were still present and whether or not there were additional conductance increases produced by EPSPs which would counteract the hyperpolarization and bring the membrane potential to some neutral level. The fact is that the membrane conductance decreased during reticular stimulation. This means a removal—not an addition—of synaptic actions. I think that the major effect is really to reduce the amount of inhibitory synchronizing activity. If there are EPSPs occuring in addition, the site of their generation must be quite remote from the site of intracelluar recording for they do not produce any observable conductance increases of the membrane, presumably, in the soma.

Bremer: I am somewhat reluctant to accept this idea that the Moruzzi and Magoun reticular activating system would be, in fact, an inhibitory system!

Purpura: Well, inhibition of inhibition has similar consequences as excitation. In addition, there is also a true excitatory drive, as we have indicated in our study.

Bremer: In the case of the lateral geniculate (LG) nucleus, there is a spectacular facilitation of transmission after stimulation of the reticular inhibition. The inhibitory tonus normally exerted on these cells would have to be extraordinarily powerful to explain that its removal could result in the enormous facilitatory effect that we have seen.

Purpura: The lateral geniculate nucleus may be a different case. There, you may have the additional problem of a significant control on presynaptic pathways. The reticular action may be extended—at least partly—by gating the presynaptic pathway.

Schlag: In all this discussion on inhibitory mechanisms in the thalamus, I think that we should stress that there are probably several types of circuits involving inhibitory neurons.

First, there is the recurrent inhibition which Dr. Andersen will certainly discuss.

Second, there are the internuclear inhibitory interactions that Dr. Purpura has described between medial and lateral thalamic cell groups.

Third, there may also be an inhibition coming from the reticularis complex which—as you know—surrounds the dorsal thalamic nucleus almost entirely. We have found that these neurons discharge at exceptionally high rates (300–450/sec) for long times (Schlag and Waszak, 1971). Other thalamic cells cannot sustain such frequency. From the Scheibels' work, we know that reticularis cells send their axons to the thalamus itself. The interesting point is that reticularis cells are particularly active during spindling activity or during thalamic low frequency stimulation (e.g., at 10/sec). From the literature (Andersen and Andersson, 1968; Purpura *et al.*, 1965), it is apparent that this coincides with a definite hyperpolarization of dorsal thalamic cells lasting as long as the whole duration of the spindle burst or the train of thalamic stimuli.

In addition to their different origins, these several types of inhibition probably are characterized by their different durations and roles. For instance, the action of reticularis cells may determine the overall duration of periods of rhythmic activity whereas the inter- and intranuclear inhibitions would determine intraspindle frequencies.

Purpura: This is possible, although the only thing we can observe at this point is the overall summated effect of such hypothetical synaptic actions.

Bremer: With respect to a possible role ascribed to reticularis neurons, it would be interesting to know what their activity is in barbiturate anesthesia inducing EEG spindle bursts.

Schlag: Yes, Waszak is looking at that. The answer does not seem to be simple. In some units, the activity is enhanced by small doses of short-acting barbiturates.

Albe-Fessard: In several cerebral structures, we have seen long rhythmic modifications of membrane potential phases of hyperpolarization underlying spindle bursts. We thought that this phenomenon was due to slow metabolic oscillations of the membrane properties.

Purpura: Do you mean that this could be a shift in the activity of an electrogenic pump?

Albe-Fessard: Possibly.

Purpura: There are now data showing long-lasting changes in membrane potential, for instance in the postseizure state of the hippocampus. At the end of the seizure, the very long increase in membrane potential is associated with an increase in membrane resistance, suggesting that an electrogenic pump has been turned on. On the other hand, Krnjevic *et al.* (1970) has shown that, in the cortex, acetylcholine—which we always thought of as acting by increasing the membrane conductance and thus inducing an EPSP—produces an excitatory event associated with an increase in membrane resistance. Presumably, this is caused by blocking potassium channels. The slow phenomenon that we see may be due to such an action.

Albe-Fessard: Another point: When an anesthetic is injected, the membrane potential of all the cells is increased.

Purpura: Now, this can be due to a disfacilitation, i.e., to a reduction of the excitatory bombardment. It would be interesting to measure the membrane resistance to test this possibility.

Albe-Fessard: Yes, I agree; but I do not think that disfacilitation is the explanation because the activity along the primary afferent pathway to the cortex is only slightly decreased under these conditions, however, the membrane of the cells in primary relay also presents an increase of membrane potential.

Purpura: The first thing one would have to do to interpret this increase in membrane potential caused by anesthetics is to establish whether or not it is accompanied by a change in membrane conductance.

CHAPTER SEVEN

Physiological Mechanism of Barbiturate Spindle Activity

PER ANDERSEN

Electrocorticographic spindles may be defined as short periods of rhythmic waves of waxing and waning amplitude and with a frequency of 6–10 per second. Because of their appearance, the cortical spindles in experimental animals have been used as models for human alpha waves and sleep spindles. In the following, particular emphasis will be put upon the type of spindle activity known as barbiturate spindles after its discovery by Derbyshire, *et al.* in 1936. It must be remembered, however, that this spindle activity is artificially simplified so that a study of it reveals the basic, anesthesia-resistant mechanisms only. In the more complex situation in awake organisms, the spindle activity is probably appreciably modified.

I. Thalamic Control of Spindle Waves

The pioneering studies by Bremer (1935, 1937, 1938a) showed that regular waves occured both during barbiturate anesthesia and also without narcosis when the brain stem was transected, leaving thalamus and all cortical areas intact in the rostral division. Furthermore, rhythmic thalamic activity (Adrian, 1941) persisted after complete decortication (Morison and Basset, 1945), indicating that the thalamic rhythmicity is not entirely dependent upon similar

127

cortical activity. On the other hand, relatively small isolated cortical slabs were reported to produce long-lasting rhythmic activity (Burns, 1950). In order to test this phenomenon, on larger cortical areas, Andersen *et al.* (1967a) isolated the entire frontal lobes in cats both acutely and chronically. Figure 7.1 shows that records taken behind the isolated section showed periodic spindle activity on both the right and left side. In front of the section, however, no normal spindle activity was obtained, neither on the chronically (left), nor on the acutely (right) denervated side. However, randomly occurring giant spikes typical of large-scale denervation were often observed. These results suggest that a rhythmic thalamocortical input is necessary for the normal spindle be-havior of the cortex. When electrically or chemically stimulated, the isolated cortex may show rhythmic activity, but of short duration and with a frequency that usually differs from that of the normal rhythmicity (Kristiansen and Courtois, 1949; Jasper, 1949; Burns, 1950, 1951; Ingvar, 1955).

Further support for the importance of thalamocortical rhythmic input was obtained by cooling experiments, fully confirming the earlier report by Bremer (1958). Local cortical cooling (Fig. 7.2B) reduced the amplitude of the cortical waves on the cooled side, but not their frequency. On systemic cooling, either by immersing the whole animal in ice water, or by extracorporeal circulation, both the amplitude and frequency were reduced, until the cortical response was very similar to that of the denervated cortex (Fig. 7.2C). Similar "denervation" records could be obtained after injection of various drugs in the thalamus

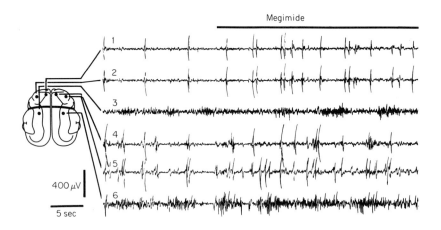

Fig. 7.1. Spontaneous cortical activity recorded from the indicated sites (dots) rostral, and caudal to a lesion (heavy line) which isolated the frontal poles completely from the rest of the brain (inset). Chronic lesion (1 week) on the left, acute to the right. The horizontal line above in-dicates the intravenous injection of 50 mg Megimide (pentylene tetrazol glutarimide), made to optimize the condition for appearance of rhythmic cortical activity.

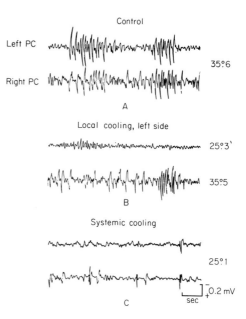

Fig. 7.2. Effect of cooling on the amplitude and frequency of cortical spindle waves recorded from the left and right postcruciate gyrus as indicated (PC). A. Control records taken at a normal cortical temperature. B. The left cortex was cooled to a temperature of 25.3°, whereas the right cortex remained at normal temperature. Note the reduction in amplitude but unchanged frequency. C. Systemic cooling through extracorporeal circulation to a thalamic temperature of 25.1°.

(Ralston and Ajmone-Marsan, 1956), or by edema inflicted by ischemia or surgical manipulation of the thalamus (Andersen *et al.*, 1967a).

II. Thalamic Recurrent Inhibition

The major feature of the model for rhythmic spindle activity given in the present communication is the recurrent inhibition in the thalamus. Following a single afferent volley to the ventrobasal complex (VBC), there was an initial discharge of thalamic relay cells (Fig. 7.3A, filled circle). The upward deflection of the lower trace was recorded from the white matter underlying the cortex and signifies that the discharging cells send their impulses toward the cortex (cross). Following the initial discharge there was a large positive wave (P-wave) in the VBC record which was terminated by the near synchronous discharge of many cells, including some of those taking part in the initial discharge but with other cells in addition (filled triangle). This secondary discharge was also associated with thalamocortical impulses as seen by the deflection in the lower trace (arrow). Following this discharge there was a new P-wave which, after another 120 msec, was terminated by a new group of synchronous cell discharges (filled square) and with a thalamocortical deflection (diamond). Thus, under these experimental conditions a single afferent volley is capable of initiating a series of discharges along thalamocortical axons, separated in time by about 120 msec.

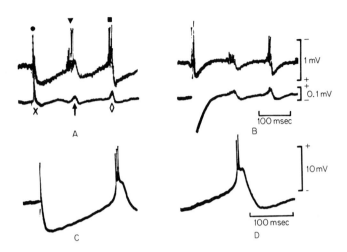

Fig. 7.3. Rhythmic activity evoked by a single afferent volley. In A and B, the upper traces are recordings from the ventrobasal complex in response to a superficial radial volley (A) or an antidromic volley from the radial receiving area of the postcruciate cortex (B). The lower traces are white matter recording in which the upward deflection signifies a thalamocortical volley. C. Intracellular record of a VBC cell response to antidromic stimulation. D. Spontaneous oscillation of the same cell recorded during a spindle period.

Figure 7.3B shows a similar response produced by cortical stimulation. Antidromic and corticothalamic synaptic activation of thalamic cells were able to initiate the same type of repetitive discharges along thalamocortical axons, the former leading to the postulate of recurrent thalamic inhibition (Andersen and Eccles, 1962). Figure 7.3C shows an intracellular record from a ventrobasal complex cell in response to antidromic stimulation of the appropriate cortex. Following the antidromic activation there was a large and long-lasting hyperpolarization which satisfies the criteria for being an inhibitory postsynaptic potential (IPSP). Without any additional stimulation, the IPSP was terminated after about 150 msec by a sudden large depolarization, on top of which are three spikes. This late depolarization has a slower rise time and a longer duration than the EPSPs following orthodromic activation to lemniscal fibers (Maekawa and Purpura, 1967a). Because of its frequent occurrence after an inhibitory potential, this response is called a postinhibitory rebound potential, earlier called postanodal exaltation (Andersen and Eccles, 1962). Figure 7.3D was taken during a series of spontaneous spindle oscillations where the cell is shown to recover from a spontaneous IPSP and to develop a large postinhibitory rebound deplorization with two superimposed spikes. Thus, the postinhibitory rebound reaction may be seen both after induced and spontaneous IPSPs.

In order to test the excitability changes of thalamic cells during such rhythmic behavior, Andersen *et al.* (1964a) delivered small test pulses to the ventrobasal complex and recorded the response from the white matter under-lying the appropriate part of the sensory cortex. The initial deflection is due to the direct excitation of thalamic cells. It is followed by a second volley caused by the excitation of afferent fibers inside the thalamic nucleus and the resulting transsynaptic discharge. A conditioning shock was delivered to the peripheral nerve. The size of the direct volley is a measure of the excitability, or membrane potential, of the relay cells. The amplitude of the subsequent wave from the white matter recording is also influenced by any presynaptic excitability changes. Figure 7.4 summarizes the results from one such experiment where the response from the VPL to a superficial radial volley is seen below and the excitability graph is plotted on top of it. The filled squares give the size of the direct volley, indicating the excitability of the postsynaptic elements, whereas the open circles give the transsynaptic response. During the P-wave there is a definite reduced excitability of the thalamic cells. However, during the post-inhibitory rebound period, signalled by the burst discharge of a single cell in

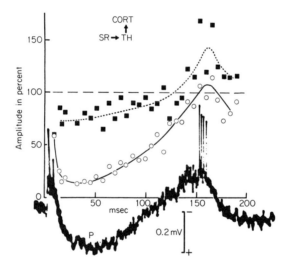

Fig. 7.4. Excitability changes of a thalamic nucleus following a single afferent volley. The analog signal shows the response of a VBC cell to a superficial radial volley. The initial N-wave with superimposed discharges is followed by a large P-wave (P) which gave way to another negative wave with a burst discharge (four spikes) of the same cell. The size of the direct (filled squares) and transsynaptic volley (open circles) recorded from the white matter in response to a test stimulus delivered to the ventrobasal complex is plotted against the time between a conditioning superficial radial volley and the test shock. Note the large excitability increase of both elements at about 150 msec after the initial shock.

the analog record, there is a definite increase of excitability of the same cells. This excitability clearly overshoots the 100% level, some observations lying very much higher. The great variability at this time probably reflects the all-or-nothing appearance of the post-inhibitory rebound phenomenon which may be seen in individual cells. It is likely that the reaction is triggered by an afferent impulse, but may, under certain conditions, be released by hyperpolarization of the membrane only (Maekawa and Purpura, 1967b).

Figure 7.5 gives a summary of the mechanism underlying the thalamic rhythmic activity in response to an afferent volley. A is a diagrammatic representation of the sequence of membrane events following an afferent volley (arrow). After the conduction latency, there is a large EPSP which discharges the cell, often with a single or double spike (Maekawa and Purpura, 1967a). Following the initial excitation there is a large IPSP which is terminated abruptly by the postinhibitory rebound depolarization giving rise to a series of spikes. Because of the intense depolarization, the sodium carrier is partly decoupled so that the last spikes have reduced amplitudes in relation to the first one. The rebound discharge is followed by a new IPSP which is terminated by a further burst discharge, and so on. Figure 7.5B shows the simplest diagram which could explain such a behavior. Each afferent fiber makes synaptic contact with a single relay cell. Two of these are excited by afferent volleys (thick lines). The thalamocortical fibers are presumed to have axon collaterals which may excite an inhibitory interneuron (black). This cell produces inhibition of a number of cells surrounding the initially excited ones. This is an example of a

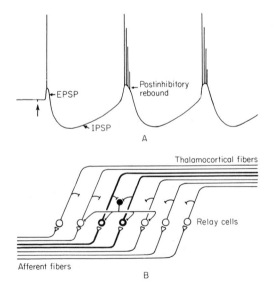

Fig. 7.5. A. Diagram of the sequence of events elicited in a thalamic cell by a single afferent volley. B. Diagram of the recurrent thalamic inhibitory pathway which may be responsible for the rhythmic activity described in the text.

recurrent inhibitory pathway which was proposed because antidromic invasion along thalamocortical fibers is as effective as orthodromic impulses in producing rhythmic activity.

III. Spontaneous Thalamic Activity

The scheme envisaged for triggering rhythmic activity by an afferent impulse can also be used to explain spontaneous rhythmic behavior of thalamic neurons. Both extra- and intracellular records of spontaneous rhythmic activity of thalamic cells appear remarkably similar to the rhythmic responses to a single afferent volley. Extracellular records show sequences of bursts separated by large P-waves, the series lasting for about 1–2 sec. The P-waves have waxing and waning amplitude giving rise to the notification of thalamic spindle for the whole period. The elements of such a spontaneous spindle seem identical to those produced by an afferent volley. Recorded intracellularly (Fig. 7.6), the spindle is associated with a series of IPSPs in a thalamic relay cell. The random discharge before the spindle is transformed to a rhythmic discharge in which the cell discharges on top of the crest between two successive IPSPs. Thus, the IPSPs are seen as phasing devices allowing the cell to discharge at a particular time only. However, because of the postinhibitory rebound phenomenon, the IPSPs are also indirectly triggers in that they provide the background for the oscillating excitability of the neuronal membrane. It should be noted that the postinhibitory rebound does not need to occur in all cells in a group. Because of the effective spread of the inhibition, probably due to an extensive ramification of the axons of the inhibitory cells, only a fraction of the relay cells need to show postinhibitory discharge in order to maintain the inhibitory oscillation.

The presence of axon collaterals of thalamic cells, originally shown by Cajal (1911) and O'Leary (1940), has recently been confirmed by Tömböl (1967). Admittedly, they are scarce, so one would like to see additional possibilities for recurrent inhibitory coupling. The recently described dendro-

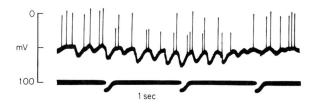

Fig. 7.6. Intracellular recording from a thalamic cell during a spontaneous spindle. The sequence of IPSPs phases the cell to discharge on the crest between two successive waves. During the spindle period the spike often shows the small A fraction only.

dendritic synaptic structures are suitably arranged to perform such a function (Lund, 1969; Famaglietti, 1970; Morest, 1971; Ralston, 1971). If the dendro-dendritic coupling is between relay cells and Golgi type II neurons, it could be an extremely efficient way to bring interneurons to discharge subsequent to relay cells' firing. If, on the other hand, the dendro-dendritic connections are between relay cells, this would be a suitable morphological substrate for the near synchronous discharge of many relay cells following the recurrent inhibition. The cell that first recovers from its depression during the P-wave could synaptically influence a considerable number of neighboring neurons and probably bring many of them to discharge.

IV. Thalamocortical Synchrony

When a thalamic microelectrode and a cortical surface electrode are placed "on-line," there is a remarkable synchrony between the rhythmic spindle waves recorded by the two electrodes. The on-line configuration is one which has a direct thalamocortical connection between the two recording sites. An example of such a situation is illustrated in Fig. 7.7. The electrode in the posterolateral ventral nucleus (VPL) shows discharges and P-waves in synchrony with the deflections of the appropriate point in the postcruciate cortex (PC). Other thalamic areas, like the posteromedial part of the ventral nucleus (VPM) also show rhythmic activity at about the same time. However, close scrutiny of the records shows that the VPM and the VPL electrode do not show perfect synchronization, the VPM trace lagging behind the other after two cycles. Further, the VPM rhythmic activity continues after the cessation of the VPL spindle and then shows a drop in frequency. Thus, spindle activity from various thalamic areas differs in precise times of start and stop, and in the shape and frequency of the spindle waves.

Further evidence for a closer connection between two sites lying "on-line" than between other thalamic and cortical areas is provided by the so-called

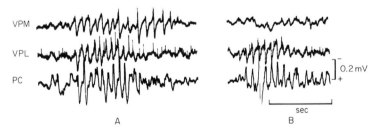

A   B

Fig. 7.7. A. Simultaneous records by two microelectrodes located in the thalamic receiving areas for the face (VPM) and the foreleg (VPL) and surface record from the cortical foreleg receiving area (PC). B. Local spindle, recorded from the same electrode positions.

local spindles (Fig. 7.7B). In such circumstances synchronous rhythmic activity may be seen in the appropriate on-line thalamic and cortical sites but not in neighboring thalamic and cortical areas.

Records of this type and records with multiple recording from closely spaced cortical regions have shown that the localization of the cortical electrode is critical. It must be placed within an area less than 1 mm in order to show perfect synchrony with a given thalamic spot. These data have given rise to the notion that the basic substrate for rhythmic activity is a little group of thalamic cells (with a diameter of about 200 μ) and those cortical cells to which this group projects, probably in the form of a cortical column (Andersen et al., 1967b). Obviously, except in the deliberately simplified experimental conditions, more cells than those of the minimal substrate will be operating. Under such circumstances the simple pattern of the on-line rhythmic activity will be masked by the additional active cells.

V. Pacemakers for Thalamic Rhythmic Activity

Since rhythmic thalamic activity of the spindle variety can be recorded from many thalamic nuclei, it is a possibility that one or several of these may serve as pacemaker for the others. Based upon their own observation of the greater ease with which rhythmic activity could be recorded from the thalamic midline structures, and the dramatic effect produced by 8/sec stimulation of that area, giving widespread recruiting potentials mimicking the spontaneous EEG waves, Morison and his co-workers (Morison and Dempsey, 1942, 1943; Dempsey and Morison, 1942a,b; Morison, et al., 1943) developed the concept of a midline thalamic pacemaker area. However, subsequent studies have shown that typical rhythmic spindle activity can be recorded also from laterally situated nuclei, including the sensory relay nuclei. In fact, the regularity of the spindles from the relay nuclei is better, and their spindle frequency higher than in more medial regions (Andersen and Andersson, 1968; Andersson and Manson, 1971). Using simultaneous recording with multiple microelectrodes from various thalamic nuclei, no thalamic nucleus was found to be pre-ponderant over any other with regard to initiation of rhythmic discharges during barbiturate anesthesia (Andersen and Andersson, 1968). Direct test of the midline pacemaker idea was made by removing the medial 3 mm of the thalamus on both sides in a series of cats. In such cats the pericruciate spindle activity was roughly unchanged both with regard to occurrence, duration, interval, internal frequency, and amplitude of the waves. However, when the lateral areas of the thalamus were removed, the cortical activity showed the typical denervation pattern described above. Therefore, during these conditions the appropriate relay cells seemed of greater importance for appropriate cortical rhythmic activity than the medially located thalamic areas. This should not be taken to mean that the midline areas are not important in influencing other areas, for example the lateral lying nuclei. Such a mechanism may be particularly important during more alert stages found during light anesthesia or in awake animals.

An alternative hypothesis is that several thalamic areas have the ability to control a given cortical area but that their influence varies in intensity during different sleep–wakefulness stages. Thus, midline thalamic areas might influence large cortical areas, including those under specific control from a relay nucleus. Under conditions of greatly diminished synaptic coupling, such as barbiturate anesthesia, the relay cells may have the strongest ability to influence the appropriate cortical area. Under lighter anesthesia or awake conditions, however, the nonspecific system may contribute to the complex electrocortico-gram recorded. Recent work by Andersson *et al.* (1971) seems to indicate that in the decorticate, nonanesthetized animal, the rhythmic activity of the midline nuclei is more prominent than during barbiturate anesthesia. Further, they postulate that the midline thalamic activity affects or modulates the rhythmic activity in lateral lying nuclei. In this context, one might say that the midline activity is necessary to produce a well-developed activity of the more lateral lying nuclei. An important part of the hypothesis invokes control of the postulated inhibitory interneuron. The midline areas are supposed to be able to influence the activity of these neurons, thereby increasing or reducing the rhythmic activity.

Further experimentation with advanced microelectrode recording from nonanesthetized free-moving animals is probably necessary to assess the relative importance of the simplest pathways necessary for rhythmic activity as they have been reviewed here, and the more elaborate machinery operating in intact organisms. In this endeavor, microelectrode recording from human thalami may yield significant results.

Discussion

Schlag: We shall certainly have an interesting discussion after this excellent presentation by Dr. Andersen. Dr. Andersen was not here yesterday for commenting on Dr. Purpura's lecture. We are now faced with two different systems of interpretation of rhythmic electrical activity in thalamocortical systems, and I wish that we might enlarge the scope of today's debate to cope with the whole problem. On one hand, we have a model based essentially on recurrent inhibition and postanodal exaltation in the thalamus. On the other hand, we have an explanation stressing the role of interneuronal interplay.

Dement: I get a little confused. I understand that postinhibitory exaltation is a descriptive term for some membrane phenomenon which causes cellular firing. Does it imply also that axon collateral recurrent inhibition is necessary for obtaining it?

Andersen: Postanodal exaltation (or postinhibitory rebound) was a term coined by Coombs *et al.* (1955) when they observed rebound firing in motoneurons that they had hyperpolarized. In thalamic cells, intracellular recording shows that IPSPs are followed by a large depolarization with high frequency spiking. Extracellularly, many cells are seen to fire simultaneously during the rebound. Recurrent inhibition is not essential to start the process. Any kind of inhibition will do, and the cells discharge as a rebound phenomenon probably assisted by background excitation.

Steriade: I would like to add that one can easily obtain evidence for the postanodal exaltation phenomenon in unanesthetized animals, by extracellular recording of spikes without any sign of injury. It is not rare to simultaneously record several VL thalamic neurons and see them going together with a series of rhythmic spike clusters superimposed on focal slow negative waves, following long-lasting slow positive waves associated with suppressed firing. It is difficult, however, to explain the rebound activity exclusively on the basis of the preceding inhibition. A delayed, powerful excitatory impingement exerted on VL neurons when they recover from inhibition has to be envisaged, thus triggering the burst of high frequency discharges. When both events (the hyperexcitable membrane at the end of the inhibitory period *and* the depolarizing pressure exerted by other elements) are eclectically considered, the rebound will be perhaps better understood. In experiments from our laboratory, the best candidates to exert this late *excitatory* drive on VL relay cells and, thus, to sculpture their rhythmic activity were found to be the VL intrinsic interneurons (synaptically engaged by direct corticofugal fibers), exhibiting a striking rhythmicity at 10/sec, each spike barrage being related to each wave of the EEG spindle sequence, an activity which, to such an extent, was not observed in other types of neurons.

Albe-Fessard: I think you need an addition to your model, Dr. Andersen. You postulate that the inhibition is due to the previous firing and is itself the cause of rebound firing which restarts the cyclic activity again. But, in spontaneous spindles, cellular discharges do not appear obligatory between successive phases of hyperpolarization. It seems that some other mechanism can modulate the membrane potential.

Andersen: It is true that in many cells, particularly in the midline region of the thalamus, the spindles occur as a succession of pure IPSPs. But, this is just what you would expect in a population where this system works and where the background activity is different from place to place. Let us assume a group of thalamic neurons which have recurrent inhibitory circuits influencing each other. If the excitatory drive on some neurons is bigger than on others, their membrane potential will be closer to the discharge level, thus leading to firing at each rebound depolarization. In contrast, cells that receive a smaller drive may never reach the discharge level, but will be hyperpolarized by the inhibitory circuit triggered by the neighboring active cells. The further away the cells are from the focus of high background excitation, the less spiking will occur.

Schlag: The level of background activity is probably an important factor in controlling the appearance of spindles. Some years ago, while measuring this activity with a technique of multiunit recording in the cerebral cortex, we observed that the background level was systematically lowered before the occurrence of spindles (Schlag and Balvin, 1963). In fact, this index could be safely used to predict their occurrence. I have no doubt that spindling depends on a certain balance between tonic influences, excitatory and inhibitory.

Purpura: I have great trouble with the recurrent hypothesis and I have even greater trouble in resolving our own data with the postulate of postanodal exaltation. The important thing—as you realize—is the period of recovery from hyperpolarization. The hyperpolarization itself lasts for tens of milliseconds during which the membrane potential comes back progressively to base line, although sometimes not quite reaching it. Our conductance measurements during that period have shown an early peak. In the late part of the hyperpolarization, the conductance is already reduced; at the end, there may still be a 5% change from resting conditions. And then, the next thing that occurs is an EPSP which is not associated with a significant increase in membrane conductance, because this EPSP is probably generated too far from the soma.

Now what about direct measurements of postanodal exaltation? What happens if we put a square wave of hyperpolarizing current into the cell? We have done these experiments. The current produced an increase in membrane potential and, at the end of the pulse, there was perhaps a little bit of depolarization in very good thalamic cells. I do not know how much conductance change there was. There might be a little bit. If the cell was a little depolarized— and this is what Dr. Andersen was talking about earlier—we see during this period a rebound. No question about it. But the point is that the square current pulse has an abrupt termination. The shape of imposed hyperpolarization is quite different from that obtained by an inhibitory input. We now must go back and repeat this experiment using a ramp current stimulation. This is the real test that we have to apply if we want to study the system under realistic conditions.

And so far as the recurrent inhibition is concerned, I think I have always been able to explain the data by involving interneurons in the operation. Some people do not like the idea but I believe that interactions between brain-stem, cortical, and thalamic activity will develop as the product of an interneuronal machine, whether we like it or not. This interneuronal machine is probably extremely complicated. In the spinal cord, the Renshaw phenomenon was initially thought to be very simple. It turns out that Renshaw cells inhibit other Renshaw cells and we have inhibition of inhibition there. And the entire story, also from a morphological point of view is no longer clear: Even the existence of Renshaw cells has been questioned. In the thalamus, the circuitry may still be more complex.

Andersen: My good friend Dr. Purpura and I disagree on the interpretation of this experiment. He mimics an IPSP by applying an hyperpolarizing current, and what happens when the IPSP is terminated? His prediction is that anything can happen. My prediction is that there will be a large depolarization. And then he sees a depolarization but does not trust it.

Let me try to give you a possible mechanism for postanodal exaltation. The first experiments were performed by Hodgkin and Huxley (1952) on the squid axon. They asked the question: How leaky is the membrane for sodium ions? If the cell was artificially depolarized, it opened its sodium channels. But if the depolarization lasted for some time, and a short depolarizing test pulse was applied, the cell was no longer able to open its sodium channels. This, they call sodium inactivation and it is the reason why the cells and axons have re-fractoriness. On the other hand, if the cell was hyperpolarized, it opened its sodium channels much more readily when the test depolarizing pulse was applied.

A similar process may occur in rhythmic thalamic cells were the recurrent inhibition is strong and long-lasting. Because of the hyperpolarization during the IPSP, the membrane of thalamic cells becomes hyperexcitable, just like the hyperpolarized axons of Hodgkin and Huxley. The cells overreact to afferent impulses. Instead of opening their sodium channels moderately, they open them widely; the sodium ions rush in and create a large depolarization with several spikes on top.

Purpura: What sort of impulses triggers it?

Andersen: They can be any impulses.

Purpura: But this is a different story now. I was under the impression that you postulated a spontaneous increase of sodium conductance which then produced an autonomous response?

Andersen: Indeed, it can be spontaneous. Or it can be triggered by a discharge, orthodromic, antidromic, or coming from an interneuronal bar-rage. But the point is that, whatever the case, the occurrence of the postinhibi-tory rebound is primarily dependent on the membrane properties.

Purpura: We have recorded from hundreds of neurons from the rostral brain and many times the IPSPs terminate without rebound. If you would just take away this magical property of postanodal exaltation and assume the existence of excitation at the end of the IPSP, there would not be any dis-agreement between us.

Bremer: My preference for Andersen and Eccles's recurrent inhibition hypothesis over Purpura's interneuronal machinery stems from the fact that Andersen and Eccles provide a sufficient explanation of autorhythmicity, whereas Purpura invokes ancillary mechanisms that he never explains.

Purpura: Well, I can. While looking at the activities of some thalamic cells in the ventrobasal region and in interconnected nuclear groups, we now see unfolding the possibility that, as EPSP and IPSP sequences develop, neurons in the nonspecific and related nuclei start showing bigger additions early or late and so participate in the interneuronal activities. Stimulation in the ventrolateral system induces very powerful and rapid IPSPs that turn off the system. There is a flip-flop mechanism in this internuclear interaction. Now we also suspect that similar flip-flop mechanisms of interneurons are operating within each nuclear group. But I am not going to draw the diagrams because I do not want to be confined to a particular scheme which I would have to change as new data are gathered. I agree that one must define a rigidly logical system. If I do not want to get into that yet, is it because I think I have another 10 years to work it out.

Bremer: This interneuronal network looks like a *deus ex machina*. Anything can be explained by invoking an interneuronal network.

Purpura: Is it better to look at the neuron itself as the *deus ex machina*?

Andersen: I have put up an hypothesis for all of you to know when you go home: At least this hypothesis is here to be shot down. This is perhaps the best thing that I learned from Eccles: The greatest fun is to try to shoot your ideas down yourself. Otherwise you are in the position of self-defense.

Schlag: A major difficulty with the idea that the rebound can be driven is that there is practically no phasic firing to be seen anywhere in the thalamus with a timing adequate for triggering the postinhibitory discharges, unless it is the firing of other thalamic cells rebounding sooner. Some of us may have difficulty with a mechanism of spontaneous postanodal exaltation. But if they reject it, it is up to them to explain where the mysterious inputs causing the reboundlike bursts come from.

The alternative is to assume that thalamic neurons are under a rather constant bombardment which applies a sustained depolarizing pressure. It may come from the brain-stem reticular formation, or the cortex, or else the reticularis nucleus (if these neurons are excitatory contrary to what we have postulated). But, whatever the case, the reboundlike activity could not be triggered by such a tonic excitatory bombardment. The real trigger must be in the state of the membrane at the end of the IPSP. When the rebound occurs, it appears as a long burst of high frequency discharges. The cell is then suddenly more active than it was any time before the appearance of the IPSP and there is no evidence that the depolarizing pressure is different. As far as VL cells are concerned, there is no better way to make them fire intensively than to reduce an inhibition. It is a paradoxical situation but the data show that consistently (Schlag and Villablanca, 1968).

Question: Do glial cells play a role with regard to cyclic potential changes, for instance in the mechanism of spindling?

Andersen: This is difficult to answer because we know so little about glia in the vertebrate brain. It seems that glial cells change their membrane potential in relation to the activity of the neurons that they cover.

Purpura: Probably the glial cells recorded in invertebrates are not the same as those of the mammalian cerebral cortex. For instance, in the cortex, the glial response to potassium concentration is not as good as in the leech cells. But I am not ready to discount some of Castellucci and Goldring data (1970) indicating some participation of glial potentials in cerebral electrogenesis, for instance in the case of recruiting responses.

Andersen: We cannot exclude it, but I think that the evidence is rather weak.

Purpura: Anyway, I would say that, in this stage of development of neurophysiology, there is little disagreement with the idea that evoked potentials and brain waves in general are rather the reflection of synaptic potential changes with their typical summation characteristics and field distributions. The most detailed studies have been able to disprove the possibility of spikes themselves contributing much to the slow wave activity. In a beautiful analysis, Humphrey (1968b) has compared the distribution of postsynaptic potentials evoked by antidromic invasion of pyramidal tract neurons, showing that this distribution suffices to account for the extracellular generator of the evoked potential. And Professor Bremer reminded me just before this session of something to which, of course, we all ought to pay attention: the reflection of the electrotonus which is built up as a result of the ionic fluxes occurring in the dendrites. We have to pay attention to them because, when we see the effects of these catelectrotonus and anelectrotonus in intracellular records, we tend to regard them as depolarizing, hyperpolarizing, or repolarizing postsynaptic activities.

As far as EEG activity is concerned (and I think this is the main interest of the audience in this course), let us recall that it represents—if you wish—the "visible part" of a much larger spectrum, a window which runs from something like 1/sec to maybe 30–40/sec. This also corresponds largely to the frequency range of synaptic potentials. Spikes are in the ultra-range and are not seen in EEG recordings. Now if we look at the infra-spectrum, we find very slow changes that occur over minutes, maybe hours. This is where metabolic events take place. The whole field of EEG has developed by just looking into a particular window. On either sides are dark areas but they are nevertheless important.

CHAPTER EIGHT

Input-Output Organization of the Motor Cortex and Its Alterations during Sleep and Waking[1]

MIRCEA STERIADE
MARTIN DESCHENES[2]
PETER WYZINSKI[3]
JACQUES-YVES HALLE[2]

The analysis of alterations in the reactivity of various brain structures during different stages of sleep and waking might be considered as an ancillary experimental approach, since it does not answer the major question "why," but only "how." However, provided that the analytical techniques of recording single units and identifying their input-output synaptic organization by means of testing stimuli can be married with the complex condition of a behaving preparation falling naturally into sleep, such a work may give useful indications not only about the phenomenology of sleep, but also about its nature. Even the adequate use of the evoked potential (for which some investigators show a reluctance which goes far beyond the still persisting difficulties of bridging the gap between mass responses and unitary events) and the study of its fluctuation during sleep and waking have offered important clues to change the key concepts on sleep. Suffice it to say, for example, that the puzzling

[1]Supported by grants from the Medical Research Council of Canada (MA-3689) and the Ministère de l'Education du Gouvernement du Québec (Subvention pour formation de chercheurs).
[2]Holder of a postgraduate MRC fellowship.
[3]Holder of a Centennial Scholarship (NRC).

increased responsiveness of all (sensory and motor) thalamic specific relay nuclei during the deepest sleep, which is of opposite sign as compared with the obliteration of the same centrally evoked thalamic responses during light sleep, added basic arguments for the duality of structures and mechanisms underlying these two stages of sleep and for the qualitative distinction between them. When the experimental effort, already started, has succeeded in identifying simple relay cells, complex units integrating converging inputs, and small interneurons, in dissociating their peculiar spontaneous firing, and in testing at various levels of vigilance the excitatory and inhibitory sequences triggered in different cell populations by stringently controlled testing stimulation, this completed mosaic will transcend the limits of "how" to a better understanding of the sleep determinism. This will be achieved since sleep is not associated with unpredictable neuronal activities, but with rather well-defined patterns of both spontaneous and evoked discharges, and of subsequent inhibitory events, thus allowing the disclosure of the causality in the chain of phenomena.

I. Background

The concept of ascending systems exerting a widespread control on higher cerebral structures has evolved in close relation with studies on changes in brain reactivity during sleep and waking. At first, the diffuse EEG activation of cortical areas during reticular arousal (Moruzzi and Magoun, 1949) found its corollary in the global facilitation of centrally evoked responses in sensory and associative cortices when the *encéphale isolé* was awakened by high frequency pulses to the reticular core (Bremer and Stoupel, 1959; Dumont and Dell, 1960). Although a simultaneous reticular-induced enhancement was observed by analysis of relayed responses in the appropriate thalamic nuclei, the principal target of these facilitatory influences appeared to be the neocortical mantle, as seen by changes in cortical responses to postsynaptic thalamic stimulation at the level of all sensory specific—visual, auditory, and somesthetic—radiations (see review by Steriade, 1970).

Such alterations of mass potentials evoked by central electrical stimuli in the rather crude conditions of reticular arousal in paralyzed animals could not be originally translated without hazards in terms of natural events occurring during the sleep–wakefulness cycle. However, further studies using convenient parameters of more natural (peripheral) stimuli, unit recordings and chronically implanted preparations could essentially reinforce the pioneering data of Bremer and Dell. Thus, enhancement of fast rhythmic photically evoked responses in the cortical visual area was induced by nonspecific thalamic stimulation (Creutzfeldt and Grüsser, 1959) and during reticular-elicited arousal (Steriade and Demetrescu, 1960). A retinal factor was excluded in this potentiation by recording unaltered responses from the optic tract, but a concomitant facilitation was found in the synaptic transmission of the specific thalamic (lateral geniculate) relay (Steriade and Demetrescu, 1960). These findings were confirmed by Bremer (1961) who regarded the facilitation, during arousal, of the thalamocortical events evoked by peripheral stimuli as the electrophysiological correlate of improvement, during brain-stem stimulation, of tachistoscopic perception in the monkey (Fuster, 1958; see also Fuster and Uyeda, 1962). Besides, the probability of long-latency discharges evoked by flashes in visual cortex neurons was increased during natural waking in behaving animals (Evarts, 1963), which was supported by enhancement during reticular arousal of comparable late ("post-primary") components of photically elicited fast afterdischarge (Steriade et al., 1968). The elective augmentation at an increased level of awareness of sensory-elicited postprimary waves, shown to be elaborated in cortical neuronal aggregates (Steriade, 1968), may be related to the specific enhancement of such components during conditioning in both auditory (Galambos et al., 1956) and visual (Hackett and Marczinski, 1969) systems.

Several research directions followed the usual manner of dissecting and nuancing the original findings. (1) Some results on fluctuations of sensory cortical responsiveness during sleep and waking in behaving animals, in apparent contradiction with data from acute experiments, have been understood when different stages of waking were recognized and the temporal course from the arousal reaction to the subsequent steady state of wakefulness was analyzed. Thus, the responsiveness of both visual (Walsh and Cordeau, 1965) and somesthetic (Allison and Goff, 1968a) cortices was found to be considerably enhanced only during the early phase of natural waking. This short-term facilitatory effect was in confirmation of facilitation elicited during reticular arousal in acute experiments. (2) A spatial reorganization was shown in the form of a transfer or "commutation" of excitability from one point to a neighbor, implying enhanced and decreased amplitude of evoked responses in different foci of the auditory cortex during arousal (Steriade and Demetrescu, 1962), and it was confirmed by opposite changes in adjacent foci of the visual cortex at different levels of awareness (Hughes, 1964). (3) When the attempt was made to define distinct zones in the upper and lower brain stem, with antagonist ("activating" and "hypnogenic") effects (see review by Moruzzi, 1964), this functional dissection stimulated new investigation which showed that setting in motion certain discrete areas of the reticular core induces opposite changes of tested responses. Chemical or electrical stimulation of the lower brain stem induced depression of thalamocortical evoked potentials (Courville et al., 1962; Demetrescu and Demetrescu, 1962), which stood in contrast to the enhancement of the same responses during arousal induced by stimulating the rostral activating reticular system. Opposite EEG patterns in midpontine pretrigeminal and rostropontine preparations have been found later to be associated with opposite alterations in cortical enzymatic activity induced by these two types of brain stem transection (Steriade *et al.*, 1969a). (4) Finally, the advent of unit recordings in behaving animals permitted the observation that sleep is not associated with silenced neuronal firing, but with rather well-defined patterns of spontaneous discharge depending upon the explored structure and the deepness of sleep. Such studies (Hubel, 1960; Evarts, 1960, 1964; see the recent review by Hobson, 1972) gave rise to inferences concerning the fluctuations of fundamental nervous processes during the sleep–wakefulness cycle. All this complexity of changes in brain reactivity at different levels of vigilance was predicted in Jasper's (1958) view stating that: "the activating effect of the ascending reticular system upon the cerebral cortex cannot be adequately described in terms of either gross excitation or inhibition . . . activation seems better described as a reorganization of temporal and spatial patterns of neuronal discharge in a matrix of more sus tained excitatory and inhibitory patterns held in the dendritic meshwork of the cortex [p. 330–331]."

II. Objectives and Description of Experiments

The present work derives from an unexpected observation a few years old concerning the peculiar alteration in responsiveness of the motor cortical area, namely that its mass response to thalamic ventrolateral (VL) stimulation was depressed during reticular arousal in *encéphale isolé* cats, which markedly contrasted in the same conditioning situation with the enhancement of thalamically elicited specific responses in all sensory cortical areas (Steriade, 1969, 1970; Fig. 8.1). It must be emphasized that, if tested by prethalamic stimuli to the cerebello-VL pathway, the decrease of responsiveness of intracortical (precruciate) processes seemed so powerful during reticular stimulation that it appeared in spite of the increased thalamic output, as reflected by the enhanced amplitude of the simultaneously recorded VL monosynaptically relayed wave. Essentially the same events could be obtained in behaving, chronically implanted animals: enhancement of VL-relayed activity evoked by prethalamic stimulation during waking and during fast wave sleep (as compared with striking depression during slow wave sleep and especially during drowsiness with EEG spindling), and decreased amplitude of the VL-elicited motor cortex response on arousal, during the steady state of waking and fast wave sleep (as compared with synchronized sleep), which contrasted with enhancement of the simultaneously recorded response in the cortical somesthetic area by thalamic ventrobasal (VB) stimulation (Steriade

Fig. 8.1. Reticular influences on motor and somesthetic thalamocortical responses. *Encéphale isolé* cat. Motor cortex responses (A) and somesthetic cortex responses (B) evoked by single (1) and 10/sec (2) shocks to the VL and VPL nuclei, respectively. Time: 2 msec. Vertical bar: 0.5 mV. In this and all the following figures, positivity downward. Note: Enhancement of the VPL-evoked cortical somesthetic response during high rate (250/sec) reticular formation (RF) stimulation contrasts with diminution, during reticular stimulation, of VL-evoked motor cortex response to a single shock (1); enhancement, during reticular stimulation, of initial augmenting responses of cortical somesthetic area to 10/sec VPL shock contrasts with reduction, during reticular stimulation, of the second positive wave developing in the motor cortex during augmenting elicited by 10/sec VL shocks (2). [Modified from Steriade, 1970]

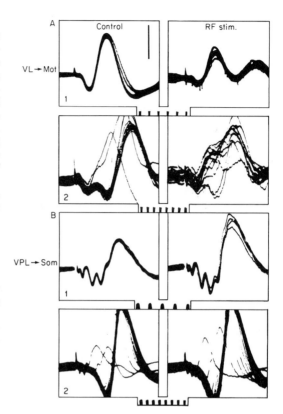

et al., 1969b; Fig. 8.2). Besides, recordings from the pyramidal tract (PT) revealed that relayed (R_1 and R_2) waves following a VL stimulus (Amassian and Weiner, 1966) were obviously reduced during reticular arousal in acute experiments (Steriade, 1969), and that indirect (I) relayed waves evoked by direct cortical stimulation (Patton and Amassian, 1954) were similarly reduced both during reticular arousal (Steriade, 1969) and natural waking as compared to behavioral slow sleep in chronic preparations (Steriade *et al.*, 1969b). The decreased responsiveness during waking of motor cortex neuronal aggregates receiving the VL output and projecting into the PT seems paradoxical not only from a teleological standpoint, but also when considering the enhanced excitability of PT neurons during waking compared to slow sleep, as was inferred from the fluctuations in the integrated fiber (Arduini *et al.*, 1963) and single-cell (Evarts, 1964)[4] spontaneous activity. The above data have been

---

[4] In a subsequent paper, Evarts (1965) dissociated the behavior of large PT neurons from that of small PT units. This will be discussed later, in the section devoted to the spontaneous firing.

obtained by recording either the spontaneous discharges of PT cells or the VL-evoked motor cortex and PT mass response during sleep and arousal. Thus, in the former case (Evarts, 1964) there was no indication to reveal the ability of single neurons to relay a message, that is, to transfer it into the efferent pathway, while in the latter approach (Steriade, 1969; Steriade *et al.*, 1969b) the spontaneous activity of the cell population under observation remained unexplored. Therefore, further investigation was required *to have simultaneous information on fluctuations in both the background activity and evoked discharges of the same identified neuron during sleep and waking.* This was the first aim of the present experiments.

The PT neurons receive, in addition to the specific input from the VL thalamus, messages from multiple sources. Polysensory neurons, responding to somatic, visual, and auditory stimuli, have been described in the motor cortex (Buser and Imbert, 1961), and work has been done on the activation of

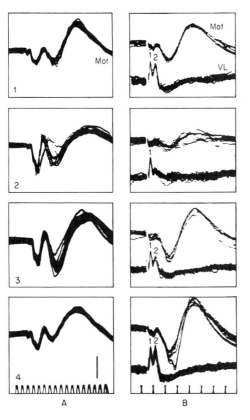

Fig. 8.2. Modifications undergone by the VL-evoked motor cortex response (A) and by rubrally evoked VL and motor cortex responses (B) during wakefulness (1), drowsiness with EEG spindles (2), slow wave sleep (3) and paradoxical sleep (4) in chronically implanted, behaving cat. Time: 2 msec. Vertical bar: 0.3 mV. Note in A the decreased amplitude of the monosynaptic (early surface-positive) cortical response to VL stimulation during waking and paradoxical sleep as compared with both stages of synchronized sleep. Note in B almost complete obliteration of the rubrally evoked VL monosynaptic response (marked by 2) during drowsiness, and clear-cut reduction during slow wave sleep, without alterations of the presynaptic component (marked by 1); increased amplitude to the cortical response during slow wave sleep in spite of the reduction of VL output. Note also the differences in fluctuations of cortical responses during sleep when tested with prethalamic (B) and VL (A) stimuli, which have to be ascribed to the changes occurring in the intercalated VL synapses when the testing shock is applied to the red nucleus. [A. Unpublished. B. From Steriade *et al.*, 1969b]

PT or unidentified cells by stimulating the joint capsules, deep tissues or skin (Brooks *et al.*, 1961; Patton *et al.*, 1962; Towe *et al.*, 1963; Oscarsson and Rosen, 1963; Albe-Fessard and Liebeskind, 1966; Nyquist and Towe, 1970). Consequently, it was of interest, as a second aim of this study, *to investigate possible differences in changes undergone during sleep and waking between "simple" neurons receiving the VL messages and those receiving convergent inputs from both the VL and the specific somesthetic thalamic (VB) complex.*

Finally, when looking at the data in the literature, one is impressed by the great amount of work devoted to the analysis of responses reflecting cortical and thalamic excitability and by the scarcity of information concerning changes in inhibitory events during sleep and waking. Some workers used the recovery cycle of thalamically elicited mass responses in visual (Evarts *et al.*, 1960; Rossi *et al.*, 1965; Demetrescu *et al.*, 1966) and motor (Steriade *et al.*, 1969b) cortices to study inhibition during the sleep–waking cycle, but the difficulty of speculating on inhibition with results obtained by means of gross surface-potential technique cannot be emphasized enough (see Section VI). Evarts (1960) analyzed the suppression of spontaneous firing in visual cortex units following stimulation of lateral geniculate radiation during natural sleep and waking in the unrestrained cat, and he concluded that inhibition is reduced during sleep with EEG slowing. A similar inference was drawn by him (1964) from analysis of temporal patterns of spontaneous discharge in PT neurons in chronically implanted monkeys, and clustered firing during sleep was believed to occur by depression of the recurrent inhibition of PT cells which may act as a frequency-limiting mechanism. On the other hand, recent works have shown that the slow positive (P) wave (reflecting hyperpolarization in a pool of neurons) induced in the VL nucleus by motor cortex stimulation (Bremer, 1970b) and the duration of the silent period following antidromic invasion of VL units (Steriade *et al.*, 1971a) were reduced during arousing reticular stimulation, thus suggesting a decrease in thalamic inhibition by setting in motion the reticular activating system. Such data have to be related to intracellular studies done by Purpura *et al.* (1966b) showing that synchronizing IPSPs induced in VL cells by low frequency medial thalamic stimulation are greatly attenuated during high frequency reticular stimulation. Thus, the above results led to different conclusions on changes in inhibitory phenomena at thalamic and cortical levels during sleep and waking. These are the only data available. It should be pointed out that so far we have no direct evidence on changes in inhibitory sequences evoked by afferent or antidromic stimulation in motor cortex units during sleep and waking.[5] Therefore, it seemed worthwhile as a

---

[5] Since this symposium, two short communications devoted to such changes in inhibition and comprising some of the findings to be reported below have been published (Steriade *et al.*, 1971c; Steriade and Deschênes, 1973).

third objective, to enlarge the picture of motor cortex neuronal aggregates, by *studying the alterations during sleep and waking, in recurrent and feed-forward inhibitory events elicited by antidromic (PT) and afferent (VL, VB and callosal) stimulation in acute and behaving preparations.*

In one series of experiments, adult cats were initially prepared for surgical procedures with moderate doses of a short-acting barbiturate (Surital) or under gas (halothane) anesthesia. The animals were immobilized with a bulbospinal cut and gallamine triethiodide (Flaxedil), and artificially ventilated so that the CO_2 content of the expired air was $4.0 \pm 0.2\%$. The rectal temperature was maintained near $37°$ C. Protected by careful infiltration of all incised tissues and pressure points with a long-lasting anesthesic (Ephocaïne), the animals fell naturally into periods of synchronized sleep, as shown by pupillar and EEG signs. They awoke spontaneously, by sensory activation (hand clapping) or following trains of high frequency pulses at liminal intensities applied to the medial part of the mesencephalic reticular formation (RF). Small doses ($1-2$ mg/kg) of Surital were occasionally administered i.v. during the recording periods for comparison with the effect of spontaneous EEG synchronization. Such unusually low doses of Surital induced very similar changes in the interspike interval histograms and responsiveness of thalamic VL (Steriade *et al.*, 1971a), reticularis (Steriade and Wyzinski, 1972), and motor cortical (Steriade *et al.*, 1973) neurons, when compared to those appearing during natural EEG synchronization. Stainless steel microelectrodes (tip diameter: $1-2$ μ) were employed to record extracellularly in the pericruciate motor cortex, and especially in the lateral part of the precruciate gyrus where the amplitude of short-latency potentials evoked by stimulating the cerebellothalamic pathway is maximal. Coaxial testing electrodes were inserted in the thalamic VL and VB nuclei, and the medullary pyramid or the pes pedunculi, to identify the unit under observation by synaptic and antidromic invasion, and to study the excitatory and inhibitory events elicited by stimulating these structures during EEG patterns of waking and light sleep. In experiments on cats concerning inhibition following antidromic PT stimulation, an extensive lesion was made in front of the stimulating pes pedunculi electrode to destroy the lemniscal fibers up to the posterior pole of the thalamic VB complex to render as pure as possible the recurrent effects.

In another series of experiments, *Macaca mulatta* monkeys were chronically implanted with a plastic cylinder over the arm area of the precentral gyrus. The animal sat in a primate chair and could move his limbs; only his head was restrained by the plastic cylinder (cf. Lamarre *et al.*, 1971a). The cylinder was filled with paraffin oil and sealed. Stainless steel or tungsten microelectrodes ($1-2$ μ at the tip) passed through the intact dura. Coaxial stimulating electrodes were inserted in the pes pedunculi, the VL and VB nuclei, and in the white matter underlying homotopic points of the contralateral motor cortex for cell identification and for eliciting different types of excitatory-inhibitory sequences to be studied during waking and behavioral sleep with EEG spindles and slow waves. Since to our knowledge there are so far no electrophysiological studies directed to analyze the topographical arrangement and components of precentral motor cortex response evoked by specific thalamic stimulation in monkeys, and because this is the envelope of one of the major type of unit discharges tested in our work, special attention was paid to position the thalamic stimulating electrode at frontal planes 8–9, lateral 4–5, depth 6.5–7.5. The best thalamic location for short-latency activation of precentral neurons was found in the intermediate region between the rostral part of the VB and the posterior part of the nucleus ventralis oralis (VOp), part of the VL in primates (Hassler, 1959). In pilot experiments on acute *Macaca mulatta* and during chronic implantation, thalamically evoked responses were recorded from different points on the surface of the precentral arm area and several classical criteria were used to differentiate specific thalamocortical responses from other responses due to stimulation of neighboring thalamic nuclei. These criteria were: (1) the cortical distribution, with prominence or exclusiveness in the precentral gyrus; (2) the pattern, with short-latency initial positive waves, among them the first spike, with a latency of 0.7 msec, was regarded as the action potentials of thalamocortical axons; the *a* wave, with a latency of about 1.5–2 msec, the first sign of postsynaptic activity, was able to follow fast (50/sec) stimuli; the later *b* wave, at around 6 msec, was obliterated with such fast stimuli, and developed into augmenting responses with 8–10/sec shocks (Fig. 8.3). As in the cat, the location of the electrodes was checked histologically.

In both types of experiments, long periods (1–3 hr) of recording of the same unit without any or significant spike alteration were permitted by covering the exposed motor cortex and small trephine holes made to insert the stimulating electrodes with a 4% solution of agar to minimize the brain pulsations in cat, or by closed chamber in chronically implanted monkeys. Such long and stable recordings were required to identify the neuron and to study its spontaneous firing, the evoked discharges and the period of subsequent inhibition elicited by several testings stimuli during fluctuations of EEG desynchronizing and synchronizing patterns in cat, associated in monkey with observation of the behavior, the EMG, and eye movements. Unit potentials, pulses synchronous with testing stimuli, EEG waves, EMG, and ocular movements were recorded on multichannel magnetic tape. The unit activity was recorded simultaneously on a direct (50 Hz–10 kHz) and on FM (0–700 Hz) channel of the tape recorder. These activities were then examined visually on an oscilloscope and EEG machine. One beam of the oscilloscope was used for the evoked unit discharges. The spontaneous spikes were displayed on the second beam and used to deflect one pen of the ink-writing EEG recorder; thus, simultaneous

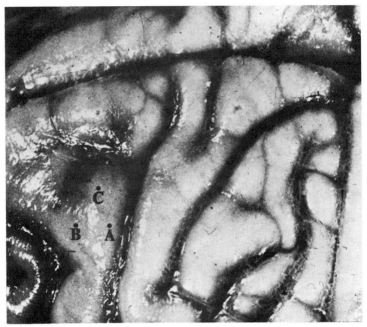

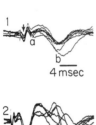

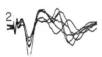

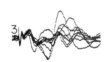

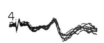

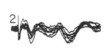

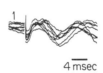

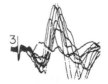

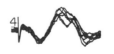

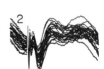

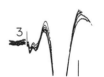

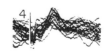

4 msec

4 msec

10 msec

10 msec

4 msec

A

B

C

information on the evoked and background unit activity could be obtained during different EEG patterns and behavioral states. Interspike intervals and poststimulus latency histograms were computed using an Intertechnique Didac 800 channel analyzer having teleprinter output of the memory contents. The data were fed into an IBM 370/APL sharing computer terminal for calculation of the probability density, mean intervals, variation, and the corresponding Poisson density.

III. Cell Identification

Before the analysis of neuronal changes during sleep and waking, the cells encountered by penetrating in the vicinity of the cat's cruciate sulcus and in the monkey's arm area of the precentral gyrus were identified by several testing stimuli. This gave us the opportunity to present some findings on the input–output organization of motor cortex neurons.

1. Antidromic invasion of *PT cells* was differentiated from synaptic activation according to classical procedures. Two main criteria were used: fixed latency and the collision phenomenon. The latencies ranged in 82 neurons between 0.8 and 5.5 msec when stimulating the medullary pyramid in cat, in another group of 29 cells between 0.5 and 4.0 msec when stimulating the pes pedunculi in cat, and in 134 neurons between 0.3 and 5.0 msec by stimulating the pes pedunculi in monkey (see the two simultaneously recorded fast and slow PT neurons of monkey in Fig. 8.4B). The second criterion was the collision between a spontaneous or synaptically elicited discharge and the antidromic spike (Fig. 8.4, A5). As to the well-known ability to follow fast stimuli without failure, it was not a *sine qua non* condition to recognize a PT cell, since complete or partial blockage of antidromic invasion could appear in some neurons following the first or the first two shocks in a train (see Fig. 8.4, A2–3). The ability to follow trains of pulses separated by intervals less than

---

Fig. 8.3. Patterns of mass responses elicited by specific thalamic stimulation (in the intermediate region between the VPL and the posterior part of the VL nuclei) in the arm area of the precentral gyrus of the *Macaca mulatta* monkey. Surface recordings in three cortical foci (A, B, and C) corresponding to the three columns with oscilloscopic traces. A–B. 1, superimposed responses to 1/sec thalamic shocks (2, the same at a lower speed) at Fr. 9, L. 4.5, D. 7.5; 3 and 4, responses evoked in the first second (3) and the third second (4) by a train of 8/sec stimuli, with the same intensity as in 1–2. C. 1, responses to 1/sec shocks at the same location as in A and B; 2, responses to 50/sec stimulation; 3, responses to 1/sec stimuli applied 0.5 mm deeper (D. 7.0) than above; 4, the same with 50/sec shocks. The first presynaptic component is indicated by the arrow. Note that the first postsynaptic component (a) is able to follow stimuli as fast as 50/sec (C2), and that the b component develops into augmenting with 8/sec stimuli (A3 and B3).

5 msec and the decreased probability of soma invasion at longer intervals (between 10 and 30 msec), as previously suggested by Suzuki and Tukahara (1963) in cat, was not a common rule for PT neurons identified by collision and fixed latency. At low frequencies of stimulation (50–120/sec), blocking of the

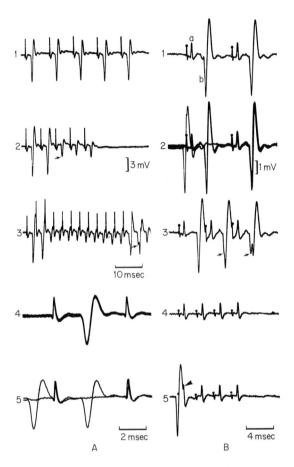

Fig. 8.4. Identification of pyramidal tract (PT) cells in the freely moving *Macaca mulatta*. Pes pedunculi was stimulated in this and subsequent figures depicting PT neurons in monkey. A slow (2 msec latency of antidromic invasion) PT cell in A, and two simultaneously recorded (fast, a, at 0.6 msec; and slow, b, at 2.6 msec) PT neurons in B. A. Stimulation at around 110/sec (1), 180/sec (2), and 310/sec (3). B. Stimulation at around 155/sec (1–2), 250/sec (3), and 385/sec (4–5); the intensity of stimulation was reduced in B4–5 to a third of that used in B1–3. IS spikes and IS-SD fragmentation indicated by small arrows. Note in A that the cell could follow a train of shocks at 110/sec, but by increasing the frequency to 180/sec and 310/sec, only the IS spikes were seen following the first two full spikes, and the IS-SD break was observed after 30–40 msec, at the end of the train; collision in 5. Note in B that the fast PT cell was discharged by a lower voltage in the absence of the other neuron (4–5). See also text.

antidromic invasion following the first shock was observed only in a few PT cells (see Fig. 8.29B) but not in other neurons (Fig. 8.5C) recorded from the cat's motor cortex. In monkey, full responsiveness of some cells was seen to all shocks in a train above 200–250/sec, but other PT neurons showed complete blocking or fragmentation between the initial segment (IS) and somadendritic (SD) spikes following the first stimulus at the same fast frequencies (Fig. 8.4). This suggests that general conclusions cannot be drawn in this respect for all PT cells and that the probability of antidromic invasion, as well as the time-course of its blocking with subsequent shocks, actually depends on different equipment of inhibitory interneurons characterizing various PT neurons.

Concerning the distinction between fast and slow conducting PT neurons, the classification of Takahashi (1965) in cat, generally admitted in literature, considered fast cells as those having conduction velocities of over 21 m/sec, and slow cells as those conducting between 11 and 18m/sec. With stimulation in the medulla, the limit between fast and slow PT neurons in cat is around an antidromic response latency of 2.0–2.2 msec, and with pes pedunculi stimulation the fast PT cells are those units invaded at latencies shorter than 1.2 msec. Comparing the highest velocities generally described in cat (around 60–70 m/sec) with those in monkey (110 m/sec), we can consider as fast PT cells in monkey those conducting above 40 m/sec (antidromic response latencies between 0.3 and 0.8 msec), which would correspond to the value of over 21 m/sec indicated by Takahashi (1965) in cat.

Identification of corticofugal neurons has been extended by studying also the antidromic invasion in 18 motor cortex neurons following VL stimulation. The latency of such spikes in the cat's pericruciate area usually ranged between 0.7 and 3.1 msec, thus suggesting a conduction velocity of about 6–30 m/sec. These values show a wider range than those reported by Uno et al. (1970). If one considers VL synaptic discharges to precruciate stimuli with latencies as short as 1.0 msec (Steriade et al., 1972), allowing 0.3 to 0.5 msec for synaptic delay, the conduction velocity in these corticothalamic fibers must be as fast as 30–40 m/sec. Only in a few instances have we identified slow PT cells in cat (5 msec latency by stimulating the medulla) giving rise to axon collaterals to the VL (1.85 msec latency of antidromic spikes by stimulating at this level). In the behaving monkey, antidromic invasion of nine precentral neurons occurred between 0.5 and 5.0 msec following thalamic stimulation at the VB–VL border, thus indicating conduction velocities of 5–50 m/sec. Only one of these corticothalamic cells was also antidromically invaded from the pes pedunculi at 1.8 msec latency. Such units (see details elsewhere: Steriade et al., 1972) are regarded as giving rise to the descending control of VL activity.

2. We conventionally call *simple relay cells* the PT units which could also be identified by synaptic activation at short latencies by stimulating the appropriate thalamic (VL) nucleus. This is to differentiate them from other neurons in cat motor cortex receiving converging VL and VB outputs, which presumably

subserve more *complex* functions and which, besides, were differently altered during sleep and waking.

The latency of the earliest spike was found in 53 VL-driven PT neurons between 1 and 4 msec. Latencies longer than 1–1.5 msec do not necessarily imply plurisynaptic activation, since: (a) there are slow conducting VL-motor cortex fibers as seen by long-latency (3.5–4 msec) antidromic spikes in VL following precruciate stimulation (Uno *et al.*, 1970; Steriade *et al.*, 1971a), and (b) a shortening of the latency of dispersed spikes from 1–3 msec to nearly a fixed 1 msec could be elicited by using twin shocks (Fig. 8.5B). Significant changes in latency of evoked discharges was observed during the different stages of sleep and waking (see Fig. 8.17). Such short-latency (1–3.5 msec)

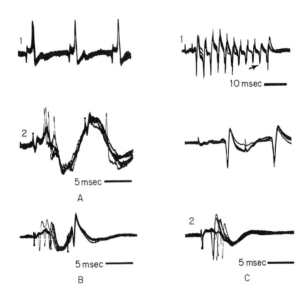

Fig. 8.5. Identification of pyramidal tract (PT) and VL-driven neurons (simple relay cells) in the *encéphale isolé* cat. Stimulation of the PT in cat was performed in the medulla. A–C. Three different cells. In A, a fast PT cell (1.2 msec latency of the antidromic spikes, 1), synaptically driven by VL stimuli at a shortest latency of 1.8 msec (2); the VL-elicited spikes are superimposed on the depth (1200 μ) primary slow negativity of the evoked potential, subsequent to the positive, presynaptic component; decrease in the probability of firing and increase in latency of spikes driven by the second shock. B. Spikes evoked by two VL shocks (this cell was also antidromically invaded by PT stimulation with a latency of 1.3 msec, not depicted). Note facilitation of the evoked firing and decrease of latency induced by a preceding VL stimulus. C. PT (1) and VL-evoked (2) cell. Note that this neuron, synaptically driven at short latencies (below 1.8 msec) by thalamic stimulation (2) is a small PT neuron, as shown by the long latency (5 msec) of the antidromic spikes (1, two different frequencies of PT shocks, at about 220/sec in the first trace, and 110/sec in the second trace; IS-SD break indicated by arrow). [Modified from Steriade *et al.*, 1973]

spikes began on the crest of the primary depth negativity of the VL-evoked potential recorded by the same microelectrode (Fig. 8.5,A$_2$), corresponding to the primary intracellularly recorded EPSP (Purpura *et al.*, 1964; Creutzfeldt *et al.*, 1966), but in some neurons they continued to be superimposed on the subsequent depth positivity (Fig. 8.29A). It is to be emphasized that the linkage between VL efferent fibers and large PT cells (Yoshida *et al.*, 1966; see also Fig. 8.5A) was not a general finding. Many PT cells monosynaptically driven by VL stimulation in cat were very small judging by the long latency (around 5 msec) of their antidromic spikes (Fig. 8.5C). This holds true in monkey: From the 17 PT neurons receiving the specific thalamic input at latencies indicating monosynaptic excitation, 6 were slow conducting (antidromic response latencies: 0.9–3.5 msec). Both in the cat (Fig. 8.5) and monkey (Fig. 8.8,D2) monosynaptically VL-driven neurons usually discharged with one impulse to one single shock at juxtathreshold intensity, and with repetitive discharges only by increasing the intensity of the VL testing shock or to the second of short-delayed stimuli. On the other hand, in both species responses of PT neurons to VL shocks at latencies ranging from 4 to 6 msec generally took the form of a burst of high frequency spikes (Fig. 8.6), thus suggesting synaptic activation through internuncial cortical excitatory neurons.

3. We call *complex relay cells* the 13 cat PT neurons which received converging inputs from the VL and the VB nuclei (Figs. 8.7, 8.20–8.21). Another population of 11 neurons was identified by their converging VL–VB inputs, but they were not antidromically invaded from the PT. The possible objection of spread of current from one thalamic point to another can be refuted since the same cell was always driven with at least 1 msec longer latency by VB than by VL testing shocks.[6] The shortest latency for the VL-evoked spikes in the cell depicted in Fig. 8.7A was around 1.4 msec, while it was around 2.5 msec for VB-elicited discharges in the same neuron. Our data are the unitary correlate at the level of motor cortex neurons of previous findings by Amassian and Weiner (1966) which recorded VB-evoked relayed population response in the bulbar PT at a longer latency (ranging between 2.9–3.7 msec) than responses elicited by VL-VA stimulation.

Three possibilities may explain the longer latency of VB-evoked discharges in such cells: (a) a slower conducting direct pathway from VB to the motor cortical area; however, at least for the cat, fibers arising in the VB do not

---

[6] Besides, the cortical distribution of mass potentials elicited by stimulating the two thalamic sites showed that VL-evoked responses were most prominent in the motor cortex (the much smaller response in the postcruciate area presumably reflecting volume conductor recording from the precruciate gyrus) which was in sharp contrast with the VB-evoked potentials; the dissimilar patterns of VL and VB-evoked potentials also showed that different pathways were set in motion (Fig. 8.7B).

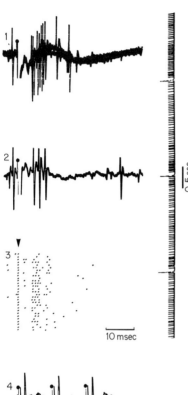

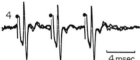

Fig. 8.6. Fast PT neuron in the monkey (0.75 msec latency of antidromic spikes in 4), synaptically modulated by VL stimulation with a high frequency burst of 2–4 spikes at 5 msec latency (superimposition in 1, single sweep in 2, and 30-sweeps dotgram in 3; the dots indicated by the arrow in 3 represent the testing VL shock). At the right of the figure, the background firing of this cell during quiet waking is depicted by using the spontaneous spikes displayed on the oscilloscope to deflect one pen of the ink-writing machine; note the tonic discharges during relaxed waking, at around 25/sec, of this fast PT neuron; three testing PT shock trains are seen to interrupt the spontaneous firing for about 100 msec.

overlap with VL-fugal projections to the motor cortex (Strick, personal communication); (b) an intermediate relay in the VL; such an explanation is not entirely satisfactory since the VB-elicited PT response survived, although reduced, following a massive thalamic lesion of VL, VA, and adjoining nucleus reticularis (Amassian and Weiner, 1966); (c) most probably, the intercalated relay lies in the somesthetic cortex; actually, the pattern of degeneration of axon terminals in motor area following restricted lesions in the somatosensory cortex indicated a somatotopical arrangement of such corticocortical associative connections (Jones and Powell, 1968) and the technique of intracortical microstimulation supported this intracortical organization of projections from the somesthetic to motor cortices (Thompson et al., 1970). That such convergent units represent a special class of neurons was shown by the opposite behavior of their evoked discharges during synchronized and desynchronized

EEG patterns as compared with those of purely VL-modulated cells (compare Figs. 8.16–8.17 and 8.20–8.21).

Such PT neurons receiving messages from both the VL and VB nuclei have not been found in monkeys at the intensities used. The reason for not increasing the stimulation intensity much above was that the two electrodes for specific thalamic stimulation were placed in areas too adjacent to exclude the spread of current.

4. *Callosal* neurons (42 units) have been identified in the monkey following stimulation in the white matter underlying contralateral cortical foci. The latency of antidromic spikes (Fig. 8.8A) ranged between 0.8 and 2.5 msec in different cells, thus indicating conduction velocities between 15 and 40 m/sec in the callosal conduction of the behaving *Macaca mulatta*, much faster than that reported by Asanuma and Okamoto (1959) in cats under Nembutal (not more

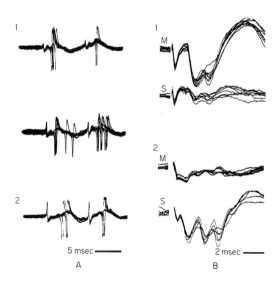

Fig. 8.7. A. Converging inputs from the ventrolateral (VL) and ventrobasal (VB) thalamus onto a single precruciate neuron in cat. Two testing, shortly delayed (8 msec) shocks applied to the VL (1) and VB (2) thalamic nuclei; two different voltages for VL stimulation (1). The shortest latency was around 1.4 msec for the VL-evoked spikes, and around 2.5 msec for VB-elicited discharges. Note in A1 the decrease in the probability of firing with increase of latency at the second shock at liminal voltage (first trace), and facilitation of evoked discharges with repetitive firing by increasing the voltage of stimulation (second trace). B. Surface-recorded mass responses in the precruciate motor cortex (M) and postcruciate somesthetic area (S) by VL (1) and VB (2) shocks with the same location as used in A. Note the different patterns of VL-evoked potentials in M and VB-evoked responses in S; striking dissimilarities in cortical distribution of the VL and VB- evoked potentials. See also text.

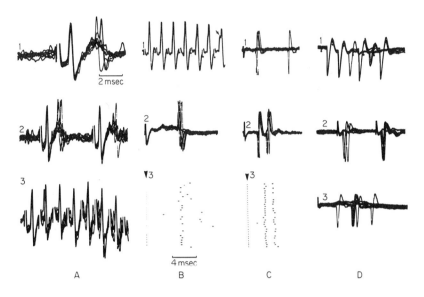

Fig. 8.8. Identification of the monkey's precentral neurons by callosal volleys. Four different neurons (A–D). A. Antidromic spikes (0.85 msec latency) in association with synaptically elicited discharges (around 3 msec latency) in A1–2; in 3, high frequency shocks to elicit only antidromic spikes. B. Thalamic stimulation in the posterior part of the VL (in 1) elicited antidromic spikes (at 0.8 msec latency; see IS-SD break at the arrow) in a cell which was synaptically driven (at around 6 msec latency) by stimulating the homotopic contralateral precentral point (superimposed spikes in 2; 30-sweeps dotgram in 3, arrow indicating the testing shock). Monosynaptic convergences seen by VL (C1) and callosal (C2–3) volleys onto a single cell; note the different patterns of discharge evoked by the two testing stimuli (in 3, a 30-sweeps dotgram to show the constancy of grouped spikes elicited by transcallosal stimulation). The fast PT cell in D (antidromic spikes at 0.85 msec latency following shocks to the pes pedunculi, in 1) was driven synaptically both by VL shocks (at 0.8 msec latency, in 2; note the facilitation induced by the preceding shock as seen in the discharges evoked by the second volley) and callosal stimulation (in 3); this spike diminished in amplitude when the callosal testing stimulation was used. The time scale (4 msec) is valid for the entire figure, except A1. [From Steriade and Hallé, unpublished observations]

than 5 m/sec). That the anesthesia was not the main reason to account for such differences is suggested by the long latency (about 7 msec) of synaptic excitation in PT cells following stimulation of the opposite cortex, which only slightly exceeds conduction time between the two cortices through callosal fibers and which was obtained by Asanuma and Okuda (1962) in unanesthetized cats. Even if the fastest (mean conduction 10.3 m/sec) callosal fibers recently found by Naito et al. (1970) in cat sensorimotor cortex are taken into consideration, these values are much lower than those we obtained in *Macaca mulatta*, thus emphasizing species differences. In agreement with the above figures for anti-dromic invasion in the monkey, the latency of monosynaptic discharges evoked by transcallosal volleys in both superficial and deep layers (which is in agreement with anatomical data of Nauta, 1954) of the precentral gyrus was as short as 2.3 msec (Fig. 8.8,C2–3), longer latencies (above 5 msec, the neuron depicted in Fig. 8.8B) implying perhaps cortical intercalated neurons. However, the concentration of some evoked discharges at a peak latency of 6–7 msec (Fig. 8.19, during sleep), without the dispersion commonly seen for plurisynaptic activation, suggests that such a firing may be also considered as due to monosynaptic activation and that it might reflect slower conduction velocities as usually detected in our measurements of antidromic response latencies. In some instances, antidromic invasion (0.85 msec latency) and short-latency (around 3 msec) synaptic excitation were obtained in the same precentral unit by stimulating the contralateral homotopic point (Fig. 8.8,A1–2), thus indicating that the two areas are reciprocally linked through a corticocortical loop.

Some units were identified as receiving a converging callosal and VL input, which was monosynaptic for both stimuli in the cell depicted in Fig. 8.8C. Such units were sometimes also identified as PT cells, but in these cases only the VL-evoked discharges were monosynaptic, while callosally elicited spikes usually occurred at latencies longer than 5 msec (Fig. 8.8,D3), supporting the idea of elements interposed in the callosal-corticospinal pathway (Purpura and Girado, 1959). This is also true for the callosal-corticothalamic pathway, as resulted from synaptic activation at latencies longer than 3–4 msec (Fig. 8.8, B2–3) in precentral neurons antidromically invaded by VL shocks (Fig. 8.8,B1). The latter type of neurons, which are common for primates and felines (see also Steriade et al., 1972) may assist the feedback regulation of the VL from the contralateral motor cortical area.

5. *Short-axoned (Golgi II)* cells have been recognized by (besides the obligatory negative evidence of the lack of their antidromic invasion following PT, thalamic, and callosal stimuli) their patterns of synaptically evoked discharges, consisting of barrages of high frequency (200–800/sec) repetitive spikes. This is a common feature of the presumed interneurons, wherever they have been found: in the spinal cord, cerebellum, hippocampus and thalamic nuclei (see review by Eccles, 1969). In addition, such units were characterized by peculiar patterns in their spontaneous firing, exhibiting spike clusters separated by long periods of silence, with a distribution of intervals which clearly differentiated them from PT or other long-axoned elements (see Section IV). The responses of motor cortical interneurons to PT antidromic and specific thalamic stimulation were also studied in the cat by Stefanis (1969). His study was not concerned with changes in spontaneous and evoked discharges of such elements during sleep and waking; besides, he reported rather long-latency (7–10 msec) responses which did not provide evidence of direct activation through the recurrent collateral pathway of PT axons and of the thalamocortical fibers. Such evidence is provided in the present work.

No qualitative difference has been found between the type of responses of 18 putative interneurons found in the cat precruciate cortex and that of 35 interneurons recorded in the monkey precentral area. Figure 8.9A shows such a cortical element synaptically driven by VL stimulation in the cat, with progressively increased number of spikes, higher frequency and shorter latency by increasing the stimulation strength. The interesting finding was that the same interneuron could be synaptically modulated in freely moving monkeys

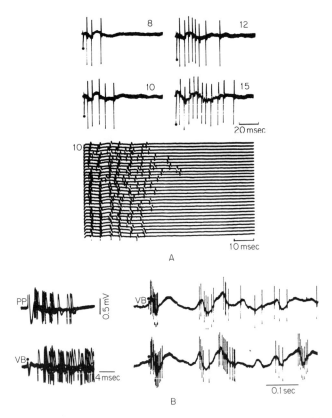

Fig. 8.9. Patterns of interneuronal responses in cat and monkey. A. A presumed short-axoned cell recorded in the cat's precruciate gyrus, synaptically modulated by VL shocks (dots) with increasing intensities (from 8 to 15 V). Below, a 30-sweeps wavegram shows the responses to 10 V stimulation. Note the progressively increasing number of spikes in the barrage (from 3 to 11), shortening of latency (from 4 msec to 2 msec) and increased frequency of repetitive spikes (up to 250/sec) by increasing the voltage of stimulation; note also the remarkable constancy in grouping of repetitive discharges seen in the wavegram. B. An interneuron recorded in monkey precentral motor cortex, synaptically driven by both antidromic PT stimulation in the pes pedunculi (PP) and by afferent stimulation of the thalamocortical pathway in the rostral part of the VB complex. Full description of latencies and intraburst frequencies in text. [B is modified from Steriade and Deschênes, 1973]

by both antidromic PT and afferent VB-VL stimulation at latencies implying monosynaptic excitation. The cell depicted in Fig. 8.9B (taken from a period of behavioral slow sleep) discharged 3–5 spikes at around 500/sec to pes pedunculi stimulation, the latency of the first discharge being 1.2 msec. The same unit was modulated by a shock to the rostral border of the thalamic VB complex with a barrage of 10–13 spikes at 500/sec; the first discharge in the burst occasionally had a latency of 2.2 msec, but usually it appeared at 3.5 msec. Similar latencies seen in the high frequency (400/sec) responses of the interneuron depicted in Fig. 8.22 (2.2 msec for VB-VL stimulation, and 0.9 msec for antidromic PT stimuli) undoubtedly show that *these interneurons are directly driven by both recurrent collaterals of PT (most probably fast) fibers and by the specific thalamocortical axons.* The longer latencies of thalamically elicited discharges in both interneurons found in the monkey and depicted in Figs. 8.9B and 8.22 preclude spread of current from the thalamus to the internal capsule. Latencies as short as 0.9–1.2 msec for responses evoked by antidromic PT stimuli exclude spread of current to other (medial lemniscus or red nucleus) mesencephalic structures. We do not have crucial evidence for the excitatory or inhibitory nature of such short-axoned elements. In some cases (Fig. 8.9B), the good time-relation between the evoked or spontaneous spike barrage and the simultaneously recorded focal slow positive wave (likely reflecting summated IPSPs of neighboring elements) allows the assumption, common in literature, that such interneurons are inhibitory. However, this may be a tenuous inference in view of complex interactions between different (likely opposite: inhibitory *and* excitatory) elements in the interneuronal pool (see Section VI).

IV. Spontaneous Firing

A. Projection (Relay) Neurons

A common feature distinguishing the neurons antidromically invaded by PT stimuli and synaptically modulated at short latencies by specific thalamic stimulation was their sustained, single-spike discharges during EEG desynchronization in the cat (Figs. 8.10 and 8.16). The probability of interspike intervals increased above the 10–20 msec class, showed a histogram peak around 30–40 msec, and decreased progressively after the 40–50 msec class, to 150 msec (Steriade *et al.*, 1973). This parallels data on cerebello-VL projection neurons (Steriade *et al.*, 1971b) and on VL relay cells (Steriade *et al.*, 1971a; Lamarre *et al.*, 1971b; Dormont, 1972). Such a distribution is very similar to that previously described during wakefulness by Evarts (1964) in monkey precentral PT neurons, and it was also found during quiet waking in both slow and fast PT cells in our experiments on freely moving monkeys (see Fig. 8.11).

EEG synchronization occurring spontaneously (Fig. 8.10,A2) or induced

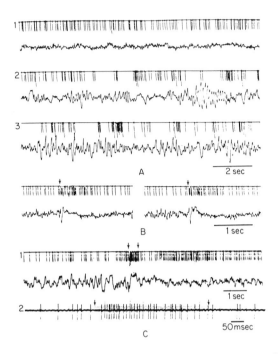

Fig. 8.10. Spontaneous discharges of relay cells during EEG patterns of waking and slow sleep, and on reticular arousal from slow sleep in cat. A–C. Three different PT neurons (antidromic response latencies from the medulla: 1.2 msec in A, the same cell as depicted in Fig. 8.5A; 4 msec in B; and 2 msec in C), synaptically driven at 1.3–2 msec latencies (earliest spikes) by VL stimulation. In this and other similar figures, EEG rhythms were recorded from the ipsilateral pericruciate area (or precentral area in monkey) and unit spikes displayed on the oscilloscope where used to deflect one pen of the ink-writing machine; each deflection exceeding the common level (especially visible in A2–3) represents a group of 2–6 high frequency spikes at 300–350/sec. A. 1, Steady state of waking; 2, spontaneously occurring EEG patterns of sleep with spindles and slow waves; 3, EEG synchronization induced by 2 mg/kg Surital i.v. Note sustained discharges during waking and high frequency spike clusters interspersed with long periods of silence both during natural and barbiturate-induced EEG synchronization. B. Transient increase of discharge frequency (from 7.5/sec to 22–23/sec) elicited by a 25-msec train of 300/sec reticular pulses (arrows). C. EEG arousal reaction associated with three-or fourfold increase in the spontaneous unit firing elicited by a long train of 300/sec reticular shocks (between arrows). The same spikes photographed on the oscilloscope and corresponding to the same period of reticular stimulation shown between arrows on the above (1) EEG record are depicted in 2. Note *phasic* increase of unit firing during reticular stimulation, occurring with a latency of about 25 msec. [From Steriade *et al.*, 1973]

by very small doses of Surital (1–2 mg/kg i.v.) in cat (Fig. 8.10,A3), and behavioral drowsiness or sleep with EEG slowing in the monkey (Figs. 8.12–8.13), resulted essentially in the same changes in spontaneous activity of PT relay cells, that is high frequency (usually 100–200/sec, but sometimes 300–350/sec) bursts of spikes[7] and long periods of silence, sometimes exceeding 1–2 sec, something not seen during waking. This pattern, originally seen by Adrian and Moruzzi (1939) in PT neurons of cats under Dial anesthesia, was reflected in the interspike interval distribution for EEG synchronization in the cat and behavioral drowsiness or slow sleep in monkey, showing very short intervals, between 1 and 10 msec, a histogram peak at 15–25 msec, and the obvious increase in the fraction of measured intervals falling outside the depicted time range of 200 msec (Fig. 8.11).

Concerning the changes in mean rates of discharge of PT neurons in cat, it was significantly lower during EEG patterns of slow sleep compared with waking, and this was valid for both small and large PT cells. In only 8 PT neurons from the group of 82 cells antidromically invaded from the medulla, and in only 3 elements from the group of 29 cells identified from the pes pedunculi, the background firing was richer during EEG synchronization and, again, this was seen not only for large, but also for slow conducting PT cells. Therefore, 90% of PT neurons (slow as well as fast) of both (simple and complex) relay types were tonically active during waking and decreased their mean rate of firing during slow sleep. A dramatic facilitation of background firing was obtained by arousing high frequency reticular stimulation in the cat, which regularized (see also Creutzfeldt and Jung, 1961) and increased the mean rate of discharge three times as compared to periods of EEG synchronization (Fig. 8.10B–C; see also Fig. 8.23). It must be noted that, as a rule, the facilitatory effect of reticular stimulation on spontaneous firing of PT cells was phasic in nature, and that subsequent depression with reexcitation could be also seen (Fig. 8.10C). These data are in general agreement with the reticular-elicited membrane depolarization and increased firing rate in PT neurons reported by Akimoto and Saito (1966).

In a study performed on chronically implanted monkeys, Evarts (1965) dissociated small size ("tonic, regular discharge during waking") from large PT cells ("relatively inactive during waking"). In fact, his experiments showed that the discharge frequencies increased during waking for cells with latencies of antidromic invasion (from the medulla) as short as 1 msec, the opposite becoming evident only for neurons with latencies between 0.7 and 0.9 msec (see Table 1 in that paper). A tonic, regular activity with a frequency as high as 20–25/sec, could be seen in our experiments in fast PT neurons, with

---

[7] Such a temporal pattern of discharge is commonly designated in literature as "clustered firing." This term masks, however, very dissimilar durations and configurations of spike clusters in various cerebral structures resulting from the frequency and organization of spikes within a burst, as well as different intercluster periods of silence, together reflecting different mechanisms underlying these patterns in cortical, medial, and lateral thalamic, and cerebellar neurons (see details in the discussion on the significance of discharge patterns during sleep in Section VI).

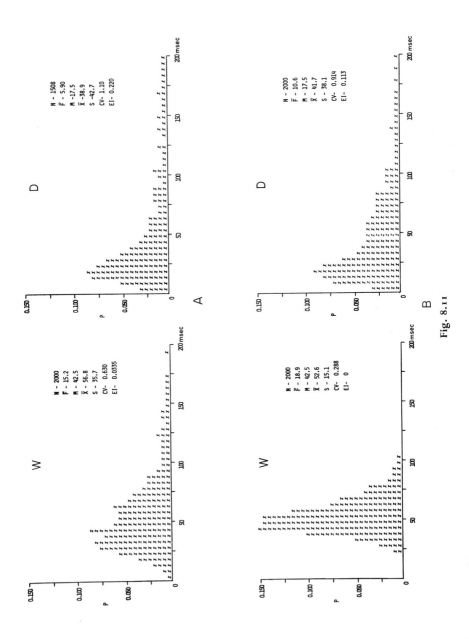

Fig. 8.11

latencies shorter than 0.8 msec by stimulating the pes pedunculi, provided that the animal was in a state of quiet waking (see Fig. 8.6). The changes in background firing of slow and fast PT neurons during the period of transition from slow sleep to wakefulness in behaving monkeys were recently further analyzed, in order to dissociate the short-lasting arousal reaction and the orienting reactions (excited wakefulness) from the stable state of quiet waking (Steriade, Deschênes, and Oakson, in preparation). The sudden increased firing in 33 of 36 slow conducting PT cells (antidromic response latencies above 0.9 msec when stimulating the pes pedunculi) from the very beginning of arousal (Fig. 8.12) could be spectacularly differentiated from the neuronal silence seen in 27 of 31 fast PT cells, lasting in different units from 4 to 33 sec (Fig. 8.13; the period of silence on arousal, marked by arrows, lasted in these three units between 7.5 and 14 sec). After this short period of arousal, the fast PT cells resumed their spontaneous discharges, but usually at a lower level than earlier seen during slow sleep (Fig. 8.13B–C). If precautions were taken to prevent an uncommon excitement of the animal, the rate of spontaneous firing increased after 1–2 min over that seen during sleep (Fig. 8.13,A2). The striking difference between the firing rate of fast PT cells during alertness and during quiet wakefulness was evident and it is depicted in Fig. 8.13C. On arousal, this neuron stopped firing for 7.5 sec; after that, the firing rate was lower than during sleep for about 30 sec. In C2, the experimenter kept the animal fully alert by moving the fingers in front of his eyes, while in C3 the experimenter was still present in the monkey's room but motionless, and the animal was relaxed (see the difference between the amount of eye movements in C2 and C3). It is obvious that the tonic discharge, at much higher rate than during slow sleep, occurred only when the animal was in a state of quiet waking. Such an increase in the mean rate of discharge during the steady state of quiet waking, compared to drowsiness or slow sleep, can be also seen in the statis-

---

Fig. 8.11. Interspike interval histograms of fast (A) and slow (B) PT neurons during behavioral state of quiet waking (W) and drowsiness (D) in monkey. Antidromic response latencies by stimulating the pes pedunculi: 0.5 msec (A) and 1.7 msec (B). The histograms show on the ordinate the probability (P) of different classes of intervals, as indicated in milliseconds on the abscissa. Symbols: N, number of counts; $\overline{F}$, mean frequency; M, modal interval; $\overline{X}$, mean interval; S, standard deviation; CV, coefficient of variation; EI, intervals in excess of the depicted time range. The distribution of intervals in the histograms depicted here during drowsiness was very similar to that seen during slow wave sleep. Note the same distribution during D of intervals in both fast and slow PT cells, and decreased firing rate during D compared with W in both neurons. Note also, during W, more dispersed intervals (with greater number of intervals in excess of the depicted time range) in the fast, than in the slow, PT neuron. Other comments in text. [From Steriade, Deschênes, and Oakson, unpublished observations]

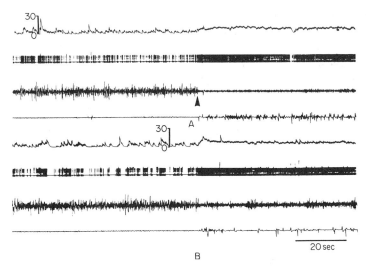

Fig. 8.12. Background firing of slow PT neurons during synchronized sleep and waking in the monkey. A–B. Two different units; antidromic response latencies of 1.8 msec (A) and 2.5 msec (B). The four ink-written traces represent in each case, from top to bottom the integrated unit activity (figures on the ordinate in A indicate number of spikes per second), unit spikes, EEG perirolandic rhythms, and ocular movements. Arousal was induced by the experimenter in A; in B, spontaneous awakening, clearly indicated by EEG desynchronization and eye movements. Note in both cases the grouped discharges interspersed with periods of silence during sleep (especially visible in B); increase of the mean rate of discharge from the very beginning of arousal. In some slow PT cells, a short-lasting, dramatic increase in the mean rate of discharge was seen during the first 2–3 sec of arousal, then followed by a plateau at a lower level (this peak can be observed at the beginning of awakening in B). [From Steriade, Deschênes, and Oakson, unpublished observations]

tical figures given in the histograms of the fast PT cell depicted in Fig. 8.11A. The apparent discrepancy between the present results and those of Evarts (1965) is probably due to the differences between excited and relaxed wakefulness in fast PT cells, two states which were not dissociated in his study. Summing up, the present data on freely moving monkeys show that the great majority of slow as well as fast PT cells are tonically active during *quiet* waking, with higher mean rates of discharge than those seen during drowsiness and slow sleep.

The above statement may appear as oversimplified since it hides a more complex reality. Indeed, the higher amount of spontaneous discharge during waking resulted from comparison of mean rates of discharge between long periods of waking and long periods of slow sleep. When dissociating during synchronized sleep different patterns of EEG activity, it became evident that spontaneous firing was minimal during interspindle lulls and reached a maximum during EEG spindles[8], when it could sometimes attain an even higher level than during waking. Bursts of activity in single PT cells or in the integrated pyramidal activity in coincidence with EEG spindle trains represent common findings in the literature. They were seen both in acute experiments on cats with midbrain lesions sparing the cerebral peduncles (Whitlock *et al.*, 1953; Martin and Branch, 1958) and in chronically implanted, unrestrained cats (Morrison and Pompeiano, 1965c; Rougeul *et al.*, 1966). Intracellular studies of Jasper and Stefanis on *cerveau isolé* cats leaving intact the PT (1965) have also shown the greater tendency to spontaneous spike discharge during spindles and they have disclosed the close relationship between spindles and large oscillations (composed of excitatory and inhibitory components) in the membrane potential of PT neurons. That a simple quantitative comparison of the discharge during long periods of "waking" and "slow sleep" does not reflect the nuanced reality of these periods came in most instances when recording projection neurons in the precentral gyrus of the chronically implanted monkey. The decrease in the mean rate of discharge during behavioral slow sleep (8.35/sec) as compared with quiet waking (13.9/sec) was revealed by statistical measurements of spontaneous firing of the corticothalamic neuron synaptically driven by callosal volleys, depicted in Fig. 8.14B (see its identification in Fig. 8.8B). The same unit, however, showed during high amplitude spindles and slow waves periodic bursts of discharges whose frequencies were 2–3 times higher (30–40/sec) than the regular firing during waking (Fig. 8.14B). This was a common finding for other precentral units and especially for callosal neurons (Fig. 8.14A and C), and it corroborates the data of Berlucchi (1965) by recording with macroelectrodes the integrated fiber activity in the rostrum of the corpus callosum of the cat.

The significance of temporal patterns of unitary discharges associated with different behavioral and/or EEG states, implying changes in excitation and inhibition according to the level of vigilance, will be discussed in the last section of this work when the evidence from analysis of excitatory and inhibitory events tested during waking and sleep will better allow a confrontation between various possible inferences.

B. SHORT-AXONED INTERNEURONS AND UNIDENTIFIED CELLS

Cortical interneurons (see criteria for recognizing these cells in Section III) were particularly active during slow sleep, discharging spike barrages separated by periods of silence, and exhibiting during this period of sleep a sharply

---

[8]The time relation between increased or suppressed spontaneous firing and pure EEG slow (2–4/sec) waves could not be accurately estimated (see for such relations of the unitary activity with spindles versus slow waves the work of Calvet *et al.*, 1964).

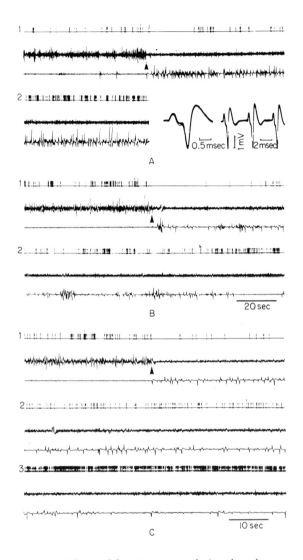

Fig. 8.13. Background firing of fast PT neurons during slow sleep, arousal, and steady wakefulness in the monkey. A–C. Three different cells; antidromic response latencies of 0.4 msec (A and B) and 0.5 msec (C). The inserts in A show the patterns of antidromic invasion of the neuron (A with a single shock and with a train of three shocks at around 250/sec). In all cases, the three ink-written traces represent from top to bottom unit spikes (displayed on the oscilloscope and used to deflect one pen of the EEG machine; each deflection exceeding the common level represents a group of several high frequency discharges), EEG rhythms recorded from the perirolandic region, and eye movements. In A, 1 and 2 are separated by about 1 min. In B, 2 is the direct continuation of 1. In C, 2 is the direct continuation of 1, and 3 is separated from 2 by about 2 min. In all cases, arousal was induced by the experimenter who entered the monkey's

defined modal interval at 2–3 msec in some units or at 4 msec in another cells.

Without exception, behavioral and EEG arousal in freely moving monkeys, and reticular-induced EEG desynchronization in *encéphale isolé* cats, were associated with striking decreased firing rate or, more often, with complete arrest of spontaneous firing in motor cortical interneurons, electrophysiologically identified by their high frequency repetitive responses to PT antidromic and/or specific thalamic stimulation. This is depicted in Fig. 8.22 for a precentral unit in the monkey. The silence in neuronal firing could be studied only when the behaving animal quietly opened the eyes, before appearance of limb movements which were accompanied by rich interneuronal activity, probably due to proprioceptive drive (see Fig. 8.22). After variable time intervals of arrest of firing on arousal from sleep (from 6 to 25 sec in different units), such elements resumed, during steady state of waking, their spontaneous discharges which remained, however, at a lower level than those seen during slow sleep. The difference was dramatic in a single case (30.45/sec during sleep, and 1.10/sec during quiet waking), while in other units the decrease in mean frequencies was from 35 to 45/sec during sleep to 25–30/sec during wakefulness.

Concerning the entity of the "unidentified cell," this certainly comprised a very heterogenous group of neurons. Among them many units might have been activated by stimuli applied to structures other than those investigated in this study, or by stimuli in other locations within the structures explored. However, a great proportion showed quite opposite behavior during sleep and waking as compared to projection (relay) cells and behavior rather similar to that of identified interneurons. Actually, such unidentified elements discharged in short (Fig. 8.15A) or long (Fig. 8.15B) bursts of 300–500/sec spikes, thus showing the same type of interval distribution seen in electrophysiologically identified short-axoned neurons, and they were much less active during

---

room (arrow). In both A and B, 2 represents quiet waking. In C, after the arousal reaction the experimenter tried to keep the animal in full alertness by moving his fingers in front of the monkey's eyes (2); in 3, the experimenter was still in the room but immobile, and the state of the monkey's vigilance was that of relaxed wakefulness (see the differences between the amount of eye movements in 2 and 3). Note the neuronal silence on arousal from sleep (arrows), lasting 11.5 sec (A), 14 sec (B), and 7.5 sec (C); immediately after this period of silence, the background firing resumed the mean rate observed during slow sleep (A1) or remained at a lower level compared to that of sleep (B1 and C1); subsequently, during quiet waking, the mean rate of discharge became higher than during slow sleep (A2 and C3). Note especially the striking increased frequency with regular discharges when the animal was left quiet in C3, compared to C2 when orienting reactions were continuously induced by the experimenter; in B, the increase in the mean rate of discharge during quiet waking compared with sleep appeared after a long period (about 3 min following arousal). [From Steriade, Deschênes, and Oakson, unpublished observations]

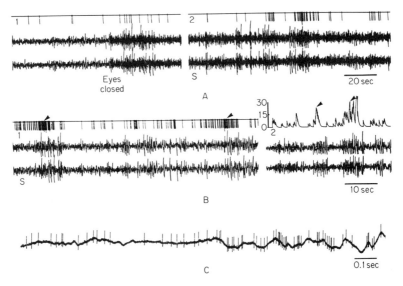

Fig. 8.14. Fluctuations in the spontaneous firing of precentral neurons modulated by callosal volleys during drowsiness and slow sleep in the monkey. A–C. Three different neurons (A, the same cell as depicted in Fig. 8.8D; B, the same cell as depicted in Figs. 8.8B and 8.19; C, a neuron synaptically driven at around 6 msec by transcallosal stimuli). In A is depicted the transitional period from waking to slow sleep (S), 1 being separated by 30 sec from 2. In B, unit firing during slow sleep (1) and integrated activity of the same unit several minutes later, during the same functional state (2, the number of spikes per second is indicated on the ordinate); note the periods of complete silence, and the bursts of neuronal activity (arrows) occurring in good time-relation with sequences of high amplitude EEG spindles and slow waves at an even higher level than during waking (the mean frequency of this cell during sleep was 8.35/sec, while it was 13.9/sec during waking). In C (original spikes of another neuron), note the increase of spontaneous discharges occurring in association with focal slow waves during drowsiness. See details and comments in text. [From Steriade and Hallé, unpublished observations]

behavioral waking than during slow sleep in the monkey. In some instances, high frequency spike barrages were seen in close time-relation with the simultaneously recorded focal positivities of EEG waves (Fig. 8.15C, arrows). In the cat, the effects of short trains of fast reticular pulses were more spectacular than those of natural arousal reaction and led to a clear-cut decrease or arrest of the spontaneous unit firing, simultaneous with classical changes in the EEG rhythms. The reticular depressing influence was particularly evident in each case when it was exerted on the spontaneous activity of cells exhibiting short (5–15 msec) or long (50–60 msec) high frequency (200–500/sec) spike barrages. This pattern also occurred during relaxed waking, something which was not encountered in PT neurons. In contrast to the behavior of PT cells (see Fig. 8.10B–C), spontaneous discharges of unidentified elements (interneurons?)

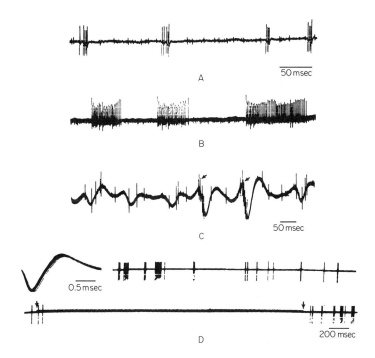

Fig. 8.15. Patterns of spontaneous discharges of unidentified, bursting neurons in monkey and cat. A–C. Three different units in the monkey's precentral gyrus. D. A precruciate unit in the cat. Note the short (A) and long (B) high frequency spike barrages occurring during behavioral slow sleep in the monkey; the close time-relation between clustered unitary firing and focal slow positivity is recorded by the same microelectrode (C, arrows). D. Cell discharging in high frequency (200–350/sec) spike barrages interspersed with periods of silence, completely stopped by reticular stimulation (between arrows), with immediate recovery of the previous pattern following stimulation; configuration of superimposed spikes in a burst was depicted (with double amplitude and at fast speed) to show that this pattern of discharge (interneuron?) was not due to injury of the cell. [D is from Steriade *et al.*, 1971c]

were completely arrested during increased vigilance induced by high frequency reticular pulses (Fig. 8.15D).

V. Evoked Discharges

A. VL AND CALLOSALLY EVOKED NEURONS

The increase in the rate of background firing of projection neurons upon spontaneous or reticular arousal was paradoxically associated in the *encéphale isolé* cat with a decrease in the probability of purely VL-evoked discharges (simple relay cells), as compared with synchronized sleep. This was a constant finding; it is depicted in Figs. 8.16–8.17 and 8.29 for three typical relay cells. Despite the fact that spontaneous discharges of such neurons dropped significantly when EEG exhibited patterns of synchronized sleep (see Fig. 8.16), during these periods the cells could be modulated by 85–100% of the testing VL shocks, while during natural or reticular-induced waking they were synaptically driven only at 10–40%. This was obvious both for single stimuli and multiple testing stimuli (Fig. 8.16).

The above data concerned obvious differences between EEG patterns of sychronized sleep and waking as found in the majority of simple relay cells. In a few neurons the changes became evident only by analyzing the post-stimulus histograms of the VL-evoked discharges during various functional states. Such a neuron is depicted in Fig. 8.17. During EEG rhythms of steady

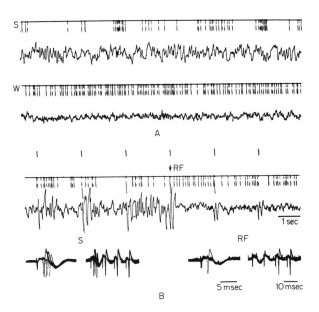

Fig. 8.16. Changes in spontaneous and VL-evoked discharges of a simple relay cell on arousal from naturally occurring EEG synchronization in an *encéphale isolé* cat. Small PT cell (antidromic latency of 5 msec), the same as depicted in Fig. 8.5C. A. Background activity during EEG patterns of slow sleep (S) and waking (W). In B, the ink-written record shows a typical example of transition from S to reticular (RF) arousal: application of VL testing shock trains at 0.5/sec (first trace), unit activity (second trace) and motor cortex EEG waves (third trace). Below, seven superimposed sweeps show the discharges evoked by both single and four stimuli (at 115/sec) applied to the VL during slow sleep (left), and by the same VL testing stimulations with short (50 msec) conditioning trains of high frequency (320/sec) RF shocks (right). Note RF-induced decrease in probability of the evoked discharges, simultaneous with regularization and increase of spontaneous firing. Further comments in text. [From Steriade *et al.*, 1973]

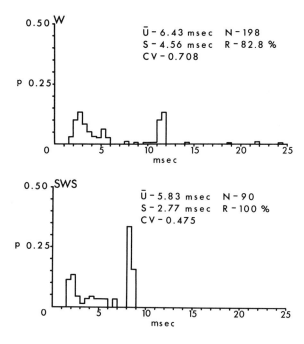

Fig. 8.17. Poststimulus histograms of a simple relay cell in cat motor cortex for single shock (0.5/sec) stimulation of VL during EEG patterns of steady waking (W) and slow sleep (SWS). Symbols: $\overline{U}$, mean latency; S, standard deviation; CV, coefficient of variation; N, number of counts; R, percentage of evoked discharges; p, probability of response for each class. Note during slow sleep: increase in the probability of firing and decrease in response latencies both for the early and especially for the late evoked discharges. See comments in text.

waking it was modulated 82.8% with one impulse discharge to one VL shock, at latencies widely dispersed between 1.5 and 12 msec, with an early and a late peak of probability at 2–3.5 msec and 11–12 msec, respectively. During natural EEG patterns of slow sleep, the cell was driven 100%, the early peak moved to 1.5–2.5 msec, and the late one to 8.0–8.5 msec. Concerning the 500% higher probability of discharges in the class of intervals between 1.5 and 2.0 msec during sleep than during waking, it is reasonable to conclude that the summit time of the VL-evoked EPSP was shorter during synchronized sleep. Comparing of early VL-evoked discharges with responses at longer latencies (the latter being likely attributable to intercalated relays through excitatory internuncial cells) reveals that the most powerful alterations occurred in the late (5–10 msec) discharges. This may be ascribed to inhibition of cortical excitatory interneurons relaying VL-fugal messages before they reach the PT neurons. An elective decrease in amplitude of the *second* I wave in the PT was observed both during reticular arousal in acute experiments (see Fig. 3 in Steriade, 1969) and during behavioral waking and desynchronized sleep in chronically implanted preparations (see Fig. 10 in Steriade *et al.*, 1969b), and the assumption was made that arousal is associated with depression of activity in motor cortical interneurons (Steriade, 1969), which are known to mediate the late I components of the cortically elicited PT response (Patton and Amassian, 1954). Summing up, in simple relay cells both the VL-evoked discharges at latencies suggesting monosynaptic excitation (1.0–2.0 msec, see Figs. 8.16–8.17 and 8.29) and especially the responses elicited by VL stimuli at longer latencies (5–10 msec) were depressed during EEG desynchronization compared to slow sleep. The increased probability of VL-evoked monosynaptic discharges elicited in motor cortical neurons has been also observed during behavioral slow sleep in monkey, compared with waking (Fig. 8.18). Other precentral neurons, synaptically driven by shocks at the level of the VB-VL border in the monkey, have been, however, clearly facilitated during waking (Steriade, Deschênes, and Oakson, in preparation). Since the distinction between simple and complex cells was not possible to make in the monkey, in view of technical difficulties resulting from the critical location of specific thalamic stimulating electrodes (too adjacent to exclude spread of current), we retain only the dissociation between the cat's simple relay cells, depressed in their synaptic responsiveness during waking, and complex relay cells, exhibiting an opposite behavior (see the following).

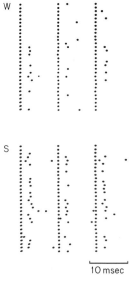

Fig. 8.18. Changes in VL-evoked discharges of a precentral neuron during behavioral waking (W) and slow sleep (S) in monkey. Dotgrams (30 sweeps) depict the train of three testing shocks (arrows) and the increased probability of evoked discharges during sleep as compared with waking.

10 msec

The neurons modulated synaptically at short latencies (2.5–6 msec) by callosal volleys in the freely moving monkey, whether or not they were identified as PT cells, behave similarly to the VL-evoked PT neurons, showing the same puzzling discrepancy between the increase of spontaneous firing and the depressed responsiveness during waking. Besides the cells which decreased the probability of their evoked spikes during waking (see also Steriade and Lamarre, 1969), the facilitation of the callosally evoked activity during behavioral sleep with slow waves was expressed in other neurons by decreased latencies and concentration of discharges, whereas the spikes were dispersed at greater latencies during waking (Fig. 8.19).

Such findings show that the responsiveness of cortical cells relaying the major synaptic input to the motor cortex, arising in the VL, is depressed during waking and they are in line with our previous data showing the reduction in amplitude, during reticular arousal of the *encéphale isolé* cat or natural waking in the behaving preparation, of motor cortex mass responses to single or repetitive (8–10/sec) VL stimuli (Steriade, 1969, 1970; Steriade *et al.*, 1969b; see also Figs. 8.1–8.2). They also indicate the common alterations undergone during sleep and waking by cells modulated by VL and callosal volleys in the motor cortical area,[9] concerning both their spontaneous firing and their ability to be evoked by such stimuli.

Several possibilities may be advanced to explain the discrepancy between the responsiveness and the spontaneous firing of such cells which represent a puzzling exception to the rule of parallel behavior, during sleep and waking, in spontaneous and evoked firing of thalamic and cortical neurons.

First one could assume that the decreased probability of the evoked discharges (Figs. 8.16–8.18) and/or their dispersion at longer latencies (Fig. 8.19) during waking are the effect of the increased background noise which might interfere with the evoked firing. That this was actually not the case was evident by careful analysis of long samples of simultaneously recorded background and evoked unit activities: (a) The increase in spontaneous firing of some cells during waking, reaching only 10–12/sec (Fig. 8.16) or 14/sec (Fig. 8.19) *regular* discharge can hardly account for the cell's relative unresponsiveness to testing shocks delivered every 2 sec. (b) In other cells, the decrease or even disappearance of VL-evoked discharges by conditioning trains of reticular arousing stimuli was not associated with significant changes in the spontaneous firing of the same unit (Fig. 8.29). (c) The increase during waking of spontaneous firing in cortical cells receiving converging VL and VB output (complex

---

[9] Decreased responsiveness during waking of cells driven by callosal volleys in the motor cortex, as revealed in the present unitary study, may be related to similar modifications in mass responses evoked by transcallosal stimulation in somatosensory (Faval *et al.*, 1964) and visual (Baldissera *et al.*, 1966b) cortices.

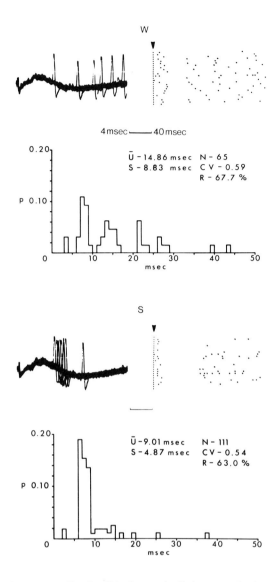

Fig. 8.19. Changes in callosally elicited synaptic discharges and subsequent inhibition in a precentral corticothalamic neuron of monkey during behavioral waking (W) and slow sleep (S). Same unit as depicted in Fig. 8.8B (see in that figure the antidromic invasion of this neuron from the thalamus). Discharges evoked by a shock to the contralateral motor cortex are depicted with original spikes in superimposition. Dotgrams (25 sweeps) are depicted at lower speed to show the changes in the early evoked discharges and the changes in the subsequent silent period, respectively. The symbols in the poststimulus histograms are the same as in Fig. 8.17. This unit discharged spontaneously at 13.9/sec during W, and at 8.35/sec during S, exhibiting a very similar distribution of intervals during W and S as that seen for PT cells in Fig. 8.11. Note the concentration of evoked discharges during sleep as opposed to dispersed activity during waking; increased duration of the inhibitory period during sleep (seen in dotgrams). [From Steriade and Hallé, unpublished observations]

relay cells) did not prevent this type of neuron from being simultaneously facilitated in their evoked discharges, which is a common property of principal cells in other cerebral areas. In this respect, it has to be mentioned that the VL relay neurons (to take only a single example from the specific thalamic nuclei) show a much greater increase in background firing during wakefulness (as compared to that seen in the motor cortex) which does not prevent these cells from being simultaneously enhanced in their responsivenss tested by shocks to the cerebellothalamic pathway (Steriade *et al.*, 1971a; Filion *et al.*, 1971).

It can be thought that a certain synaptic organization, peculiar for fibers arising in the ascending activating systems and for VL-fugal fibers,[10] both reaching PT neurons, can favor this picture of decreased thalamically elicited discharges in cells showing an increased firing rate. The increase in spontaneous neuronal discharges during natural waking in the monkey or during reticular arousing stimulation in the cat is likely owing to the effect mainly exerted on the distal apical dendrites of PT cells by fibers of reticular origin, relayed in more rostral structures, and consisting of membrane depolarization transmitted through the dendritic tree to the soma. The early surface-positive wave of the VL-evoked motor cortex mass response is believed to arise from summation in proximal apical dendrites of individual EPSPs due to specific influxes. Thus, the reduction in the field response during waking or reticular stimulation (see again Figs. 8.1–8.2) could be ascribed to the diminution of EPSP amplitude of the less polarized subsynaptic membrane. On the unitary level, the decreased reactivity of motor cortex "simple" relay cells during waking is clear but not as striking as in the case of field responses, possibly because the decrease in EPSP amplitude is partially compensated by a tonic increase of soma excitation. Anyhow, the diminution of EPSP amplitude could be so great that electrotonic spread of the dendritic depolarization to the axon hillock becomes ineffective, with the result that a testing volley arriving along the specific input pathway is less likely to cause a discharge in spite of the fact that neuron polarization is somewhat closer to the firing level. The importance of partial spikes conducted with decrement through large dendrites has been discussed by many researchers. The initial magnitude and efficiency of conduction of these "traveling impulses," if they exist in the dendrites of simple relay neurons, could be very sensitive to the state of polarization of the proximal dendritic membrane.

Finally, another possibility of this paradoxical depression in evoked dis-

---

[10] The difference between the decreased probability of evoked firing in "simple" VL-modulated PT cells during waking, and the increased responsiveness of cells receiving converging VL and VB inputs (see Figs. 8.20–8.21) might be due to different synaptic arrangements in these two types of cells. However, complete lack of anatomical evidence in this respect would make tenuous any further inference, this difference still remaining a mystery.

charges during waking might be a presynaptic depolarization induced by facilitatory impulses of the ascending activating systems at VL and callosal terminal fibers on PT cells. Despite the fact that extensive searches did not disclose axo-axonic synapses in neocortical areas, this mechanism might exist and it may submit to future investigation.

B. Cells Receiving Converging VL and VB Inputs (Complex Relay Neurons)

The differences in latency and pattern between VL- and VB-evoked discharges of the same neuron (Figs. 8.7A, 8.20, and 8.21) exclude the physical spread of current from one thalamic nucleus to another at the testing intensities of stimulation used (see other details in Section III). Furthermore, the opposite changes, during EEG patterns of waking and slow sleep in cat, in evoked discharges of such neurons, when compared with simply VL-driven cells, differentiated "simple" from "complex" pericruciate neurons. Actually, during waking the latter type showed an increase in both the spontaneous firing, which

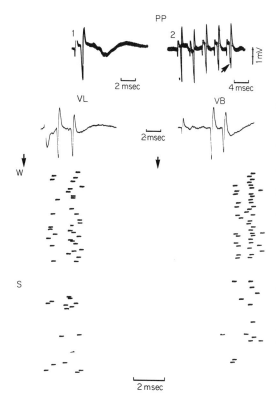

Fig. 8.20. Synaptic responsiveness of a complex relay cell during EEG patterns of waking (W) and synchronized sleep (S). This neuron was antidromically invaded from the pes pedunculi (PP) at 1.25 msec (1) and could follow 250/sec shocks (2) with progressive IS-SD fragmentation at successive shocks (arrow). It was also modulated synaptically with an identical pattern of discharge by both VL and VB shocks, at 1.5 msec and 3.5 msec, respectively. Four dotgrams, each consisting of 30 successive sweeps, show the VL-evoked (left) and the VB-evoked (right) responses during W and S (the "dots" are actually small bars, because of the fast speed; note different time scales for the dotgrams and for the above depicted original spikes). Testing VL and VB shocks indicated by arrows. Comments in text. [From Steriade et al., 1973]

was common for all projection cells, and in the discharges evoked by VL and VB shocks. The facilitation of evoked discharges (contrasting with decrease, during waking, in synaptic responsiveness of simple relay cells) was expressed by increase in the probability of firing to testing stimuli (Fig. 8.20), and occasionally by decrease in discharge latencies. In some PT cells, the decreased probability of VL-induced and VB-induced discharges (from around 90–95% during EEG desynchronization to around 35–40% during synchronizing EEG patterns) was associated for most of the testing stimuli with reduction of double spike responses during waking to one single discharge during slow sleep (Fig. 8.20). In the majority of complex relay neurons, poststimulus histograms showed an unequal decreased probability of responses to VL shocks compared to VB-evoked discharges during synchronized sleep (Fig. 8.21).

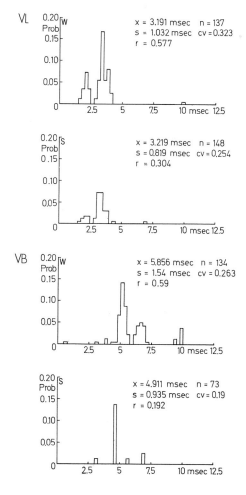

Fig. 8.21. Poststimulus histograms of VL-evoked and VB-evoked discharges in a complex PT cell during EEG patterns of waking (W) and slow sleep (S). Symbols: x, mean latency; s, standard deviation; r, fractional response (probability), indicating the total number of times that the neuron responded to the stimulation in the time interval shown divided by the total number of stimulations; n, number of counts; cv, coefficient of variation. [From Steriade *et al.*, 1973]

The opposite alterations disclosed in this work between the synaptic responsiveness of simple relay cells (Figs. 8.16, 8.17, 8.29) and that of complex PT neurons (Figs. 8.20, 8.21) during the investigated states of EEG synchronization and desynchronization emphasize the importance of careful identification of different inputs acting on a given neuronal class, when characterizing its changes in reponsiveness at various levels of vigilance. Lack of complete identification of several synaptic inputs acting on PT neurons may lead to some results reporting reticular-induced facilitation in thalamically evoked discharges of some neurons and depression in other units recorded from the cat's motor cortex (Spehlmann and Downes, 1972). Such differences between responsiveness of various investigated units are likely ascribable to their different synaptic inputs of thalamic origin, as described in the present work. It is now reasonable to assume that the previously reported reticular facilitation in the VL-evoked discharges of a PT neuron (seen in Fig. 6D of Akimoto and Saito, 1966) actually dealt with a complex PT cell which was tested by only one of its thalamic imputs.

It can now be inferred that the increased output from the VL during waking in both paralyzed (Frigyesi and Purpura, 1964; Purpura *et al.*, 1966b; Steriade, 1969; Steriade *et al.*, 1971a; Filion *et al.*, 1971) and behaving (Steriade *et al.*, 1969b; Favale *et al.*, 1971) preparations, which could not be understood when only the decreased responsiveness during waking of purely VL-driven PT cells was considered (see the first part of this section), may subserve high integrative processes governing motor performances and requiring converging thalamic inputs acting on the source of the cortical outflow.

C. Short-Axoned Interneurons

Synaptically evoked spike barrages following antidromic PT and/or afferent specific thalamic stimulation were profoundly depressed on arousal from slow sleep in monkey (Fig. 8.22) and during reticular-elicited EEG desynchronization in cat. This paralleled the drop in spontaneous activity of internuncial elements. The depression of evoked activity on arousal was expressed by longer latency and especially reduction of number of spikes in the barrage. Such a dramatic inhibition of both spontaneous and evoked activities on arousal, as seen in Fig. 8.22, was followed during the steady state of waking by resumption of interneuronal activity. As mentioned in the preceding section, the rates of spontaneous discharges were lower during steady waking compared to slow sleep. Poststimulus histograms in two identified interneurons of monkey, driven monosynaptically by both recurrent collaterals of PT fibers and by specific thalamocortical axons (one of them is the unit depicted in Fig. 8.22, the other is depicted in Fig. 8.9B), showed, however, that the total number of spikes discharged by these cells to 100 antidromic PT shocks was not different

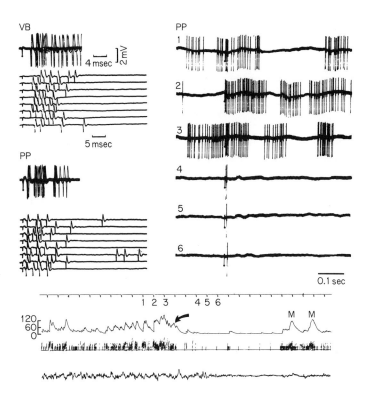

Fig. 8.22. Spontaneous and evoked discharges of a precentral interneuron during behavioral slow sleep and arousal in freely moving monkey. This cell discharged monosynaptically with high frequency (400/sec) spike barrages to both pes pedunculi (PP) and thalamic ventrobasal (VB) stimuli (0.9 msec latency for PP stimuli, 2.2 msec for VB stimuli). Left column shows the discharges elicited by single shocks to the VB and PP (superimposition of several sweeps and eight successive sweeps in the wavegrams). Note differences in latencies of responses evoked by antidromic PP and afferent VB stimuli. The time scales depicted for the superimposition and wavegram in VB are also valid for the PP stimulation. Right column shows six testing shocks dots to the PP; the first three (1–3) were delivered during slow sleep (and correspond to the number indicated on the ink-written record at the bottom), while the last three (4–6) were delivered after the arousal elicited at the arrow, but before any detectable movements of the animal, which appear only later (see M). At the bottom of this figure, the ink-written record shows testing PP shocks (first trace), the integrated unit activity (second trace; figures on the ordinate indicate spikes per second), unit activity (third trace), and EEG waves (last trace). Note that the rich spontaneous firing and the PP-evoked spike barrage during sleep develop into double or single evoked spikes during arousal, simultaneous with the drop in spontaneous discharge; unitary changes occurred before changes in EEG waves. [From Steriade and Deschênes, 1973]

during behavioral slow sleep and during steady state of quiet waking. In both neurons, the probability of the first discharge in the barrage (bin 0–1 msec in the interneuron depicted in Fig. 8.22, bin 1–2 msec in the interneuron illustrated in Fig. 8.9B) was greater during steady waking. This emphasizes that the striking inhibition of interneuronal activities is confined in the behaving preparation to the short-lasting period of arousal.

VI. Inhibitory Events

The motor cortex is a place of choice to study fluctuations of inhibitory events during different behavioral states, since intensive intracellular studies and laminar analysis of field responses at this level have disclosed reproducible patterns of activity whose alterations can be submitted to investigation during sleep and waking.

Backfiring antidromic response elicited by PT stimulation is followed by prolonged inhibition in cells giving rise to corticospinal axons, as shown by intracellularly recorded IPSPs (Phillips, 1956; Stefanis and Jasper, 1964a,b; Armstrong, 1965), by focal depth positivity (maximum at 1.4–1.6 mm) of the field potential reflecting IPSPs in a pool of neighboring neurons (Kubota *et al.*, 1965b; Humphrey, 1968a,b), and by depression of extracellularly recorded unit responses evoked by stimuli to the skin when preceded by antidromic stimuli, thus leading to constriction in the receptive field of PT cells (Brooks and Asanuma, 1965; Kameda *et al.*, 1969). The latencies of IPSPs, at least 1.4 msec but sometimes 4.8 msec (with a mean of 2.5 msec) longer than those of the antidromic spikes, suggested that the recurrent collaterals of PT axons engage one or several local inhibitory interneurons to complete the circuit (Stefanis and Jasper, 1964a).

The difficulty of dissociating between afferent (feedforward) and recurrent (feedback) inhibition was pointed out by Eccles (1969): "it is not yet known how far these IPSPs are generated by the discharge of pyramidal cells and the consequent activation of the axon collateral pathways . . . , and how far these are inhibitory pathways directly activated from the afferent pathways [p. 67]." Nonetheless, there are some evidences by Oscarsson *et al.*, (1966) on inhibitory interneurons in the primary sensorimotor cortex monosynaptically excited by thalamocortical fibers. That the same cortical interneuron may be directly driven by both the recurrent collaterals of PT fibers and the specific thalamo-cortical fibers was recently shown by Steriade and Deschênes (1973; see also Figs. 8.9B and 8.22). An obvious difference in rhythmicity, duration, and amplitude has been observed in the same cortical focus between powerful cyclic sequences (with excitatory and inhibitory components) reflected in 8–12/sec spindle waves elicited in the motor cortex by VL stimuli, and the much less pronounced rhythmic events following antidromic PT stimulation with the same parameters, although, at convenient intervals, the two types of stimuli may be additive in their interaction (unpublished data from this laboratory).

In the present experiments concerned with sleep and waking, the degree of inhibition was estimated from the duration of neuronal silence following

antidromic (PT) and afferent (specific thalamic and callosal) stimuli, the duration and amplitude of related focal slow positive waves reflecting hyperpolarization in a pool of neurons, and from the unit responsiveness to successive
shocks in a train or preceded at different delays by a conditioning stimulation.
The data reported below essentially show the reduced duration, during
reticular-elicited or spontaneous EEG arousal in cat and during behavioral
waking in monkey (compared to slow sleep), of the inhibitory period following
antidromic PT and afferent (thalamic and callosal) volleys.

Figure 8.23 depicts a fast PT cell in the cat precruciate gyrus which, following

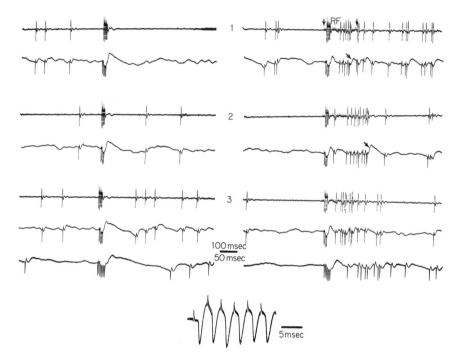

Fig. 8.23. Changes, during reticular arousal, in inhibition following PT-elicited antidromic
invasion in the motor cortex of the *encéphale isolé* cat. A train of seven shocks at 320/sec, applied
to the medullary pyramid, evoked antidromic spikes without failure at 1.2 msec latency (the
bottom part of the figure depicts superimposed responses to the first six shocks in the train).
Left column: control periods during EEG synchronization. Right column: effects of reticular (RF)
stimulation (between arrows). 1, 2, and 3 show three typical records in these two functional
states; recordings with handwidths of 50–10,000 Hz (upper trace) and 1–700 Hz (lower trace),
respectively; lack of shock artefacts in the lower traces is due to attenuation of high frequency
components. Note the obvious reduction, during reticular stimulation, of the duration of the slow
negativity following antidromic invasion (likely reflecting the IPSP of the same cell, as suggested
by interruption of the spontaneous discharges in this juxtacellular recording; see oblique
arrows) and the increased spontaneous firing. Time calibration is at a double speed in the third
trace of 3.

antidromic spikes elicited by a train of seven shocks to the bulbar pyramid, exhibited a long-lasting (140–200 msec) slow negative wave during periods of spontaneous EEG synchronization. As judged by the large amplitude (4 mV) of the spike and its initial positivity, the recording must have been juxtacellular and, thus, the subsequent slow negativity may be regarded as reflecting the IPSP of the same cell. Actually, slow negative shifts of this cell (oblique arrows in 1 and 2) were invariably observed to interrupt the spontaneous firing. During spontaneous EEG desynchronization or, more efficiently, during high frequency stimulation of the mesencephalic reticular formation, the duration of the inhibitory period subsequent to the antidromic invasion was reduced to 50 msec and the spontaneous discharges were increased above the mean rate observed prior to stimulation.

Stimulation of the PT in the medulla without taking the precaution of isolating the pyramid from the adjacent medial lemniscus might cause spread of current to the specific ascending pathway and, thus, to complicate the interpretation because of intermingled recurrent and afferent inhibitory effects. Therefore, other experiments were performed on *encéphale isolé* cats in which the mesencephalic medial lemniscus was destroyed, the pes pedunculi was stimulated, and the fluctuations of the evoked recurrent inhibition (reflected by the laminar analysis of different components in the antidromic field response) were studied during periods of EEG synchronization and desynchronization. The negative wave following α and β components of the antidromic response recorded at the surface of the precruciate gyrus, and the reversed (positive) wave in deep layers following α, N_1 and N_2 components,[11] were both significantly reduced in duration during spontaneous or reticular-elicited EEG desynchronization as compared with periods of EEG synchronization occurring spontaneously or induced by very small amounts (1–2 mg/kg i.v.) of a short-acting barbiturate (Fig. 8.24). The reduction in duration of such waves, believed to derive from IPSPs in deep-lying somata and proximal dendrites (Humphrey, 1968a,b), was not dependent upon alterations in the preceding components of the antidromic response. During EEG patterns of synchronized sleep, the slow waves following the early fast components lasted without interruption for 50–60 msec, in agreement with figures previously reported by Humphrey (1968a) working with deeply barbiturized preparations. During EEG patterns of waking, a surface-positive wave (which reversed its polarity beginning at a depth of 0.8 mm) cut off at around 20–25 msec the slow wave which reflects recurrent inhibition of PT cells; a second surface-positive (depth-negative)

---

[11] See for a detailed discussion on the significance of these components, respectively reflecting the volume conductor recording of PT axons (α) and the antidromic invasion of fast (N_1) and slow PT cells (N_2, which probably includes at a depth of 800 μ also recurrent EPSPs), the paper by Humphrey (1968a).

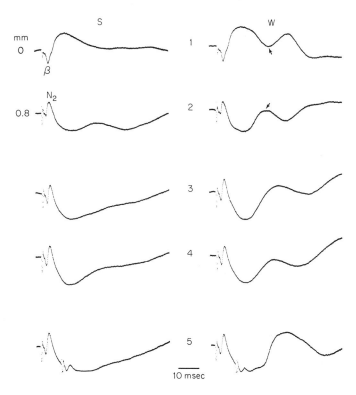

Fig. 8.24. Changes, during EEG patterns of slow sleep (S) and waking (W), of recurrent inhibition in the motor cortex, as reflected by field responses evoked by pes pedunculi stimulation in the *encéphale isolé* cat (with destruction of the mesencephalic medial lemnicus). Averaged responses (20 sweeps). 1, Surface recording in the lateral part of the precruciate gyrus; 2, depth recording (0.8 mm) in the same focus; 3 and 4, recordings at the same depth, with an intensity 50% higher than that used in 1 and 2; 5, paired shocks with the same intensity as in 3–4 (note diminution in amplitude of the N_2 wave evoked by the second shock). Full explanations in text.

wave appeared at the end of the inhibitory period, with a latency of about 40–45 msec. These two "depolarizing" waves (the first is indicated by an arrow in Fig. 8.24), which differentiated in our experiments the waking from the sleeping state and which split the long-lasting inhibition seen during naturally occurring or barbiturate-induced synchronization, are to be related to the data of Asanuma and Brooks (1965) showing two peaks of facilitation interrupting at approximately the same latencies (20 and 40 msec) the recurrent inhibition induced by capsular stimulation in the vigilant cat.

Similar reduced duration, during waking, of periods of neuronal silence or of related slow waves, was observed when testing with afferent stimuli. In the cat, reticular arousing stimulation greatly reduced or even abolished the silent period elicited in PT neurons by specific (VL or VB) thalamic stimuli (see below, Fig. 8.29C). In the behaving monkey, when little spontaneous firing was seen in the VL-driven cell, the changes in the subsequent inhibition could be inferred only from the simultaneously recorded depth-positive slow shift following a train of thalamic shocks. This slow positivity and subsequent negativity, the latter being sometimes associated with a rebound in the form of a group of unit discharges, became more and more accentuated as the animal fell into sleep (Fig. 8.25). In other neurons, with richer background activity, the increased inhibition during sleep with EEG synchronization could be estimated both from the changes in spontaneous firing of the cell under observation and from the focal slow positive waves suggesting hyperpolariza-tion undergone by neighboring units. Reduction or suppression of unit firing associated with rhythmic positive slow waves (120–150 msec in duration) and followed by spike clusters superimposed on negative slow waves was partic-ularly evident during the period of falling into sleep. This contrasted with much less pronounced inhibitory events during waking. The inhibitory phenomena occurring during transient periods of closing and reopening the eyes peculiar to sleepiness, sometimes preceded the clear-cut EEG signs of sleep by 1–2 min (Figs. 8.26 and 8.27, stage D). These findings are consistent with our previous data on behaving cats showing that the synaptically relayed activity in the VL nucleus is inhibited to the highest degree during falling into sleep (drowsiness)

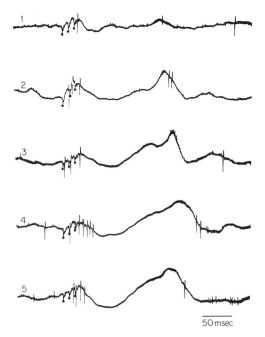

Fig. 8.25. Changes in VL-elicited slow focal waves during quiet waking (1), drowsiness (2), and sleep with slow waves (3–5). Three testing VL shocks. Note progressive increase in duration and amplitude of the slow positivity reflecting hyperpolarization in a pool of neighboring neurons as the monkey fell into sleep; note also the increased number of the early VL-evoked dis-charges of the neuron under observa-tion (the large, biphasic spike) during slow sleep as compared with waking.

50 msec

and related EEG spindles (Steriade *et al.*, 1969b). At deepened stages of slow sleep, VL-induced repetitive positive waves and subsequent rebound unit activities were less pronounced, whereas the first period of inhibition of the

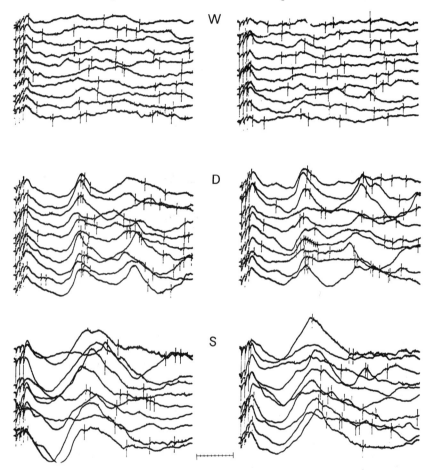

Fig. 8.26. Changes in afferent inhibition induced in monkey's precentral cortex by VL stimulation during the steady state of waking (W), drowsiness (D), and sleep with EEG slowing (S). Two simultaneously recorded neurons (positive-negative and negative-positive spikes). Recordings of unit discharges and slow waves using a bandwidth of 1–10,000 Hz. In each of these three functional states (W, D, S), two examples of successive activities elicited by VL stimuli at the left of each sweep (from top to bottom). Time: 100 msec. Note increased inhibition during D and S as compared to W, inferred from both spontaneous unit firing and patterns of slow waves; note especially during D double or triple positive waves, the first followed by rebound (spike clusters), and during S the increased first slow positivity associated with complete silence of the neuronal firing. See also the following figure depicting the dotgrams of the positive-negative spike. [Modified from Steriade *et al.*, 1971c]

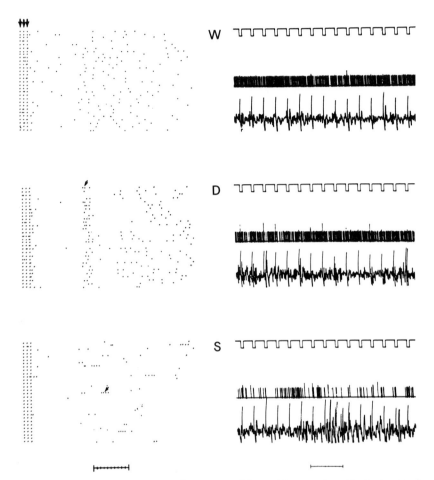

Fig. 8.27. Dotgrams showing the fluctuations of the positive-negative spike depicted in the preceding figure (left column), and the associated EEG signs (right column), during waking (W), drowsiness (D), and sleep with EEG slowing (S). The ink-written records in the right column show the testing VL shock train (first trace), the unit activity (second trace) and the EEG waves from the precentral gyrus (third trace). The VL three testing shocks are indicated by arrows at the left of each sweep in the left column. Thirty sweeps in each dotgram. Time: 100 msec (left column) and 6 sec (right column). Especially note the increased inhibition of neuronal discharges following the VL train shock during D (as compared to W) in spite of no significant changes in the background firing of the cell and in the EEG gross waves; postinhibitory rebound in D and spontaneous spike clusters in S indicated by oblique arrows. See further comments in text.

spontaneous firing and the simultaneous slow positive wave were more powerful (Figs. 8.26 and 8.27, stage S). The same increase in the inhibitory period during slow wave sleep, as compared to waking, was seen when testing with transcallosal stimulation (see dotgrams in Fig. 8.19). Conversely, spontaneous or sensory induced arousal and the subsequent steady state of waking were associated with obvious reduction of the cortical cyclic inhibitory phenomena elicited by afferent VL stimulation, depressing the positive-negative slow waves and practically erasing the unit rebound (spike clusters), restoring and regularizing the spontaneous firing and, usually, increasing the mean rate of discharge (Fig. 8.28). This was observed prior to any detectable movements.

The depression during arousal of the inhibitory mechanisms was also shown by comparing the lack of antidromic spikes to PT shocks after the first response in a train and, on the other hand, the ability of the cell to follow without failure the testing shocks when preceded by arousing reticular pulses (Fig. 8.29B). This was seen in simple relay cells which interestingly showed that full responsiveness to antidromic PT volleys during reticular-elicited arousal, compared to inhibition following the first shock in the train seen during EEG synchronization (Fig. 8.29B), contrasted with depressed synaptic responsiveness of the same unit to VL shocks when preceded by the same conditioning reticular stimulation (Fig. 8.29A; see again possible explanations for the latter effect in Section V). It is, however, to be emphasized that this additional experimental clue (recovery from inhibition following the first antidromic PT shock by reticular stimulation in cat or during behavioral waking in

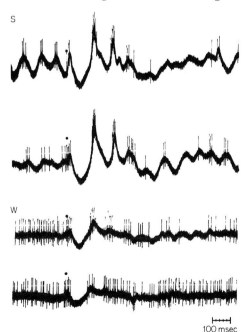

S

Fig. 8.28. Patterns of spontaneous unit discharges in the motor cortex of monkey during behavioral slow sleep (S) and waking (W), and the VL-elicited events during these functional states. The VL shock marked by dot. Note during S the spike clusters superimposed on slow negative waves following slow positive shifts, and regular discharges with increased frequency during W; note similarities between spontaneous slow waves with superimposed spike clusters and VL-evoked rhythmic events; reduction during W of rhythmic slow positive waves and of rebound sequences following VL stimulation.

W

├───┤
100 msec

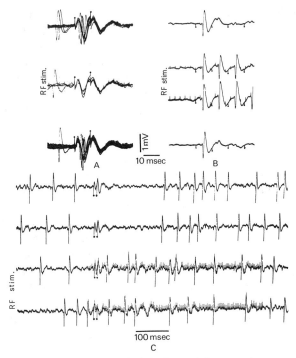

Fig. 8.29. Reticular effects on VL-evoked discharges (A), responsiveness to PT antidromic invasion (B) and VB-elicited inhibition (C) in a precruciate cell of the *encéphale isolé* cat. A. As in other simple relay units (see Fig. 8.16), reticular stimulation decreased the probability of VL-evoked discharges. B. Antidromic spike (4 msec latency) evoked by the first shock in a train of four stimuli at 100/sec applied to the medullary pyramid, followed by no responses to the subsequent shocks, and full responsiveness to all four antidromic stimuli when preceded by high frequency 320/sec reticular pulses (two intensities of reticular stimulation). C. Erasure of VB-evoked silent period and restoration of spontaneous firing by reticular stimulation.

monkey) could be found in only a few (10%) neurons in cat and monkey, since the great majority of PT cells did not show differences between waking and slow sleep in the ability to follow the shocks subsequent to the first in a train. This supports prior observations on the high safety factor of antidromic invasion of these cells (Phillips, 1956) and the data indicating that even the strongest inhibition, elicited by surface cortical shocks, may not block the backfiring elicited in Betz cells by antidromic PT stimuli (Krnjević et al., 1966).

The change in recurrent inhibition during sleep and waking was further analyzed by studying the effects exerted by a conditioning antidromic PT stimulation upon antidromically and synaptically elicited testing responses. This was done both in cats (with extensive lesion of the medial lemniscus in the mesencephalon) and in freely moving monkeys. From this work, still in progress, it can shortly be reported that the time course of inhibition induced by a preceding antidromic PT single shock or three-shock train on the subsequent testing antidromic invasion of the same unit showed much faster recovery of the testing response during waking than during slow sleep (Fig. 8.30). The time required for recovery was variable in different PT units, and this can be seen by comparing the effects of a single antidromic conditioning shock in the two curves depicted in Fig. 8.30A–B. As expected, the inhibition of the antidromically

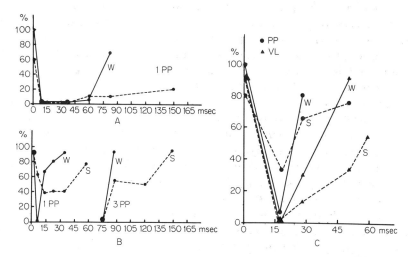

Fig. 8.30. Recurrent inhibition of antidromically and synaptically elicited discharges during EEG patterns of waking (W) and slow sleep (S) in cat. A–C. Three different PT units (antidromic response latencies of 3.8 msec, 1.5 msec, and 0.7 msec in A, B and C, respectively; the fast PT cell in C was also synaptically driven by VL stimulation at around 2 msec). EEG patterns of waking (W), and spontaneously occurring (in A and C) or Surital-induced (in B) synchronization (S). The testing shocks (antidromic in A–B, antidromic and synaptic in C) were preceded by a single shock or three-shock trains to the pes pedunculi (PP), as indicated in each graph (1 PP or 3 PP); in B, both conditioning procedures were used; a three-shock PP train was used in C. Testing PP shock was delivered at the same intensity as the conditioning one in A and C, and it was at 60% of the intensity used for the conditioning stimulation in B. Note in A the deep inhibition during both W and S below a 60-msec interval, and faster recovery during W; note also the decreased probability of the test antidromic response during S compared to W. Note in B the much longer inhibition with 3 PP conditioning shocks than with a single one; when a single PP shock was used to elicit inhibition, this was deeper during W than during S in this particular neuron; with both conditioning procedures (1 PP and 3 PP), the recovery was slower during S. Note in C the decreased probability of the antidromic PP test (control) response during S (80%) compared to W (100%); deeper inhibition during W of an antidromically elicited spike at an 18 msec interval and shorter recovery during W; deeper recurrent inhibition of VL-elicited synaptic discharges compared to antidromically (PP) elicited ones at the same intervals; faster recovery of synaptically elicited responses during W compared to S, as was also the case when testing with antidromic volleys. [From Steriade and Deschênes, in preparation]

elicited testing spike was much longer with a conditioning shock train than with a single shock (Fig. 8.30B). At short delays (10–15 msec) between the conditioning and the testing antidromic PT stimulation, the inhibition of the testing response was deeper during waking in some units (Fig. 8.30B, single conditioning shock; see also Fig. 8.30C, the procedure with the testing antidromic volley), but in other PT neurons it was equally developed or even deeper during slow sleep. However, the constant finding for all investigated units came from analysis of longer delays, when recovery was invariably faster during waking (at about 20–70 msec) than during slow sleep (at 50–150 msec, and sometimes longer than 200 msec). As expected, VL-elicited synaptic discharges were much more susceptible to recurrent inhibition than the antidromically elicited spike, but the same finding holds true, namely much longer recurrent inhibition during slow sleep than during waking (Fig. 8.30C).

The above results showed decreased duration of inhibitory effects during waking compared to sleep. It seemed worthwhile to check the level of polarization of PT cell membranes at different levels of vigilance. Intracellular recordings in freely moving animals, to show removal, during behavioral waking, of strong hyperpolarization in PT neurons during slow sleep, still seems to be an insurmountable task. In spite of this, we tried to record juxtacellularly the pattern of antidromic invasion in monkey, and to analyze the changes, during sleep and waking, in the degree of IS-SD fragmentation. The fast PT cell, depicted in Fig. 8.31, antidromically invaded from the pes pedunculi at 0.5 msec, was recorded juxtacellularly as suggested by the large (5 mV) spike amplitude. During behavioral slow sleep, even the first antidromic spike showed fragmentation between the IS and the SD spikes, while the responses to subsequent antidromic volleys exhibited progressive augmentation of the IS-SD break, although the cell was not damaged, as seen by lack of notches in the spontaneous spikes. During waking, the first antidromic spike was fully recovered, with no sign of IS-SD break, and subsequent responses showed less pronounced fragmentation than during sleep. It is known from intracellular studies on spinal cord motoneurons that the degree of IS-SD splitting occurs in relation to the increased hyperpolarization of the cell (Coombs et al., 1955). It appears, thus, that the transition from sleep to waking is associated with decrease in the hyperpolarization of PT neurons.

Here are some general remarks on different problems discussed throughout this work, in the light of the findings reported in the final section on inhibitory events.

The pattern of spontaneous discharges seen in motor cortical neurons during behavioral sleep with EEG slowing (see Fig. 8.28) is usually termed "clustered firing," and it consists of bursts of high frequency spikes inter-

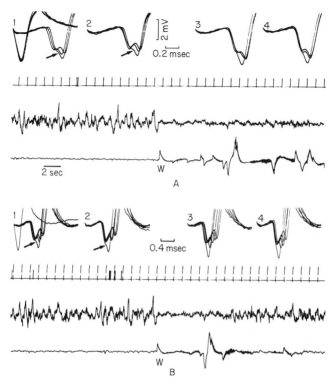

Fig. 8.31. Changes in antidromic invasion of a pyramidal tract (PT) neuron on arousal from sleep in the freely moving monkey. A and B. Two different cycles showing the awakening reaction (W) elicited during a period of slow sleep. Three shocks at 110/sec (in A) and five shocks at 350/sec (in B) were applied every second to the pes pedunculi. The oscilloscopic traces (1–4 in both A and B) show the superimposed antidromic spikes to all shocks in the train. Sweeps were triggered by both the shock artefacts and the spontaneous discharges (see 1 in A and B). 1 and 2, typical responses during sleep; 3 and 4, typical responses during waking. Below, the ink-written records depict the testing stimuli and the evoked discharges, and occasionally spontaneous discharges (top trace), EEG waves (middle trace), and ocular movements (bottom trace). The arrows indicate the IS–SD break of the first spike in the train, which occurs during sleep in spite of the fact that spontaneous spikes (see 1) do not present such notches, thus showing that the cell was not damaged. Note that full recovery of the first spike and diminution in the IS–SD break of successive spikes during waking were *not* associated in this fast PT cell with an increase of spontaneous discharges. Other comments in text. [From Steriade and Deschênes, 1973]

spersed with periods of silence. The assumption of Evarts (1964) was that changes in impulse frequency and in temporal patterns of discharge from regular firing during waking to spike clusters and periods of silence during sleep may be ascribed to both a decrease in the excitatory drive and a failure in recurrent inhibition acting as a frequency-limiting mechanism of PT neurons (see also the discussion in Martin and Branch, 1958). Evarts noted that the transitional periods between waking and sleep had not been analyzed in his experiments. When looking at such periods of falling into sleep, recording unit firing with related slow waves, and testing inhibitory sequences elicited by VL stimuli, it became evident that clusters of high frequency spikes (super-imposed on negative slow waves) always followed long-lasting slow positive waves associated with reduction or disappearance of spontaneous dis-charges and likely reflecting periods of increased afferent inhibition during drowsiness (see Fig. 8.26, stage D). At this initial stage of sleep, this was often seen as a first electrographic sign, without alteration in the mean discharge rate of cortical neurons or even in the gross EEG waves (Fig. 8.27, same stage D), thus suggesting that an increased efficiency of inhibitory mechanisms may favor the falling into sleep before any reduction in the excitatory drive.

Clustered firing thus follows long periods of neuronal inhibition, and this was seen not only in motor cortical neurons, but also at the VL level (Steriade et al., 1971a; Lamarre et al., 1971b). It may be argued that such a pattern was observed by testing changes in cortical inhibition with artificial (electrical) stimulation and that this might not be the case with spontaneously occurring sleep patterns. However, if the neuronal patterns of discharge during spontan-eous EEG spindle waves in a sleeping behaving monkey are compared with those induced by a VL shock on this background of activity, it is obvious that the VL-evoked spindlelike sequence is a caricature of the spontaneous back-ground waves, consisting of hyperpolarizing and depolarizing (with super-imposed spike clusters) components, but that the two (spontaneous and evoked) events are essentially similar (Fig. 8.28). Thus, the testing shock seems only to reveal and enhance basic properties of the cortical neuronal network during the initial stage of drowsiness, as well as later, at deeper stages of sleep with EEG synchronization. It has to be stressed that the rhythmic spike clusters of VL relay cells following long-lasting positive shifts and superimposed on negative waves, belonging to 8–12/sec EEG spindle sequences occurring naturally, were also found to be almost identical in rhythmicity and configur-ation with the cyclic events elicited by setting in motion the same VL neuronal population with corticothalamic orthodromic volleys (Steriade et al., 1972).

Spike clusters follow long-lasting inhibition reflected in extracellularly recorded slow positive waves, but they are not entirely dependent upon these periods of preceding inhibition, i.e., they are *not* to be regarded exclusively as postanodal exaltation. An additional, delayed, and powerful excitatory impingement from VL intrinsic interneurons has been found to be exerted on VL principal cells when they recover from the long-lasting inhibition, thus allowing initiation of the so-called rebound activity (Steriade, 1972; Steriade et al., 1972). Similar phenomena may account for the clustered firing in cortical neurons, but no direct evidence is available in this respect. Some differences can be seen when comparing the clustered firing of VL relay cells (Lamarre et al., 1971b; Steriade et al., 1971a)[12] with that of PT cells (Evarts, 1964; present work), mainly consisting of the lower intraburst frequency and the lack of a late modal interval in the latter case. It may be advanced that the appearance of spike clusters with high intraburst frequency, with successive intervals increasing progressively towards the end of the burst, and with a certain rhythmicity (as seen from the small, but evident late modal interval at around 300 msec showing the constancy of silent periods), as described during slow sleep in the specific thalamic nuclei (Steriade et al., 1971a), reflect powerful and rhythmic inhibitory sequences. The VL especially has been found to be the target of such influences arising in the medial thalamus (Purpura et al., 1965). That this may be actually the case was confirmed by disappearance or obvious reduction in the rhythmicity of VL clusters in midline thalamic lesioned animals (Steriade et al., 1971a). The existence within the thalamus of such a system, combined with projections from intrinsic VL inhibitory interneurons (Steriade et al., 1972) and perhaps with projections arising in the reticularis complex (the Scheibels, 1966; Massion, 1968; Schlag and Waszak, 1971; Lamarre et al., 1971b), may account for the more powerful synchronizing thalamic sequences (as compared with cortical events), reflected in longer inhibitory periods with richer post-inhibitory rebound activities.

On the other hand, a dissimilar, irregular "clustered firing" was observed during slow sleep in deep cerebellar nuclei, with much longer duration of clusters (150–250 msec, as compared to 10–25 msec seen in VL and motor cortex spike clusters) and with a lower intraburst frequency than in VL clusters (Steriade et al., 1971a,b). The shortness of the VL spike clusters might be explained by the existence of a powerful equipment of inhibitory interneurons within this nucleus, which cut off the bursts of spikes. The same mechanism may act within the cerebral cortex. On the other hand, the long duration of cerebellar clusters might be ascribed to the fact that such inhibitory cells with short axons are doubtful in deep cerebellar nuclei (Jansen and Jansen, 1955), thus explaining the ability of cells in these nuclei to follow fast (above 500/sec) antidromic VL stimuli for periods exceeding 30–50 msec, while in VL neurons inhibition is seen for a few msec following the initial sign of antidromic invasion by cortical stimulation (Steriade et al., 1971a,b). Very long duration of reticularis clusters during slow sleep (Massion, 1968; Schlag and Waszak, 1971; Lamarre et al., 1971b; Steriade and Wyzinski, 1972) may also be due to lack of a local feedback inhibitory mechanism within this nucleus.

Let us now try to discuss the arrest of firing in 27 of 31 fast PT neurons on arousal from slow sleep in the behaving monkey (Fig. 8.13, arrows), which

[12] The frequency of spikes within a burst is similar in VL to that found by Benoit (1970) in VB cells of cat during slow sleep.

contrasted with both the increase in mean rate of discharge of slow PT neurons from the very beginning of arousal (Fig. 8.12) and the increased firing rate of the same fast PT units during the subsequent period of quiet waking (see Fig. 8.13, A2 and C3). The neuronal silence was not seen in fast PT cells on reticular arousal in *encéphale isolé* cats (see Figs. 8.10C and 8.23). Two main mechanisms may be taken into account when explaining this particular behavior of fast PT cells on behavioral arousal in monkey: inhibition and/or sudden removal of some tonic excitatory impingement resulting in disfacilitation. None of these possibilities is entirely satisfactory in the light of what is already known. (1) The major excitatory synaptic input acting on fast PT cells arises in the specific thalamic (VL) nucleus. Experimental evidence in cats showed that the increased firing rate in VL relay cells is even more marked during the first few seconds of arousal than during the subsequent state of waking (Steriade *et al.*, 1971a). This must be related to powerful excitatory influences exerted by the reticulo-VL fibers on the postsynaptic membrane of VL relay cells (Purpura *et al.*, 1966b). If such findings can be extrapolated in the monkey, for which there is yet no direct evidence concerning the fluctuations in the VL output during sleep and waking, the hypothesis of cortical disfacilitation with respect to the thalamic source of excitation may be discarded. (2) Strong postsynaptic inhibition electively exerted on arousal on fast PT cells also seems to be disproved by data which, on the contrary, suggest removal, during arousal, of hyperpolarization seen during slow sleep. Such data may be summarized as follows: recovery of full antidromic spikes during arousal and waking, as opposed to obvious IS-SD break of antidromic spikes during slow sleep (Fig. 8.31) and increased probability of antidromic invasion during arousal and waking compared to sleep. Besides, as already stated, short-axoned inter-neurons stopped firing on arousal and no exception could be detected in this respect. Even if we do not have crucial evidence on the excitatory or inhibitory nature of these elements, both categories were presumably recorded and it is likely that many of these units were inhibitory interneurons. Arrest of firing in such internuncial elements on arousal is hardly to be reconciled with postsynaptic inhibition of fast PT cells during the same functional state. But we have to stress again that silence of spontaneous firing and striking depres-sion in responsiveness was observed on arousal in *all* investigated short-axoned elements (see Fig. 8.22). Among these interneurons, many must have been excitatory, especially stellate cells described by Ramon y Cajal as *"cellules à double bouquet dendritique"* which may secure vertical spread of excitation. We, therefore, suggest that arousal is associated with inhibition of cortical interneurons, and predominantly with inhibition of excitatory interneurons, thus leading to disfacilitation of fast PT neurons, which are possibly more susceptible than slow PT cells to this removal of depolarizing pressure. Some previous and present evidence for inhibition of excitatory interneurons on arousal is presented in the text referring to Fig. 8.17.

All of the preceding data, concerning changes in recurrent and afferent inhibition of motor cortical neurons during slow sleep and waking, show that the duration of inhibition acting on PT cells is reduced on arousal and during the subsequent steady state of waking (Figs. 8.23–8.30). These observations fit well with studies of Jasper et al. (1965) on γ-aminobutyric acid (GABA), the chemical agent believed to be the best candidate for cortical inhibition. The rate of release of GABA from the cerebral cortex is three times higher during synchronized sleep than during wakefulness.

Some data showing the recovery or even increase over control values during slow sleep of the second potential evoked by paired specific thalamic stimuli in the visual (Evarts et al., 1960; Rossi et al., 1965; Demetrescu et al., 1966) and motor (Steriade et al., 1969b) cortices might now be explained by increased hyperpolarization, during sleep, following the first response. Actually, increased extracellularly recorded slow depth-positive field potentials and reduction or suppression of unit firing reflect IPSPs in a pool of neurons (see again Figs. 8.25–8. 28, during sleep). Consequently, the EPSPs elicited by a second specific thalamic testing shock in this period of membrane hyperpolarization will be accentuated, thus enhancing the primary surface positivity of the evoked potential, considering that it is composed of EPSPs in deep layers.

The question remains as to the mechanism underlying this reduced duration of inhibition during waking. It might result from inhibition of the local inhibitory interneurons and/or by an increased excitatory drive which overwhelms inhibition. For the majority of PT neurons, the conditioning reticular stimulation or the natural awakening did not simply restore spontaneous discharges which were inhibited following testing inhibitory shocks, but even increased the discharge frequency over the control values (see Fig. 8.23). We could, therefore, postulate that powerful excitatory influences by ascending influxes on the postsynaptic membrane of PT cells may overwhelm the effect of inhibition. However, reduction or erasure of recurrent and feedforward inhibition occurred in some units during arousal and wakefulness without a simultaneous significant increase in the firing rate (see Fig. 8.29; compare also stages W and D in Fig. 8.27). Besides, the removal, on arousal, of strong hyperpolarization seen during slow sleep in PT cells, occurred without increased spontaneous firing in such cells (see Fig. 8.31). In these cases, it is conceivable that a depressed activity of the inhibitory interneuronal apparatus may be the major factor. This is supported by decreased spontaneous firing or complete arrest of high frequency spike barrages of presumed interneurons by reticular arousing stimulation in the cat (Fig. 8.15D) and with arrest of firing in identified short-axoned elements on behavioral arousal in freely moving monkeys (Fig. 8.22). Since this profound depression of interneuronal activities was seen only during arousal, we may conceive that the major factor to account for faster recovery from inhibition during the subsequent steady state of waking is an increased excitatory drive. The spectacular differences between arousal, excited wakefulness, and quiet waking may be seen in the spontaneous firing of the fast PT cell depicted in Fig. 8.13C. The reduced inhibition of motor cortex principal cells during waking may be viewed as an embarrassing result, since inhibition is known to assist in discriminatory functions implied in the vigil state. However, when analyzing the depth of recurrent inhibition on antidromically and synaptically elicited discharge, and its time course during waking and sleep (Fig. 8.30), we can see that "reduced inhibition" during waking is actually only an obvious shortening in duration, but that inhibition of the testing response at short (10–15 msec) delays may be deeper in some units during waking. The deep and short inhibition seen during wakefulness shows that this state is associated with a neuronal reorganization, leading to sharpening, accuracy, and ability to follow rapidly recurring activity in the cerebral cortex.

ACKNOWLEDGMENTS

   We are greatly indebted to G. Oakson for his continuous interest and assistance in the electronic work, and for the design of a time-ordered display of temporal patterns of evoked unit activity in both dot and analog forms [*Biomed. Eng.* **19**:244–246 (1972)]. V. Apostol, visiting investigator from the Institute of Neurology, Bucharest (Rumania), actively participated in the early stage of the experiments on the cat's motor cortex. We wish to express our thanks to Y. Lamarre of the University of Montreal for showing us the technique of chronic implantation of monkeys. G. Guano assisted technically in the chronic implantation of monkeys.

Discussion

Purpura: The report by Dr. Steriade amply illustrates the value of the extracellular unit recording technique when applied in conjunction with statistical analyses to studies of complex neuronal organizations during different behavioral states. Moreover, a proper appreciation of cellular synaptic mechanisms in the interpretation of such data can adequately compensate for the lack of intracellular observations at this stage in the analysis. This is by way of saying that much can be learned about the intimate operations of cortical neuronal networks without intracellular recording and its attendant difficulties. But I am certain that Dr. Steriade will pursue his interesting studies in this direction and it is likely that much of what has been suggested from the present extracellular unit analyses will be confirmed in general and in detail.

   There are several new findings in the present report which have greatly expanded our awareness of the complexities of interneuronal operations in sensorimotor cortex during sleep–wakefulness activities. To begin with, Dr. Steriade has shown that there is no general correlation between the spontaneous changes in discharge frequency of cortical neurons during sleep and wakefulness (or reticular stimulation) and the responsiveness of cortical neurons to stimulation of specific thalamic relay nuclei. His discovery of contrasting changes in what he has designated as "simple" and "complex" relay cells is of particular interest since it indicates the operation of different intracortical neuronal organizations interposed between VL pathways eliciting short latency relay activity and VL and VB pathways converging onto more complexly organized interneurons subserving relay discharges of pyramidal tract neurons. As yet, the explanation is not available for the finding that simple relay cells show a reduced responsiveness during the time they exhibit an increased spontaneous activity in waking. However, in view of the complex interactions that can be expected at thalamic and cortical sites by increased inputs from reticular activating systems, as indicated in my report elsewhere in this volume, such differences may not be surprising. Further analysis of this intriguing phenomenon is certainly in order.

Dr. Steriade has also pointed to the operation of a number of additional synaptic events occurring in sensorimotor cortical organisations during reticular activation, notably the reduction in recurrent inhibition and increase in excitatory synaptic drives onto pyramidal tract and related interneurons. The suggestion of inhibition here is in keeping with observations on intracellular recordings from thalamic neurons which have been discussed elsewhere. The importance of Dr. Steriade's observations should be underscored particularly as they relate to the findings in the behaving animal. His studies cast doubt on the importance of the postanodal exaltation mechanism in the production of "clustered firing" and this calls attention to the necessity for a more detailed analysis of the temporal factors involved in conjoint excitatory and inhibitory effects modulating pyramidal tract discharges during sleep and wakefulness. Dr. Steriade's concern that the demonstrated reduced inhibition of motor cortex principal cells during waking may not assist discriminatory functions can hardly be championed at this stage in our knowledge of motor control systems. His evidence for this is impressive and it therefore falls to those who would be so inclined to consider this suggestion in any future attempts to hypothesize on the functional significance of different patterns of pyramidal tract discharges on motor performance.

Bremer: Dr. Steriade and his collaborators must be congratulated for this very thorough analysis of the modifications of spontaneous and reactional thalamocortical activities corresponding to variations in the level of vigilance of the brain.

The identification of different categories of cortical neurons in itself represents a beautiful performance in microphysiology.

I was also delighted by the confirmation of the participation of the process of intrathalamic inhibition in the determinism of slow wave sleep. It seems to me that the demonstration of such a relationship concerning the intracortical inhibitory processes is an important generalization.

The intimate mechanism of the self-maintenance of inhibition raises difficult problems. This mechanism is probably not unique. Undoubtedly the authors are right to be eclectic and to admit the coexistence of the kind of recurrent inhibition described by Eccles and Andersen with the classical "feed forward" type. I have already given the reasons behind my conviction that the first type is more important functionally. It has, in my opinion, the advantage of offering an explanation for the self-maintenance of the thalamocortical synchronized rhythms without recourse to the somewhat mysterious interplay of the "interneuronal machinery" of our colleague Purpura.

Another problem which is also approached with insight, is that of the intimate mechanism of the blockade of inhibition exerted by the ascending reticular inflow. Dr. Steriade, while recognizing that the powerful excitatory influence of this influx on the postsynaptic membrane of the PT cells can be sufficient to "overwhelm the effect of inhibition," does not exclude the intervention of a process of inhibition at the interneuronal level. He supports this possibility with original experimental arguments. The future will undoubtedly see the correctness of this eclecticism.

Steriade: As Professor Bremer remarked, the fact that the same short-axoned cortical interneuron was modulated by both recurrent collaterals of PT axons and by specific thalamocortical fibers (Figs. 8.9B and 8.22) suggests that it most likely subserves both feedback and feedforward inhibitory mechanisms. I am inclined, at least for the cerebral cortex, to consider that inhibition elicited by afferent specific thalamic stimulation is more powerful than that induced by antidromic PT volleys. This came out from the findings reported in my talk and fits well with the data of Krnjević *et al.* (1966). I do not deny that in the thalamus the recurrent collateral inhibitory mechanism may participate in sculpturing the rhythmic bursting activity seen during patterns of slow sleep. But this is particularly evident under the experimental condition of barbiturate anesthesia. When working on an unanesthetized preparation and looking, for instance, at the VL rhythmic activity (mimicking 8–12/sec spindle waves) elicited by precruciate cortical stimulation, the orthodromic corticothalamic volleys proved to be mainly responsible for setting in motion the VL rhythmic activity. Following administration of a dose of barbiturate as low as 1 mg/kg, the orthodromic cortico-VL discharges were abolished, leaving intact the antidromic invasion of VL neurons. The use of much larger doses of barbiturates in the experiments done by Andersen, Eccles and their colleagues (1964) was perhaps the main reason for dismissing the participation of orthodromic corticofugal pathways in the elicitation of rhythmic sequences of inhibition and subsequent rebounds in thalamic neuronal populations. Concerning the interneuronal affair, I think it is becoming less and less mysterious. Actually, we have been able to identify cells within the VL anatomical limits, discharging high frequency barrages following precruciate stimuli at latencies suggesting monosynaptic engagement of intrinsic VL interneurons by corticofugal fibers. Such interneurons proved to be the main elements involved in the regulation of rhythmic activity following orthodromic corticothalamic volleys. The story of cortical interneurons is covered in my report.

NEUROCHEMICAL
MECHANISMS OF SLEEP

CHAPTER NINE

The Role of Monoaminergic Neurons in the Regulation and Function of Sleep[1]

MICHEL JOUVET

Early during the ontogenesis of the central nervous system of higher vertebrates two systems of monoaminergic neurons appear (Masai *et al.*, 1965) (Fig. 9.1). The first develops from the midline of the floor of the fourth ventricle. This is the serotoninergic system which is mostly located in the raphe nuclei (Dahlstrom and Fuxe, 1964). The second develops from the sulcus limitans of Hiss which runs rostrocaudally on both lateral walls of the neural tube. This is the catecholaminergic (and mostly the noradrenergic) system.

In this essay, I will try to demonstrate that these two systems play a paramount (but probably not exclusive) role in the regulation of the sleep–waking cycle by "modulating" the activity of other neurons. Finally, some peculiar aspects of these monoaminergic neurons will enable us to speculate about some possible functions of sleep.

[1] The research of the Department of Experimental Medicine has been supported by Direction des Recherches et des Moyens d'Essais (contract 71009), Institut National de la Santé et la Recherche Médicale (Group U 52), Centre National de la Recherche Scientifique (LA 162), and Fondation pour la Recherche Médicale Francaise.

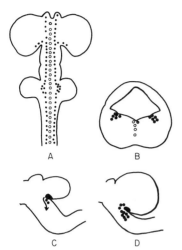

Fig. 9.1. Schematic representation of the onto-genesis of the serotoninergic system (white dots) and the catecholaminergic system (black dots). A. Horizontal section; B. frontal section of the primitive neural tube in a chick embryo. [From Masai *et al.*, 1965] C,D. Ontogenesis of the locus coeruleus complex in the rat brain (sagittal section). [From Maeda, personal communication]

I. Monoaminergic Systems and Their Experimental Approach

Thanks to the development of histochemical methods which permit visualization of the enzymes responsible for the catabolism of some monoamine (MA) neurons (Shimizu *et al.*, 1959; Maeda *et al.*, 1960), and mostly thanks to the histofluorescent technique developped by Falk *et al.* (1962), it has been possible to map out the cell bodies (Dahlstrom and Fuxe, 1964) and some of the pathways ascending from 5-hydroxytryptamine (5-HT) and catecholamine (CA) neurons in the rat (Ungerstedt, in press) or in the cat (Pin *et al.*, 1968; Maeda and Pin, 1971). Figure 9.2 summarizes the organization of some MA systems which are involved in the regulation of the sleep–waking cycle in the cat.

Thus the histochemical technique has narrowed the gap between neuropharmacology and neurophysiology and two main different strategies are now possible when studying the possible role of monoamines in sleep–waking mechanisms: (1) studying the effect of the neuropharmacological or neurophysiological alterations of the monoaminergic neurons upon the sleep–waking cycle, (2) studying the effect of the alteration of the sleep–waking cycle upon the activity of the MA-containing neurons.

Most of the data concerning the role of the MA in sleep–waking mechanisms have been provided by the first strategy in the cat. Indeed, the second approach necessitates sophisticated techniques to recognize the electrical activity of MA neurons and it is likely that the instrumental alteration of the sleep–waking cycle (i.e., sleep deprivation) would interfere with some unspecific mechanism (stress).

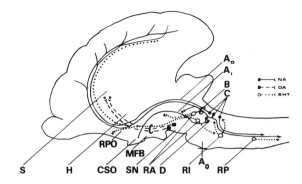

Fig. 9.2. Organization of some monoaminergic neurons in the cat brain. From the complex of the locus coeruleus (C) and subcoeruleus (D) ascend at least two pathways, the dorsal NA pathway (A_D) and the intermediary pathway (A_I) which crosses the midline at the level of the supraoptic decussation (CSO). Lesion of the dorsal NA pathway at the level of the isthmus (B) increases both SWS and PS and increases the central turnover of 5-HT neurons, probably through some interaction with the rostral group of serotoninergic neurons (RA). Lesion of the dorsal NA bundle rostrally to B induces only a decrease of waking and of NA in the forebrain. RI, intermediary group of the raphe system priming paradoxical sleep. RP, caudal group of the raphe system, SN, substantia nigra and dopaminergic neurons of the nigrostriatal (S) system ascending through the medial forebrain bundle (MFB); RPO, preoptic region; H, hypothalamus; A_0, Horsley-Clark plane anterior (frontal) zero. [From Maeda and Pin, 1971]

II. Alteration of the Serotonin (5-Hydroxytryptamine) System: The Sleep-Waking Cycle as a Dependent Variable

A. NEUROPHARMACOLOGICAL ALTERATION OF 5-HYDROXYTRYPTAMINE

It is not easy to alter cerebral 5-hydroxytryptamine (5-HT) in the adult animal since 5-HT does not cross the blood–brain barrier, and since it is not certain that, in the *normal condition*, 5-hydroxytryptophan (5-HTP) could be the physiological precursor of 5-HT. A very significant step forward was made when it was shown that p-chlorophenylalanine (PCPA) was able to inhibit the first step in the synthesis of 5-HT in the rat's brain and liver (Koe and Weisman, 1966).

I. Action of p-Chlorophenylalanine

This drug also inhibits tryptophan hydroxylase in the cat brain as shown in the following experiment (Pujol, 1970; Pujol *et al.*, 1971). Slices of cat cerebral cortex or brain stem were incubated in tritiated tryptophan (TRY) or [³H] 5-HTP and the amount of [³H] 5-HT synthesized was subsequently measured. There is a 80–90% decrease of the [³H] 5-HT synthesized from [³H] TRY in PCPA-pretreated cat (as compared with the control) whereas there is no alteration of [³H] 5-HT synthesized from [³H] 5-HTP (Fig. 9.3). The action of PCPA upon the states of sleep of the cat has been the subject of many studies (Delorme *et al.*, 1966b; Mouret *et al.*, 1968; Koella *et al.*, 1968; Pujol, 1970; Pujol *et al.*, 1971, 1972) which can be summarized briefly as follows:

After a single injection of 400 mg/kg of PCPA, no alteration of behavior or of polygraphic recording is observed during the first 14–18 hr. Thus the drug, in itself, has no *direct* pharmacological action upon the brain. Following this period, an abrupt decrease of both slow wave sleep (SWS) and paradoxical sleep (PS) occurs, and after about 30–40 hr, an almost total insomnia appears (Fig. 9.4B). The increase of waking is accompanied by the appearance of almost permanent discharges of ponto-geniculo-occipital (PGO) activity (similar to the PGO activity which is observed during SWS immediately preceding PS or during PS in normal cats). The mechanism of the appearance of PGO activity during waking after PCPA is still under discussion. It may be related to the decrease of 5-HT at some serotoninergic terminals since the same phenomenon is observed after lesion of the raphe system (see the following). The

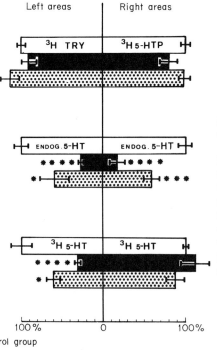

Fig. 9.3. Decrease of endogenous 5-HT and alteration of the synthesis *in vitro* of [³H] 5-HT from [³H] TRY (left areas) and [³H] 5-HTP (right areas) in the cortex of the cat after administration of PCPA (experimental group I) or destruction of the raphe system (experimental group II). Results are expressed in percentage of the mean value obtained for the control group ± S.E.M. $p < 0.05$; .... $p < 0.001$. [From Pujol *et al.*, 1971]

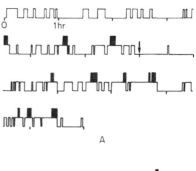

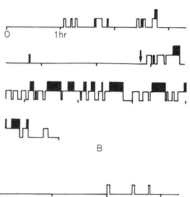

Fig. 9.4. Effect of a small dose of DL-5-HTP (5 mg/kg) (see arrows) upon sleep. A. In the normal untreated cat there is no significant effect. B. In an almost totally insomniac cat having received 400 mg/kg of PCPA 40 hr before, the injection of 5-HTP restores normal sleep. C. In a cat whose raphe system was destroyed 3 days previously, the injection has no effect and permanent insomnia persists. Time scale, 1 hr. Base line of each record, waking. White rectangles, slow wave sleep. Black rectangles, paradoxical sleep. [From Pujol *et al.*, 1971]

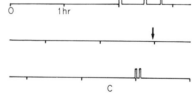

recovery of sleep begins after the 40th hour and qualitatively and quantitatively normal patterns of sleep are resumed after about 200 hr.

Under the influence of PCPA, a significant correlation has been found to exist between the decrease of SWS and the decrease of cerebral 5-HT both in the rat and in the cat (Mouret *et al.*, 1968; Koella *et al.*, 1968; Pujol *et al.*, 1971) whereas there was no alteration of catecholamine level.

Since PCPA inhibits only the first step of the synthesis of 5-HT at the level of tryptophan hydroxylase and since the synthesis of 5-HT from 5-HTP is still possible, it is possible to bypass the blocking action of PCPA and thus to re-establish a higher level of 5-HT turnover by injecting 5-HTP. With this procedure, it is possible to manipulate *at will* the states of sleep of the animal: thus a single injection (i.v. or i.p.) of a very small dose of 5-HTP (2–5 mg/kg) given when the insomnia has reached its maximum is able to restore a quantitatively and qualitatively normal pattern of both states of sleep for 6–8 hr (Fig. 9.4 B).

But if a larger dose of 5-HTP is injected (30–50 mg/kg), only cerebral synchronization accompanied by sedation reappears during the first hours and PS
is delayed for 4–6 hr. This suggests that after the inhibition of the tryptophan
hydroxylase, in the absence of endogenous substrate, the 5-HT-containing
neurons are able to rapidly synthesize 5-HT from *small* amounts of exogenous
5-HTP, whereas it appears possible that with larger quantities, exogenous
5-HTP may interfere with the normal process of PS at some other site.

B. Neurophysiological Alteration of 5-Hydroxytryptamine

*1. Destruction of 5-Hydroxytryptamine-Containing Perikarya
   of the Raphe System*

The destruction of the raphe system was performed in chronically implanted
cats (Renault, 1967; Jouvet, 1969a). Following operation, the animals were
continuously recorded for a period of 10–13 days and sacrificed (this period
being the critical duration for the voiding of the serotoninergic terminals).
With this method, the following information was obtained: a quantification of
the sleep states, a measurement of the volume of the lesion by topographical
analysis of the brain stem, and an analysis of the monoamine level in the rostral
brain.

Following a subtotal coagulation of the raphe system (Fig. 9.5), a state of
permanent behavioral and EEG arousal is observed during the first 3–4 days
(Fig. 9.6). In the following period the percentage of SWS does not exceed
10–15% of the nycthemeron. In these preparations, PS is never observed. However, continuous discharges of PGO spikes recorded from the lateral geniculate
or occipital cortex appear at least 3 hr after the destruction of the n. raphe
pontis and magnus at a rate of 30–40/min. The pattern of discharge is similar
to the one which follows injection of reserpine (Delorme *et al.*, 1965) or PCPA
in the normal cat and has been called the "reserpinic syndrome." The rate of
discharge of the PGO spikes diminishes on the third day to 10/min. The injection of a low dose (5 mg/kg) of 5-HTP which is able to restore sleep in PCPA-
treated cats does not alter the permanent arousal which follows the raphe
lesion (Fig. 9.4C).

There is a topographical organization of the raphe nuclei concerned with
sleep mechanisms (Table 9.1). The destruction of the rostral group (nucleus
raphe dorsalis and n. raphe centralis superior) is followed by an almost complete suppression of SWS, but PS may persist directly following the waking
state. The destruction of the intermediary group (n. raphe pontis, n. raphe
magnus) is followed by a selective decrease of PS and by only a slight decrease
of SWS. The biochemical analysis of these insomniac preparations revealed
also a significant decrease in cerebral 5-HT and 5-hydroxyindolacetic acid
(5-HIAA) with no variation in catecholamines, noradrenaline (NA) or dopa-

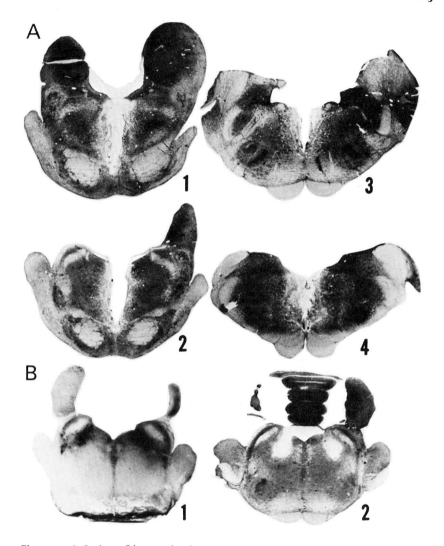

Fig. 9.5. A. Lesions of the rostral and intermediary group of the raphe nuclei which suppress both SWS and PS (see Fig. 9.6). B, 1. Concentration of MAO (coloration of Glenner) in the locus coeruleus complex and in the raphe (see Fig. 9.1B). B, 2. Lesions of both loci coerulei which selectively suppress paradoxical sleep. [From Jouvet, 1969a, Biogenetic amines and the states of sleep. *Science* **163**, 32–41. Copyright 1969 by the American Association for the Advancement of Science.]

mine (DA) in the telencephalon and diencephalon. Since the rostral group of the raphe nuclei is much larger than other groups, it was therefore demonstrated that a significant correlation exists between the amount of destruction

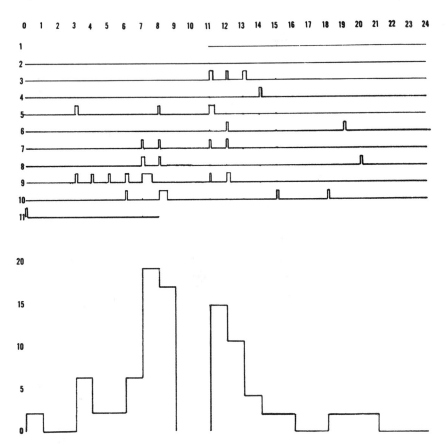

Fig. 9.6. *Top*: Almost permanent insomnia (total sleep is only 3.5% of the recording duration of 11 days) after lesion of the rostral and intermediary group of the raphe nuclei. Sleep (only cortical synchronization) is represented by the white rectangles. Time in hours. Each line represents 24 hr of continuous recording. *Bottom*: Circadian repartition of the sleep phase (in percent of the total sleep time.) Even in an almost totally insomniac cat there are still two significant peaks of sleep between 6 and 8 A.M. and between 11 and 12 A.M.

of the raphe system, the intensity of the resulting insomnia, and the selective decrease of cerebral 5-HT.

2. Metabolism of 5-Hydroxytryptamine in Raphe-Destroyed Cats

By incubating cortical or brain-stem slices in labeled precursor of 5-HT, some additional information has been obtained concerning the metabolism of 5-HT at the level of the terminals at different intervals after the destruction of the 5-HT containing perikarya (Pujol, 1970; Pujol *et al.*, 1971, 1972).

TABLE 9.1

CORRELATIONS BETWEEN THE LESION OF EACH NUCLEI OF THE RAPHE SYSTEM
AND 5-HT IN THE TELEDIENCEPHALON, SWS OR PS[a]

	5-HT [b] (N = 25)	SWS (N = 40)	PS (N = 40)
N. raphe dorsalis	0.5847	0.4687	0.30
	× × ×[c]	× × ×[c]	NS[c]
N. centralis sup.	0.4651	0.4755	0.24
	× ×[c]	× × ×[c]	NS[c]
N. raphe pontis	0.3911	0.3219	0.5251
	×[c]	×[c]	× × ×[c]
N. raphe magnus	0.006	0.3723	0.4845
	NS	×[c]	× × ×[c]
N. raphe pallidus	0.10	0.2958	0.2935
	NS[c]	NS[c]	NS[c]

[a] N. n. raphe obscurus was never destroyed.

[b] N = number of animals in each group. The Bravais-Pearson coefficient was used. It is apparent that only the rostral group (n. raphe dorsalis and centralis superior) is involved in the 5-HT innervation of the telediencephalon and in the SWS mechanism, whereas N. raphe pontis and magnus are responsible for priming PS.

[c] × × × $p < 0.01$; × × $p < 0.02$; × $p < 0.05$; NS, nonsignificant.

Eighteen hr after the lesion, there was a decrease of the synthesis of [3H] 5-HT from [3H] TRY and also a decrease of the catabolism of [3H] 5-HT since [3H] 5-HIAA is diminished. This parallel decrease of both synthesis and catabolism explains why the concentration of [3H] 5-HT is not altered. In contrast, there is a very significant (60%) decrease of the spontaneous release *in vitro* of [3H] 5-HT present in the incubation medium. This fact suggests that there might be also a significant decrease of the release of 5-HT *in vivo* at the terminal level after the destruction of the 5-HT-containing perikarya at the time of maximum insomnia.

Ten days after the lesion, there is a very significant decrease of endogenous 5-HT and 5-HIAA at the level of the terminals which is correlated with the decrease in labeled 5-HT synthesized *in vitro* from [3H] TRY. In contrast, there is no significant alteration in [3H] 5-HT synthesized *in vitro* from [3H] 5-HTP (Fig. 9.3). This can be explained by the fact that 5-HTP can be decarboxylated in other neurons, presumably catecholaminergic, or in brain capillaries, where the "nonspecific" 5-HTP-dopa decarboxylase is located.

Since low doses of 5-HTP are unable to restore physiological sleep in raphe-destroyed cats (in contrast to PCPA-pretreated cats) it is very likely that only the amount of 5-HTP which is decarboxylated in the serotoninergic neurons is physiologically active and that sleep cannot follow the possible decarboxylation of 5-HTP and the liberation of 5-HT in nonserotoninergic neurons. This fact is very important since it forces us to admit that 5-HT must be released (and possibly must be bound) at some specific central receptor in order to induce physiological sleep. Apparently exogenous 5-HTP at a very low dose is able to be decarboxylated preferentially in 5-HT-containing neurons only when endogenous 5-HTP is lacking (as after PCPA). It is thus possible that high doses of 5-HTP (50 mg/kg) (which are usually given) do not really induce a physiological state due either to exogenous 5-HTP itself or to the presence of 5-HT in other monoamine-containing neurons.

The insomnia following the destruction of the raphe system has also been obtained by a midsagittal split of the brain stem which destroys most of the raphe neurons (Michel and Roffwarg, 1967). According to Mancia (1969), the insomnia could be explained not by the destruction of the 5-HT perikarya, but by the interruption of synchronizing pathways ascending from the medulla and crossing at the level of the pons. However, even in a split brain stem, homolateral cortical synchronization can still be elicited by stimulation of the vagoaortic nerves (Puizillout and Ternaux, 1971). This latter experiment does not support Mancia's hypothesis.

C. Mechanisms of Action of 5-Hydroxytryptamine during Sleep

Different hypotheses are possible when considering the presynaptic and postsynaptic mechanisms which are involved in the serotoninergic induction of sleep.

1. Presynaptic Mechanisms: What Triggers 5-Hydroxytryptamine?

The mechanisms by which 5-HT neurons are activated in the cat are still obscure. The waking system is almost indefatigable, since a subtotal insomnia of at least 2 weeks duration may be obtained after raphe lesion. Thus the onset of sleep has to be triggered by the activity of the 5-HT sleep system (and not just by a possible circadian dampening of the turnover of the CA waking neurons). It must be recognized that almost nothing is known concerning the mechanisms which activate the 5-HT system. It is possible that 5-HT—5-HT synapses may exist from n. paragiganto cellularis to the medial raphe whereas raphe cells (but not necessarily 5-HT perikarya) may apparently also respond to iontophoretic administration of NA and ACH (Couch, 1970). Thus the 5-HT perikarya could be either serotoninoceptive, catecholaminoceptive, or cholinoceptive. In such case, the "doors of SWS" might also be opened by other transmitters or neural systems belonging to "synchronizing structures of the lower brain stem" (see review in Moruzzi, 1972).

Besides true neural mechanisms, it is also likely that the triggering of the 5-HT sleep system could be facilitated (at the perikarya or at the terminal level) by true humoral influences. Among them, the level of blood tryptophan might play a role, since tryptophan hydroxylase is not a true rate-limiting enzyme and it is possible that a study of the intimate mechanisms regulating tryptophan uptake by the synaptosomes might elucidate some forms of pathological insomnia or hypersomnia.

2. *Postsynaptic Mechanisms: Where Are the Serotoninergic Receptors, Involved in Sleep, Located?*

It is likely that the onset of sleep could be obtained through the release of 5-HT upon the neurons of the mesencephalic reticular formation, upon the CA-containing neurons responsible for the prolongation of cortical arousal (see below), or both. This would explain the persistence of the ocular behavior of slow wave sleep in the chronic decorticated or high mesencephalic cats (Villablanca, 1966b). This would also explain the striking arousal which follows the mediopontine pretrigeminal transection (Batini *et al.*, 1959). Indeed, in such a case, most activating structures are situated just in front of the transection while most raphe neurons are situated caudally to the transection. In fact, the selective destruction of the raphe system caudal to the plane of the mediopontine transection induces a similar insomnia (Renault, 1967).

It is also possible that the release of 5-HT in some forebrain structures might be involved in slow wave sleep, especially in the preoptic region. In this case the release of 5-HT would facilitate (or modulate) the postsynaptic synchronizing mechanisms which are apparently triggered from this region (Sterman and Clemente, 1962a,b). This would explain why the direct injection of 5-HT in the preoptic area may trigger SWS (Yamaguchi *et al.*, 1963) and why the pretreatment of cats with *p*-chlorophenylalanine suppresses the synchronizing action of the stimulation of the preoptic area (Wada and Terao, 1970). The secondary and mild insomnia (as compared with the immediate and total insomnia subsequent to the destruction of the raphe system) which follows the destruction of the preoptic region (McGinty and Sterman, 1968) could indicate the involvement of 5-HT mechanisms. That is, the destruction of the 5-HT terminals located in this area would secondarily affect the 5-HT perikarya of the raphe system and decrease 5-HT turnover.

Finally, one puzzling question should be asked. Is 5-HT a true neurotransmitter or a neuromodulator? The fact that 6–8 hours of physiological sleep can be restored by very small doses of 5-HTP (2–5 mg/kg) in the PCPA-pretreated cat is difficult to explain by our "classical" view of the neurotransmitter release and reuptake. On the contrary, the possible binding of 5-HT to some receptors (where it could act as a neuromodulator for other transmitters) might be more adapted to such a long action.

III. Alteration of the Catecholamine System:
The Sleep–Waking Cycle as a Dependent Variable

A. WAKING MECHANISMS[2]

The intervention of catecholaminergic mechanisms in the control of tonic cortical arousal in the cat is suggested by converging experimental evidence which can be summarized as follows (see complete bibliography in Jouvet, 1972):

1. The increase of cerebral catecholamine (after L-dopa) induces a long-lasting arousal in the cat.

2. The inhibition of the synthesis of catecholamines with α-methyl-p-tyrosine decreases waking in normal cats and totally suppresses the behavioral and EEG arousal which normally follows the injection of DL-amphetamine.

Norepinephrine, and not dopamine, seems to be involved in the maintenance of a tonic cortical arousal for the following reasons:

1. The destruction of the substantia nigra, which decreases telediencephalic (including striatal) dopamine levels by more than 90%, does not interfere significantly with cortical arousal but strongly alters behavioral waking (Jones et al., 1969) (see Fig. 9.13).

2. The destruction of the dorsal noradrenaline (NA) pathway in the mesencephalon, or of group A8 in the mesencephalic reticular formation, strongly reduces telediencephalic NA and increases cortical synchronization. There is a significant correlation between the decrease of cortical arousal, and the decrease of NA in the mesencephalon and forebrain (Jones et al., 1969) (see Fig. 9.13).

B. PARADOXICAL SLEEP

The intervention of CA and/or ACH-containing neurons of the laterodorsal pontine tegmentum in the "executory mechanisms" of PS are suggested by these neuropharmacological and neurophysiological facts (see complete bibliography in Jouvet, 1972).

1. Reserpine-pretreated cats receiving dopa (50 mg/kg) exhibit PS much earlier (2–4 hr) than animals not receiving dopa (24 hr) (Matsumoto and Jouvet, 1964). This suggests that the refilling of some pools in the CA terminals could be a condition for the reappearance of PS.

2. Alpha-receptor blocking drugs, which cross the blood–brain barrier of the rat, suppress PS (Matsumoto and Watanabe, 1967).

3. The administration of α-methyl-dopa (200 mg/kg) which results in the

---

[2] Cholinergic (ACH) mechanisms are also involved in waking and paradoxical sleep mechanisms (see references in Jouvet, 1972).

synthesis of the false transmitter α-methyl-NA, selectively suppresses PS in the cat for 12–16 hr and decreases waking.

4. The destruction of the caudal third of the nucleus locus coeruleus suppresses the motor inhibition which occurs during PS, while other ascending phenomena are still present (PGO, fast cortical activity). After such a lesion the cat presents, periodically during sleep, some peculiar hallucinatory-like behavior (rage, defense against some imaginary enemy) (Fig. 9.7) (see Jouvet,

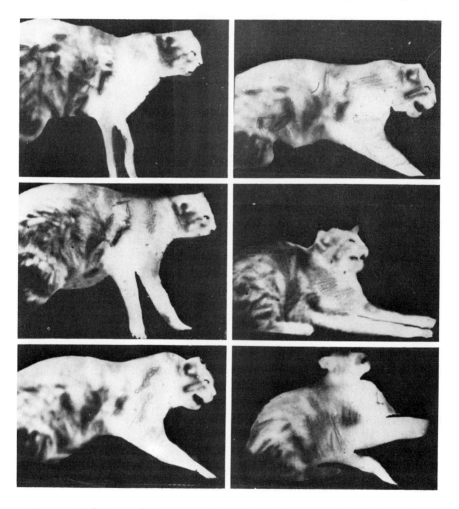

Fig. 9.7. Hallucinatory behavior occurring during sleep in a cat 2 weeks after destruction of the caudal part of the locus coeruleus. Despite this behavior, the pupils are miotic and the nictitating membranes are relaxed. The cat does not react to visual or auditory stimuli (from an 8 mm movie shown at the XXIII International Congress of physiology in Tokyo). [Jouvet, 1965a]

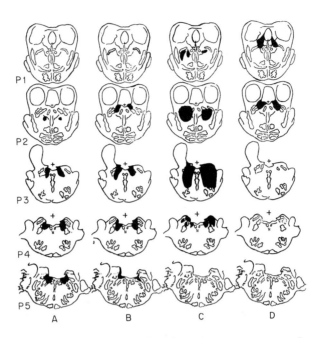

Fig. 9.8. Effects of lesions of the dorsolateral pontine tegmentum upon sleep. The lesions are represented in black upon a frontal section according the Horsley-Clark coordinates (see Fig. 9.2 for the localization of NA-containing neurons of the pontine tegmentum). A. Lesions of the caudal part of the n.locus coeruleus which suppress only muscular inhibition during paradoxical sleep. After such a lesion, the cat exhibits hallucinatory behavior during PS. (Fig. 9.7). B. Subtotal lesions of the locus coeruleus which totally suppress paradoxical sleep. PGO still occur during slow wave sleep. C. More extensive lesions which definitively suppress paradoxical sleep and PGO. D. Lesions of the most rostral part of the locus coeruleus and of the dorsal NA bundle which increase both slow wave sleep and PS (see Figs. 9.9 and 9.10). [From Jouvet, 1972]

1965a). Such behavior is a good evidence that paradoxical sleep may be accompanied by oneiric activity even in the cat. The total destruction of the caudal part of the locus coeruleus and of the nucleus subcoeruleus selectively suppresses all the central and peripheral components of PS (including PGO waves) (Fig. 9.8). This same selective suppression of PS is also obtained secondarily after microinjections of 6-hydroxydopamine (6-OHDA) which selectively destroys CA neurons (see Malmfors and Thoenen, 1971) in the laterodorsal pontine tegmentum (Buguet *et al.*, 1970).

IV. Interactions between the Serotoninergic System and the Catecholaminergic System during the Sleep–Waking Cycle

Some complex interactions exist between the two antagonistic serotoninergic systems responsible for sleep and the catecholaminergic system responsible for waking, while there is some agonistic interaction between the 5-HT and the noradrenergic mechanism which is responsible for PS. The intimate nature of these regulations is not yet understood but they may explain the dialectical interactions which exist between the increased waking and the following rebound of both SWS and PS.

A. POSSIBLE INTERACTIONS OF THE CATECHOLAMINE NEURONS INVOLVED IN WAKING UPON 5-HYDROXYTRYPTAMINE NEURONS

1. The destruction of the *rostral* third of the nucleus locus coeruleus or of the caudal part of the ascending dorsal NA pathway at the level of the isthmus in the cat induces a striking hypersomnia with increase in both SWS and PS (up to 300%) for 5–10 days (Figs. 9.9 and 9.10). The biochemical analysis of the brain shows a decrease of NA in the forebrain and mesencephalon and a significant increase of both tryptophan and 5-HIAA (Petitjean and Jouvet, 1970). Thus it is likely that the destruction of some NA fibers coming from the anterior part of the locus coeruleus has induced some increase of 5-HT turnover in the rostral raphe (as demonstrated by the increase of 5-HIAA). Many CA terminals are located in this region (Loizou, 1969) and may interfere directly or indirectly with 5-HT neurons. It is interesting to note that the possible increase of 5-HT turnover is accompanied by an increase of tryptophan. Thus the uptake of tryptophan seems to play an important role in the regulation of the biosynthesis of brain 5-HT.

2. The destruction of CA-containing neurons with 6-OHDA (injected intraventricularly or intracisternally) induces in the rat a very significant increase of the synthesis of central 5-HT as shown by the increase of 5-HIAA and by the increase of labeled 5-HT synthesized from labeled tryptophan intracisternally injected whereas endogenous 5-HT does not change (Blondaux *et al.*, 1973).

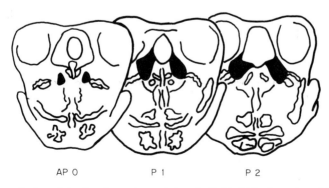

AP 0   P 1   P 2

Fig. 9.9. Lesion of the dorsal noradrenergic bundle (in black) in the region of the isthmus (frontal planes) according to Horsley-Clark coordinates—AP O–P1–P2.

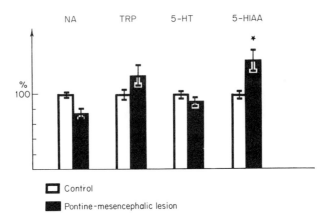

Fig. 9.10. After the lesion of the dorsal noradrenergic bundle (see Fig. 9.9) there is a temporary insomnia with increase of both SWS and PS. The biochemical analyses of the cat brain show a relative decrease of noradrenaline (NA) in the telediencephalon in the lesioned cats (black column) compared to sham operated animals (control) (white column). The decrease of NA is accompanied by an increase of both tryptophan (TRP) and 5-HIAA without any significant altera-tion of 5-HT. These results may be taken as an indirect index of the increase of 5-HT turnover. $\times$ P $<$ 0,05. (Further explanation in text.)

This phenomenon is observed as early as 40 hr after the injection of 6-OHDA and as long as 3 weeks (Juge *et al.*, 1972).

3. In the cat, the inhibition of catecholamine synthesis with α-methyl-tyrosine induces, after 8 hr, a significant increase of endogenous 5-HIAA and of labeled 5-HT synthesized from labeled tryptophan in the brain stem (pons and medulla) (Stein *et al.*, in press).

B. POSSIBLE INTERACTION OF 5-HYDROXYTRYPTAMINE NEURONS UPON THE CA NEURONS INVOLVED IN WAKING

The increased waking which follows the destruction of the raphe (mainly in its rostral part) is most probably mediated by catecholaminergic mech-anisms, as shown by the following experiment: An injection of 200 mg/kg of α-methyl-*p*-tyrosine was given to cats with raphe destruction at a time when behavioral and EEG waking was almost permanent (2–6 days after the lesion). The running movements stopped, miosis appeared, and there was an almost continuous cortical synchronization. This lasted for 24 hr, after which time there was a rapid return to behavioral and EEG insomnia (Fig. 9.11). The experiment provides some neuropharmacological evidence that the almost permanent arousal which follows the destruction of the rostral group of the 5-HT-containing neurons of the raphe system might be related to the increased turnover of central catecholaminergic neurons.

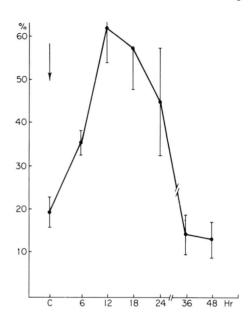

Fig. 9.11. Effects of α-methyl-p-tyrosine upon cortical synchronization after destruction of the raphe system. *Ordinates*: percentage of cortical synchronization during the experimental period (every 6 or 12 hr). *Abscissas*: time in hours. C: percentage of cortical synchronization (mean and S.E.M.) in control conditions in 8 cats whose raphe system was subtotally destroyed 2 to 6 days previously. The arrow signals the i.p. injection of 180–200 mg/kg of α-methyl-p-tyrosine methyl ester. There is a very marked increase in cortical synchronization which lasts for about 24 hr, after which there is a return to insomnia. [From Jouvet, 1972]

Thus, it is possible that under normal conditions, 5-HT neurons might exert some tonic inhibitory action directly or indirectly upon some CA-containing neurons at the onset of sleep.

C. POSSIBLE INTERACTION BETWEEN 5-HYDROXYTRYPTAMINE NEURONS AND THE CATECHOLAMINERGIC NEURONS OF THE COERULEUS COMPLEX INVOLVED IN PARADOXICAL SLEEP

The hypothesis that the 5-HT-containing neurons play a role in the priming of PS is founded upon the following facts.

1. There must exist a critical minimum of slow wave sleep in order for PS to appear (after either subtotal lesion of the raphe system or inhibition of 5-HT synthesis with PCPA). Indeed, a statistical correlation has been found between the amount of SWS and PS; for example, PS = (SWS−16)/3.2 holds true for cats subjected to lesions of the raphe system (with decrease of 5-HT turnover) and for hypersomniac cats subjected to lesions of the dorsal NA bundle (with increase of 5-HT turnover) (Fig. 9.12). Thus, a minimum of 16% of daily SWS (which is roughly one-third of the normal amount) is necessary to prime PS. Since there is some relationship between the amount of SWS and 5-HT turnover, this would suggest that any important decrease of 5-HT turnover (induced either by lesion or drug) would decrease or suppress PS, although other interpretations are possible (such as the suppression of deamin-

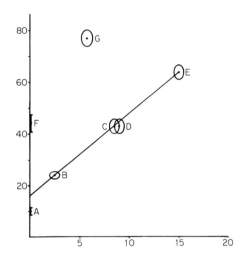

Fig. 9.12. Relationships between paradoxical sleep and slow wave sleep after different lesions of the monoamine systems. Results are expressed in mean ± S.E.M. A. Total or subtotal lesions of the raphe (16 cats). B. Partial lesions of the raphe system (13 cats). C. Control lesions of the brain stem outside monoaminergic system in the ventral pons or in the tectum. D. Sham-operated cats recorded under the same conditions as the experimental animals during 10–13 days (11 cats). E. Hypersomniac cats with increase of both SWS and PS after lesion of the isthmus destroying the dorsal NA bundle (11 cats), (see Figs. 9.9 and 9.10). F. Subtotal lesion of the locus coeruleus complex selectively suppressing paradoxical sleep (15 cats). G. Lesion of the mesencephalic tegmentum destroying CA-containing neurons (decrease of waking, but not true hypersomnia since PS is slightly decreased). In the group of cats B, C, D, and E, the correlation between PS and SWS may be obtained with the following formula:

$$\% \, PS = \frac{\% \, SWS}{3,2} - 16$$

This means that no PS can occur under a minimum amount of SWS which is equal to 16% of recording time. *Ordinates*: percentage of cortical synchronization during the 10–13 days of the postoperative survival. *Abscissas*: percentage of paradoxical sleep during the same duration. [From Jouvet, 1972]

ated metabolites of 5-HT: 5-hydroxyacetaldehyde or 5-hydroxytryptophol, which may play a physiological role (Sabelli *et al.*, 1969)). This hypothesis might explain why the inhibitors of monoamine oxidase (nialamide, phenyliso-propylhydrazine) which decrease the 5-HT turnover are very potent suppressors of PS.

2. The 5-HT neurons responsible for the priming of PS are not located in the anterior part of the raphe system since the destruction of the n. raphe dorsalis (which decreases SWS) is not followed by a similar reduction of PS. In contrast, the lesion of the pontine raphe system (n. raphe pontis and magnus)

is followed by a significant decrease in PS. Thus it is possible that some 5-HT neurons originating from these nuclei are involved, either directly or indirectly, with priming mechanisms. This could lead, in turn, to the appearance of PS triggered from the catecholamine-containing cells of the dorsolateral pontine tegmentum.

In the light of these data, one should interpret dialectically the results obtained after the "selective" inactivation of one system with a drug or a lesion. The physiological action may be the result of *both* the inactivation of one system *and* the increased turnover of the other. Thus α-methyl-paratyrosine may decrease waking through two different mechanisms: by decreasing the turnover of some CA neurons and by increasing the turnover of the 5-HT neurons. This, in turn would facilitate the 5-HT priming mechanism impinging upon the CA and ACH neurons located in the coeruleus complex. This would explain why α-methyl-paratyrosine does not suppress paradoxical sleep in the cat (King and Jewett, 1971).

It must be admitted that many of these mechanisms are still hypothetical. Direct or indirect determination of the turnover of both indolamine and catecholamine in those discrete brain regions implicated in the regulation of sleep–waking are needed. However, most of the data obtained in the cat favor the hypothesis that the sleep–waking cycle is regulated by two antagonistic ascending systems of neurons: the 5-HT neurons for inducing sleep and priming PS, the CA and ACH neurons for waking and PS (Fig. 9.13).

Depending on these antagonistic systems, the following two different kinds of insomnia are possible.

1. The first follows the decrease of central 5-HT turnover (lesion of the raphe system or inhibition of 5-HT synthesis). This insomnia is accompanied in the cat by an increase of PGO activity. Its subjective equivalent in humans is not yet known, but it might mark the border of pathological insomnia which may preceed or accompany some psychopathological disturbances. Such insomnia is almost never followed by a secondary rebound of SWS or PS during recuperation.

2. The second follows the increase of central CA turnover (stress, amphetamine). Such insomnia is either short lasting or necessitates increasing quantities of stimulation or drugs. It is not accompanied by permanent discharges of PGO activity and it is almost always followed by a rebound of both SWS and PS, the duration of which is proportional to the duration of insomnia. This suggests that in some conditions there exists a direct or indirect long-term regulation of the biosynthesis of 5-HT by some NA neurons.

Finally, both forms of insomnia share a common characteristic: They can be reversed immediately to sedation by inhibition of the synthesis of CA.

The following two different forms of decrease of waking are also possible.

1. After increase of 5-HT turnover (lesion of the dorsal NA pathway at the

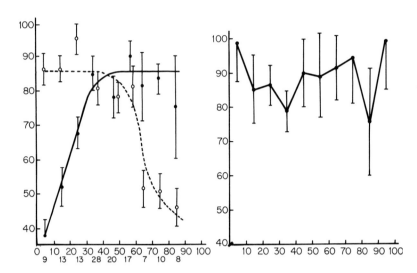

Fig. 9.13. Monoaminergic (MA) control of the cortical activity in chronic cats. Two antagonistic systems (5-HT and NA but not DA) are strongly implicated in the mechanisms of cortical synchronization and desynchronization. The figure summarizes all the biochemical data obtained from 133 cats (which were all operated, recorded, sacrificed, and biochemically analyzed by the same technique). They were subjected to lesions of the midline raphe, or of the bulbar, pontine, mesencephalic tegmentum, or of the substantia nigra. Control lesions were also made outside MA-containing neurons, and 12 sham-operated animals served as controls. (Groups of animals are classified according to the percentage of EEG synchronization during 10–13 days of the postoperative survival and the mean value of the percentage of 5-HT and noradrenaline in the telencephalon and diencephalon for each group is given.) *Left diagram*: 5-HT and noradrenaline fit two opposite curves. Cats with insomnia (less than 30% of cortical synchronization) have a decreased telediencephalic 5-HT and normal telencephalic noradrenaline content. Cats with normal or subnormal levels of synchronization (30–60%) have normal or subnormal values for both 5-HT and noradrenaline, whereas cats with increased synchronization have a decreased noradrenaline with normal or subnormal 5-HT level in the telediencephalon. *Right diagram*: there is no significant correlation of dopamine levels with the amount of cortical synchronization. *Left ordinate*: percentage of 5-HT (black circle) and NA (white circle) in the telediencephalon relative to control cats (mean and S.E.M). *Right ordinate*: percentage of dopamine (DA). *Abscissas*: percentage of cortical synchronization during the 10–13 days of survival after the lesion. The lower small figures refer to the number of cats in each group. The absolute values (100%) for 50 control cats are respectively 622 ng/g $\pm$ 22 for 5-HT, 399 ng/g $\pm$ 10 for NA, and 947 ng/g $\pm$ 41 for DA.

level of the isthmus) there is a true hypersomnia with increase of both SWS and PS. Such hypersomnia could theoretically be reversed by decreasing the 5-HT turnover with PCPA or MAO inhibition.

2. After decrease of CA turnover following the lesion of the dorsal NA bundle *rostrally* to the isthmus, the decrease of waking cannot be assimilated with a true hypersomnia since there is no increase of PS. In such case the time

originally spent in waking is occupied neither by SWS or PS but by a "deactivated EEG." This form of decrease of waking could be reversed by a drug which could increase CA turnover (amphetamine or L-dopa) provided that there exist enough active CA terminals.

V. Some Hypotheses Concerning the Function of Paradoxical Sleep

If we admit that the monoaminergic neurons play an important role in the regulation of the sleep–waking cycle, we should try to integrate some of their functional properties with the neurophysiological and developmental aspects of the states of sleep, in order to get some insight into the function of sleep. We shall concentrate mainly upon PS since it is still the most mysterious phenomenon occurring during sleep.

A. Tentative Conclusions

If we consider both the phylogenetic and ontogenetic evolution of PS we can make the following tentative conclusions.

1. PS does not exist in fishes, amphibians, or reptiles (at least as considered by the polygraphic index which serves to identify it in higher vertebrates). Thus the evolution of the central nervous system in poikilothermic animals did not require the "invention of PS." As a matter of fact, the poikilothermic central nervous system differs from the homeothermic nervous system since it has particular regenerative properties (in fact, the most successful experiments on the regeneration of the central nervous system have been done in amphibians or reptiles). Thus the nervous system of the poïkilothermic animal which is capable of some form of primitive learning seems to have some regenerative capacity which is linked to the genome.

By way of a very naive analogy which has often been used, we can consider that the brain is like a very complicated computer which may modify itself. In the poikilothermic animal, both the "hardware" and the "software" seem to depend upon the same kind of organization. The genome is both responsible for the organization of the brain during growth and for its eventual reorganization in adulthood. Such a system is relatively rigid since any mutation can act at the same time upon both the "hardware" and the "software."

2. In homeothermic animals, on the contrary, the hardware seems to be much less plastic and does not regenerate; for example, the visual system whose organization is embedded in the blueprint of the genome of visual cells necessitates external stimuli in order to perform correctly. In fact, the absence of patterned vision during a critical period after birth induces the atrophy of some lateral geniculate cell bodies, a drastic decrease of the dendritic spines in the visual cortex (Valverde, 1967), and some irreversible alteration of the

unitary activity in the occipital cortex (Hubel and Wiesel, 1963). Thus, at least in some specialized systems which might be compared with the "hardware," the interaction with the external world is necessary for performing some functions. Thus it is unlikely that the internal stimulation of the brain (through the PGO activity) during PS is sufficient to maintain the proper functioning of some types of neurons. On the other hand, the considerable increase of PS either *in utero* (Astic and Jouvet-Mounier, 1969) or during the immediate post-natal period (Jouvet-Mounier *et al.*, 1970) is an argument that the maturation of some specialized systems necessitates some endogenous activation during PS. The organization of these systems could not only be effectuated through anatomical (synaptic) contact but also through some functional mechanism of which the electrical expression might be the PGO activity. Thus some genetic coding could initiate the complex succession of PGO events. The synaptic organization of the hardware (and the hypothetical long-lasting modification which takes place during learning) would be subjected during PS to a genetic coding. Thus there would be two different possibilities for evolution to improve the brain. Mutations could affect either the organization of the hardware or the genetic coding of the software.

The software would not be responsible for learning *per se*, but for the ability to learn, the learning of learning which would be genetically programmed.

Since there is some evidence that some monoaminergic terminals may be attracted by specialized biochemical messages at the level of some synapses (see below), it is likely that numerous possibilities of interaction may exist between "nurture" (i.e., learning acquired during waking) and nature (genetic PGO coding). Thus new information which has been acquired during waking would be processed through a genetic blueprint during dreaming.

Summing up, in poikilothermic animals, both the hardware and the software of the CNS would depend upon the same genome and any mutation would act upon both organizations at the same time. In homeothermic animals, the hardware and the software would depend upon different systems. This would offer more possibilities for the evolutionary process and much more liberty to select more adaptable models. Paradoxical sleep (and dreaming) would represent the interactions between some system of neurons whose anatomical organization is genetically programmed (the hardware) and another system of neurons having much more plasticity (some MA neurons). These latter neurons would be responsible for some genetic coding through a functional system whose final electrical expression is the PGO activity.

I am quite aware of the difficulties and the pitfalls of such a theory which integrates some previous theories of dreaming (Jouvet, 1965b; Roffwarg *et al.*, 1966; Dewan, 1969). The following facts may be taken as an indirect proof in favor of this general theory.

B. Neurophysiological Facts

As considered from the point of view of neurophysiology, PS appears to be either a "genetic arousal," since it exists *in utero*, or a "brain storming" during which the firing of the great majority of cerebral cells (60–70%) (Benoit, 1970) is under the (direct or indirect) influence of the pontine pacemaker responsible for the PGO activity. Pyramidal and extrapyramidal motor neurons do not escape from this influence and it is very likely that two different mechanisms have been selected during evolution in order that such "genetic programming" could exist.

On one hand, there is a very powerful mechanism which blocks most efferent motor discharges, probably at the alpha-motor neuron level in the spinal cord. This mechanism is dependent upon the caudal part of the n. locus coeruleus. Thus, even the most potent activation of the pyramidal cells cannot induce any gross movements (other than rapid eye movements) and does not risk awakening a sleeping animal. On the other hand, it is obvious that such a periodical atonia (or paralysis) can occur only when animals are in a state of relative security (the possible cataplectic mutants must have had very few offspring). This state of "nonemergency" appears only when the waking system is no longer excited by external stimuli or stress, i.e., during sleep. Thus it is conceivable that the biochemical signals which trigger PS might be represented by serotoninergic neurons. The priming serotoninergic step is the biochemical representation of the fact that the external world is no longer harmful (neither the hare- nor anxiety-ridden neurotics dream much).

C. Histological Facts

If we admit that PS (or dreaming) is the expression of some plastic system capable of organizing the "software" of the central nervous system, we should have some proof that some MA neurons (and mostly the NA neurons) have such plastic properties or even that they are able to regenerate. In fact, there is now converging evidence that the NA neurons behave somewhat like poïkilo-thermic neurons and that they have tremendous plastic and regenerative capacities.

1. The section of a MA pathway in the rat induces first a degeneration distal to the lesion. After 8–10 days some sprouting occurs and regenerated axons may reinnervate the brain (Katzman *et al.*, 1971) [this process of sprouting of NA neurons could be responsible for the reoccurrence of fast cortical activity in the chronic *cerveau isolé* preparation (Batsel, 1960; Villablanca, 1962)].

2. The sprouting and the regeneration of NA neurons seems to be induced by specific biochemical stimuli. Thus the implantation of the iris in the brain stem of the rat is followed by its reinnervation by NA neurons from the brain

stem (coming most probably from the locus coeruleus) (Bjorklund and Stenevi, 1971).

3. Finally, in some cases the biochemical stimuli which attract the NA neurons are induced by the central nervous system itself, i.e., the hardware. Thus the denervation of some septal nuclei (provoked by the ipsilateral section of the fornix) is followed by the appearance of *new* NA terminals which seem to take the place of degenerated terminals (Moore *et al.*, 1971).

The histofluorescent technique has just provided the proof that some NA neurons are plastic and may regenerate (provided of course that the cell bodies are intact). If we accept the hypothesis that NA neurons (coming from the complex of n. coeruleus and subcoeruleus) are responsible for PS, we can speculate that these neurons may have many ways to interact with other neurons. Thus they could be attracted at the level of some synapses by some biochemical stimuli which could have been induced previously by learning and, in turn, they could interact with these synapses via some genetic coding of which the electrical aspect could be the PGO activity. Paradoxical sleep would thus act not on learning itself but on the learning to learn, which is probably genetically programmed.

D. FUNCTIONAL FACTS

There has not yet been any convincing evidence of any specific physiological or psychophysiological alterations induced by the specific suppression of PS. Most experiments have been done in adult animals or humans. All the trials in which we have attempted to suppress PS either *in utero* or in newborn animals have been unsuccessful (or have met with the death of the newborn animals, probably for "unspecific" reasons). It is likely that the suppression of PS during the maturation of the central nervous system should induce long-lasting disturbances, but no definite proof has yet been provided. In adult animals, there seems to be some interaction between learning and PS (Lucero, 1970; see review in Stern, 1970; and Greenberg, 1970) which could be the result of the induction of some new NA connections with some synaptic mechanisms involved in learning. On the other hand, there is also some evidence that the decrease of processing of information from the external world does not alter significantly the endogenous periodicity of PS and the firing of PGO waves. In fact, PS still appears regularly in the pontine cat or in normal cats almost totally deafferented (after section of the Ist, IInd, Vth, VIIIth, IXth and Xth nerves and dorsal transection of the spinal cord) (Vital-Durand and Michel, 1971).

Finally, there has not yet been any *unequivocal* data showing that the selective suppression of PS results in a specific disturbance of learning or of long-term memory since most of the experiments have used instrumental deprivation which induces many unspecific effects due to stress. In adult men, the long-term suppression of PS with MAO inhibitors or with chlorimipramine does not seem to interfere with any learning or memory processes. Nevertheless, it is still possible that the alteration of personality which is observed in patients receiving these drugs might result not only from the drug, but also from the lack of periodical coding during sleep due to the suppression of PS. Adult animals or humans can probably spend a "normal" life in laboratories or psychiatric wards with pharmacological suppression of dreaming, but we still do not know if they could survive under "normal biological conditions," i.e., under the "struggle for life condition" in which wild animals and our ancestors or "primitive" tribes were or are still living. In the actual artificial modern way of life, phenotypic programming may well take the place of the genetic coding which served during ontogeny or phylogeny.

It is even possible that the suppression of PS by drugs may sometimes have curative effects. This could be the case when dreaming is suppressed by MAO inhibitors in a case of lethal coding occurring in some severe endogenous depression which may be genetically determined.

E. Genetic Approach to PS

This approach is just beginning but seems to open an interesting field of research. Each genetic strain of mice seems to have its own EEG pattern of SWS (spindles or only slow wave during SWS) or of PS (duration-circadian rhythm). These patterns seem to be transmitted according to genetic laws (Valatx et al., 1972). When we can study more precisely the pattern of PGO activity during PS in mice, we will be able to know its correlation with the capacity of learning to learn that is genetically linked to some strain of "stupid" or "intelligent" mice (Bovet et al., 1969). It is also interesting to note that the organization of the pattern of rapid eye movement during PS seems to be altered in some mentally retarded children (Petre-Quadens, 1969). Finally, as another experimental approach, it is possible to test the hypothesis that dreaming represents the periodical processing of the brain by some genetic (or archetypic) code during sleep. Thus, if the hallucinatory behavior which is displayed by cats after lesion of the caudal part of the locus coeruleus represents the motor expression of the PGO code transmitted by NA neurons, the following experiment may test its genetic origin. Since we have been impressed by the complex stereotyped pattern of these hallucinatory behaviors (almost always rage or defense), if such a behavior can still be observed in cats raised in total isolation from time of birth (without any social contact, or patterned vision, audition, or olfaction), it will be most likely that such a behavior is genetically programmed (for teleological reasons).

VI. Summary

The sleep–waking cycle appears to be regulated by two antagonistic mono-aminergic systems. Some serotoninergic neurons are responsible for slow wave sleep and the priming of paradoxical sleep, while some catecholaminergic (and possibly cholinergic) neurons play a role in cortical arousal and in paradoxical sleep.

The most convincing evidence favoring the role of 5-HT neurons in the induction of sleep is the following: (1) The inhibition of 5-HT synthesis by *p*-chlorophenylalanine leads to a total insomnia which may be immediately reversed to sleep by the subsequent injections of low doses of 5-HTP which bypass the inhibition of synthesis. (2) Lesion of the 5-HT-containing perikarya of the rostral (n. raphe dorsalis and centralis) and intermediary group (n. raphe pontis and magnus) induces insomnia which is proportional to the decrease of 5-HT at the levels of the terminals. This insomnia is not reversed by low doses of 5-HTP. (3) Lesion of the dorsal noradrenergic pathway at the level of the isthmus induces both an hypersomnia (increase of both SWS and PS) and an increase of 5-HT turnover.

Catecholaminergic (and possibly cholinergic) neurons are involved in the maintenance of tonic cortical arousal and in the executive mechanism of paradoxical sleep.

There are some direct or indirect interactions between some 5-HT and CA neurons. Three different experimental approaches have shown that the in-activation of catecholaminergic neurons is followed by the activation of the 5-HT system.

The existence of two antagonistic systems regulating cortical activity permits one to postulate different mechanisms underlying insomnia or decrease of waking.

Finally, some speculation is made concerning the role of paradoxical sleep. It is proposed that PS represents a periodical genetic coding of the brain occurring during sleep.

Discussion

Bremer: In spite of your commendable efforts to reconcile tradition and your new neurochemical findings, there are points which are still difficult for me to understand. It has been shown by Bonvallet and Allen (1963) that a relatively small bilateral lesion, in the neighborhood of the nucleus of the solitary tract, is sufficient to produce a striking increase of the vigilance level in the *encéphale isolé* cat. This lesion is so small and its bulbar localization is such that this waking behavior could not be the destruction of the serotoninergic system. My second question refers to the slide which shows the distribution of the serotoninergic neurons in the brain stem. As far as I saw, several of them were laterally located. But your lesion was really medial. Could you explain?

Jouvet: This lateral group belongs to the nucleus paragiganto-cellularis in the caudal part of the raphe. It does not seem to contribute to the 5-HT innervation of the telediencephalon and is probably not related to sleep mechanisms.

Steriade: Does the site in the brain stem where Rossi applied stimulation to precipitate a paradoxical phase of sleep when the cat was in slow wave sleep correspond to your posterior division of the locus coeruleus? I do not think so. Perhaps Professor Moruzzi could answer this question.

Moruzzi: Rossi *et al.* (1961) reported that EEG and EMG patterns quite similar to those occurring during paradoxical sleep were precipitated by high rate reticular stimulations in behaving cats. This observation, however, could be made only when the stimuli were applied during a stage preceding immediately the natural onset of the desynchronized phase of sleep. The stimulated reticular sites were dispersed in the medulla, pons, and mesencephalon.

Steriade: Dr. Jouvet, I was delighted by your very clear systematization in an anterior, a middle, and a posterior part of the locus coeruleus, each with its corresponding functions. This nucleus does not exceed 3 mm in the caudal-rostral direction. I know that you do not like experiments using brain stimulation. In spite of your reluctance toward such a technique, I would like to ask you how one may explain the fact that high frequency, low voltage stimulation of discrete points in the dorsal part of the pontine tegmentum, including your anterior, middle, and posterior zones, does not elicit different kinds of behavior or their EEG correlates. On the contrary, stimulation of any of these points induces an awakening reaction as a rule. I think that the anterior part, where locus coeruleus neurons become embedded in the periaqueductal gray, might be included within the region of the rostral pons which, when stimulated, has a very low threshold for the arousal reaction and a long-lasting waking effect, as shown by Bonvallet (1966). But arousal, which I do not just identify with EEG desynchronization but rather with all the events characterizing waking, (i.e., temporal patterns of spontaneous firing, changes in mass and unit responsiveness, recovery cycle, etc.) is obtained by stimulating all the areas in the dorsal pontine tegmentum, including the different parts of the locus coeruleus and the surrounding zones. How can this be reconciled with your tentative differentiation in zones with different or even opposite functions related to sleep–waking behavior?

Jouvet: It is possible that noradrenergic neurons, responsible for waking, are intermixed with the neurons responsible for paradoxical sleep in the locus coeruleus and I would be surprised that electrical stimulation could differentiate between them.

Steriade: Stimulation, however, with either low or high frequency pulses, has proved to be efficient in the experiments of Clemente and Sterman in inducing behavioral and EEG signs of sleep when applied to the preoptic area and, if I remember correctly, insomnia or marked hyperactivity was elicited by Nauta, among others, when the same region was lesioned. The same may be said if one considers the slow sleep patterns triggered by stimulating the raphe system.

Koella: I have a question for Dr. Jouvet: What happens if you give 5-HTP to a raphe-lesioned cat?

Jouvet: The injection of a low dose (5 mg/kg) of 5-HTP in raphe-destroyed cats does not reverse the insomnia as it always does in PCPA-pretreated cats. This is a very strong argument favoring the specificity of the effect of 5-HT. Indeed, in raphe-destroyed cats, 5-HTP is decarboxylated in non-5-HT terminals (since the synthesis of [³H] 5-HT is still possible from [³H] 5-HTP) while it is most probably decarboxylated in 5-HT terminals in PCPA-pretreated cats.

Bremer: One could contest the expression "serotoninergic"!

Jouvet: The Swedish school has provided enough evidence that there exist 5-HT-containing neurons. Of course, there will always be some discussion concerning the term "serotoninergic," but I think that most of the criteria have been fulfilled (release, re-uptake, inactivation, enzymes, postsynaptic effect). The question which remains to be solved seems to be the following: Is 5-HT a neurotransmitter or a neuromodulator?

Question: The compound 4-hydroxybutyric acid which causes a sleeplike state in animals, also causes a selective increase in dopamine levels in the substantia nigra. This is potentiated by giving L-dopa. How does this fit in with reduced dopamine and reduced activity?

Jouvet: It is true that 4-hydroxybutyrate acts upon dopamine level but, unless the complex of the locus coeruleus contains dopamine, there is no explanation for the fact that this drug can induce paradoxical sleep in a pontine cat if we accept *only* this mechanism of action. The short-chain fatty acid may act also through different mechanisms: either by acting upon acetylcholine (Giarman and Schmidt, 1963), or by reacting with the lecithin of the membrane, as has been suggested by two different groups (Dahl, 1968; Rizzoli and Galzigna, 1970).

Question: Hydroxybutyric acid enters the metabolic cycle though?

Jouvet: This hypothesis is very unlikely since C_5 and C_6 fatty acid induce paradoxical sleep more rapidly than the C_4 in the pontine cat (Delorme *et al.*, 1966a).

Metcalf: I want to have your comments about PCPA experiments. First, how much PCPA accumulates and what is its half-life? Second, does not this induce a phenylalanine toxicity as in phenylketonuria? If this is the case, how valid are the interpretations about sleep physiology in animals rendered toxic with PCPA?

Jouvet: I do not know the figure for the half-life of PCPA. The cornerstone of the hypothesis that 5-HT is involved in sleep is *not* the insomnia induced by PCPA but *the immediate restoration* of *physiological* sleep by a low dose of 5-HTP in the insomniac cat pretreated with PCPA.

Metcalf: But 5-HTP has no effect on mice or human.

Jouvet: This is true. In normal cats, small doses of 5-HTP have no significant effect, but we do not know if exogenous 5-HTP enters 5-HT neurons in *normal* conditions.

Koella: You see at the beginning of PCPA a kind of amphetaminic reaction very early, i.e., during the first 4 hr. The effect on sleep starts much later.

Bremer: Another difficulty to meet in your synthesis is that it neglects one proven fact: that acetylcholine acts as an arousal substance.

Jouvet: This is because I did not have the time to discuss the role of cholinergic neurons in waking mechanisms. Indeed, there are many data which show that ACH plays a very important role both in waking and paradoxical sleep. These data have been reviewed at length elsewhere (Jouvet, 1972).

Bremer: The problem is the following: when you inject strong doses of atropine in the cat there is a marked slowing of the EEG with a spindlelike modulation of its waves. How is that slowing produced? The common idea is that you block the cholinergic path. But when you inject a small dose of pentobarbital in the atropinized *encéphale isolé* cat, the slow atropine waves are replaced by the briefer waves of barbiturate spindles. To me it seems that the atropine effect is a toxic one. I do not think that it is the result of a true blocking of cholinergic or cholinoceptive neurons.

Question: You made a very nice story about the role of MAO in paradoxical sleep, saying that an unknown metabolite of monoamines plays a role in paradoxical sleep. Does this hold true?

Jouvet: I do not know (MAO inhibitors could of course decrease the formation of deaminated metabolites like 5-hydroxyacetaldehyde or 5-hydroxytryptophol), and there is some evidence that these compounds may have a physiological role. But MAO inhibitors may also decrease the 5-HT turnover by some feedback mechanisms and they may also act upon catecholamine mechanisms.

Question: What is the survival time in bilateral nigral lesions?

Jouvet: About 2 weeks.

Question: What are the percentages of the stages of sleep in the hypersomnic cat?

Jouvet: Seventy percent of slow wave sleep; 16–18% of paradoxical sleep.

During the first 3 days after the lesion, paradoxical sleep may increase up to 50% of the recording time.

Question: We do not understand the effect of drugs in other species because we ignore the feedback mechanisms involved. I would like to ask you about lesion experiments and histochemical experiments in other species. Have you done some work in rats?

Jouvet: Yes, it works as far as the caudal part of the locus coeruleus is concerned but we did not work with decerebrate rats.

Question: Are all the noradrenaline pathways involved with arousal in the cat? If not, which one is related to arousal?

Jouvet: Apparently there are three ascending noradrenaline pathways in the cat which have been mapped out by Prof. Maeda in my laboratory. The first one comes from the medulla and is analogous with the *ventral NA pathway* described in the rat. The second one is the *dorsal NA pathway* which ascends from the locus coeruleus; the third one is the *intermediary NA pathway* ascending from the locus subcoeruleus. Apparently these pathways and their terminals regulate different functions. We have some converging data that the dorsal pathway is involved in cortical arousal while the intermediary pathway is possibly involved with some of the central components of paradoxical sleep (PGO activity).

Purpura: What would be your prediction on the maturational status of the raphe system versus more lateral reticular systems, both in terms of cell development, synaptic organization, etc?

Jouvet: As far as the guinea pig is concerned, Maeda (personal communication) has found catecholamine cell bodies in the brain stem as early as 30–35 days of gestational age (at a time when PS has been first recorded *in utero*).

Purpura: You are talking about histofluorescence. You are not talking about synaptology. My question is: Would a cell of the raphe system, e.g., in n. obscurus or magnus, look mature at birth, in a newborn kitten, compared to cell of the lateral reticular system?

Jouvet: I do not know.

CHAPTER TEN

Neurochemical Aspects of Sleep

WERNER P. KOELLA

In Chapter 9 Jouvet has outlined results of his far-reaching studies that strongly suggest the participation of biogenic amines in the organization of sleep and wakefulness. Our own investigations of the past 10 years have led us to similar conclusions; in particular we have been able to show that serotonin (5-hydroxytryptamine = 5-HT) seems to be, in the experimental animal (cat), an indispensible factor for the induction and maintenance of sleep, particularly slow wave sleep. (Non-REM = NREM.) In this chapter, we intend to supplement Jouvet's report in two ways: first, by describing some of our own combined biochemical–pharmacological findings obtained with 5-HT-depleting and restoring agents. These findings add further weight to the argument that in the cat the lack of brain serotonin is attended by a drastic diminution of sleep and that replenishing this amine restores sleep. In the second part of our discussion we shall describe some of our experiments in which serotonin was applied directly to various parts of the brain. They led us to assume that 5-HT, in addition to its possible role as a transmitter in the raphe system, i.e., as an information vehicle in a network subserving the active organization of sleep, also acts as a "gain enhancing" agent in a system of "antiwaking" properties.

Concerning the first aspect of this report we shall describe our experiments with PCPA (p-chlorophenylalanine) (Koella et al., 1968). This tryptophan-hydroxylase inhibitor allows depletion of the brain (and peripheral) serotonin in a graded fashion (Koe and Weissman, 1966; Loevenberg *et al.*, 1967) without altering catecholamine levels in a more than barely appreciable way.

Cats, supplied with electrodes for EEG, eye movement, and neck myogram recordings, were observed continously around the clock for as many as 21 days. After 2 to 3 control days, PCPA was injected in various doses (200, 150, 100, and 50 mg/kg i.p.) and the sleep behavior was observed for another 14–18 days. There occurred a dose-dependent loss of total sleep, which started about 24 hr and reached its peak about 3–4 days after injection. Return to control occurred about 8 days after injection of smaller doses and not before 2 weeks with the larger doses. Slow wave sleep followed a pattern similar to that of total sleep, and paradoxical sleep usually did not increase in its ratio to total sleep. With the smaller doses of PCPA there was indication of a "rebound," i.e., a transient increase in total, slow wave, and paradoxical sleep above control level with a peak on about the ninth day after injection of PCPA. After larger doses of PCPA there was also a hump in the return curve which, however, never reached control levels; these temporary elevations also peaked at about the ninth day after injection (Fig. 10.1). More will be said about these peaks later in this paper.

Figure 10.1 also depicts the time course of the serotonin levels in various brain areas after a single dose of PCPA. It is evident from these curves that total serotonin returns toward control levels considerably more slowly than does sleep. This divergence may be explained by assuming that total serotonin levels do not reflect the amount of the free amine at the receptor sites in the brain. It is not unlikely that the available serotonin returns faster toward normal levels and thus may run a time course more closely related to that of sleep.

The divergence between the time course of sleep return and brain serotonin, however, could also be viewed as an indication that the decrease of sleep is not caused by the diminution of brain serotonin but rather by a (still unknown) direct action of PCPA or of a metabolite thereof. This interpretation though is made untenable in view of the following experimental results. If at, or close to, the height of the PCPA effect, 5-hydroxytryptophan (5-HTP) (30 mg/kg i.p.) is injected, sleep, i.e., slow wave sleep, returns almost immediately (within 10 min.) to control levels or to levels even above control and only within about 24 hr does it return to those low amounts revealed by that time by animals which had received PCPA but not 5-HTP.

Figure 10.2 shows one example (823) of such 5-HTP experiments in comparison with the control (i.e., PCPA only) cats (820 and 817). Figure 10.3 illustrates the rapid return of (slow wave) sleep to almost 100% levels and the later appearance of PS. In Fig. 10.4 the sleep behavior during the last 8 hr

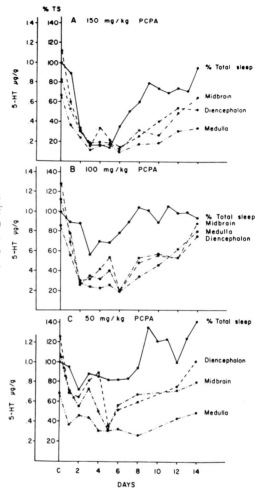

Fig. 10.1. Effects of three different doses of PCPA on percent of total sleep (mean from two animals) and on 5-HT content of three brainstem areas (means of values from two cats at each time point). [From Koella et al., 1968].

of the 48-hr span after PCPA and the effect of 5-HTP on sleep and 5-HT and 5-hydroxyindoleacetic acid (5-HIAA) content of various brain areas are depicted. Again, there is a fair parallelism between the time course of the biogenic amine concentration and the one of sleep. These data then strongly suggest that it is the lack of serotonin and not a direct action of PCPA which causes the lack of sleep.

There is, however, a third and, as it seems, most probable explanation for the difference in time course between (total) 5-HT and sleep, which is based on the assumption that overall sleep regulation includes a kind of a negative

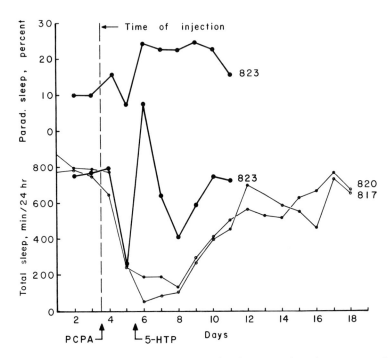

Fig. 10.2. Time course of sleep in cats injected with PCPA only and one cat treated also with 5-HTP.

feedback system. Indeed, there is evidence that such feedback regulation exists. If one imposes sleep deprivation for a given period there is a rebound; after termination of the deprivation period sleep occurs in amounts exceeding the normal level. It looks as if the temporary lack of sleep is being made up. This compensation could be explained on the basis that there is negative feedback with a number of delay components.

The divergence between the curve describing return of serotonin and the one describing the return of sleep in the later phases of the PCPA experiment may be the manifestation of such a negative feedback mechanism. With the increasing lag of sleep behind the physiological need, there is a build-up of "sleep pressure" which brings about sleep in spite of the low level of serotonin. With the assumption that there is a feedback system involved with delay components, one also could explain not only the "rebound" after small doses of PCPA but the humps in the return curve (occurring at the same time as the rebound peak) after larger doses of PCPA as well. One could view all these temporary elevations as manifestations of a slow oscillation (with a period of several days),

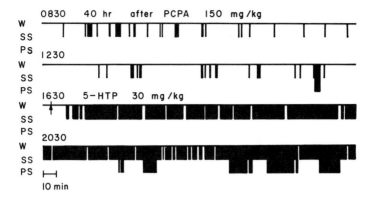

Fig. 10.3. Sleep pattern of a cat previously injected with PCPA 8 hr and 7 min before and 7 hr and 53 min after injection of 5-HTP. [From Koella *et al.*, 1968]

initiated by, and time locked to, the injection of PCPA and independent in its frequency and phase relation to the dose of the drug. This oscillation would be the consequence of an exogenous disturbance in this delayed feedback regulated system. Of interest in this connection is the observation of Dement (1973) that such oscillatory behavior (and thus evidence for negative feedback) occurs also in experiments with chronic administration of PCPA.

Notwithstanding the existence of such systemic factors which complicate the picture and thus the interpretation of the pharmacological data, there is enough evidence from Jouvet (1967b, 1969b), Torda (1967), Weitzman *et al.* (1968), Dement (1972), and from our own laboratory (Koella *et al.*, 1968) to strongly indicate that at least in the experimental animal 5-HT is a necessary factor for the proper occurrence of sleep.

Still, a pertinent question remains to be answered—the mechanisms through which 5-HT plays this important role in sleep. Jouvet in this volume has presented beautiful data which strongly suggest that this amine could be considered to be a transmitter substance in the sleep-organizing system, in particular in the raphe-forebrain system. Indeed, the observation that electrical stimulation of the raphe system induces sleep in the rat (Kostowsky *et al.* 1969) adds strength to Jouvet's interpretation (1969b) and there are no findings which could contradict the "raphe theory." We have, however, during the last 10 or so years accumulated some data which make it not unlikely that there is, in addition to the serotonergic raphe system, another mechanism through which 5-HT could play a pertinent role in the initiation and maintenance of sleep namely as an "antiwaking" agent, reducing the activity and reactivity of the brain stem reticular ascending arousal system.

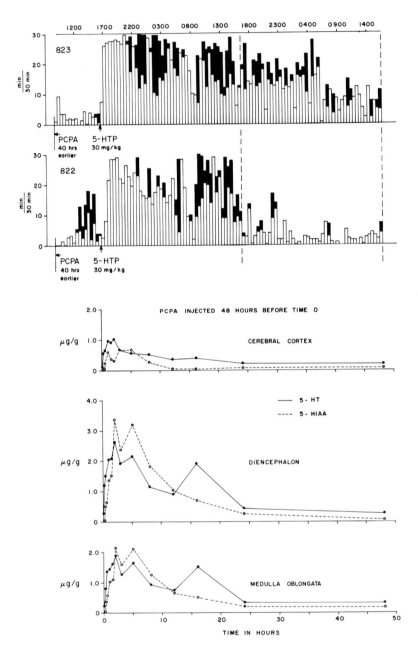

Fig. 10.4. Sleep behavior and 5-HT as well as 5-HIAA content of brain areas in PCPA-treated cats after 5-HTP. [From Koella, 1970]

A first step in developing this idea was our own (1966) as well as Bradley's (1958) and Rothballer's (1957) observation that the injection of 5-HT, particularly through the carotid route was followed, after an initial phase of arousal, by a prolonged period (up to 20 min) of hypersynchrony in the EEG, of sleep spindles, and of enhanced recruiting responses.

In an attempt to delineate the locus of action of 5-HT in bringing about this hypersynchronizing or "hypnogenic" effect, we transected the brain stem of a number of cats and injected again 5-HT in similar doses into the carotid artery. Invariably we found that after severing the posterior brain stem from the forebrain, serotonin induced signs of arousal only and there was no more indication of any hypersynchronizing effect. With these findings we corroborated Glässer and Mantegazzini's data (1960) and produced evidence that the synchronizing effect of 5-HT was due to an action of this substance somewhere in the posterior brain stem, from where the "hypnogenic" influence would be transmitted to the forebrain via nervous pathways. This interpretation was further supported by the additional observation that in intact unanesthetized immobilized cats injection of serotonin into the vertebral artery induced immediately a shift toward cortical synchrony without a preceding phase of arousal.

Locating the point of action of 5-HT in still more detail proved to be somewhat more complex, because we had to explain CNS effects of this amine although it is well known that it does not, or in very small amounts only, penetrate the blood–brain barrier. Thus we had to look for a "hole" in the blood–brain barrier somewhere in the region of the posterior brain stem or then postulate a receptor site which would be situated outside the blood–brain barrier but which has information channels leading to the intra-blood–brain barrier part of the brain. The latter assumption proved to be the correct one, as there is in the lower brain stem a structure which would satisfy these prerequisites. Weil-Malherbe et al. (1961) and Wilson and Brodie (1961) have shown that the *area postrema*, located at the caudal end of the floor of the fourth ventricle, is a place where various substances, that do not enter the brain, penetrate into the perivascular tissue to a considerable degree. This *area postrema* is not a brain structure proper but consists of blood vessels, flat ependymal cells, nerve fibers, astrocytes, oligodendroglia, glialoid cells, and nerve cells. According to Wilsocki and Putman (1920) and Faber (1955), trypan blue and Prussian blue do not penetrate into the brain tissue surrounding the area postrema. Thus, the area postrema and similar structures are not actually places of increased blood–brain permeability, but they nevertheless could be the site of accumulations of perivasal serotonin receptors that could be easily reached by blood-borne and CSF-borne substances. Neural pathways then could transmit signals elicited by such local drug action to, and modify the activity in, brain-stem structures and thus induce the synchronizing effect described above. The results of a number of experiments strongly indicated that the area postrema and/or possibly its immediately adjacent structures indeed are involved as a link in the 5-HT-induced EEG synchronization.

Following cauterization of the area postrema in 21 animals, involving occasionally the adjacent parts of the floor of the fourth ventricle, the synchronizing effect of intracarotid serotonin was always reduced and, in a few cases, completely eliminated.

Application of cotton pellets soaked with LSD_{25} (50–100 μg/ml) or methysergide (= UML, 50–100 μg/ml), two powerful 5-HT blocking agents, led to a partial or total suppression of the 5-HT-induced hypersynchronous phase; this blocking effect lasted as long as 4 hr.

Topical application of serotonin in concentrations of 5–10 μg/ml to the posterior region of the fourth ventricle induced an increase in the recruiting responses, an increase (or appearance) of spindle bursts, and an increase in slow wave output often lasting as long as 15 min. Application of solvent only (Tyrode or saline solution) ordinarily did not produce any change in the EEG.

After the experiments involving ablation of the area postrema, and the results obtained with topical application of serotonin and serotonin blockers, pointed to this structure as the receptor site for serotonin action in its EEG-synchronizing effect, the question arose as to how the 5-HT-induced activity was transmitted to hypnogenic areas of the brain. Morest (1960) had found that "nerve fibers leave the fiber plexus of the area postrema in the direction of the nucleus tractus solitarius." He observed, furthermore, in the area postrema, dendritic arborizations of neurons located in the medial edge of the nucleus of tractus solitarius. Furthermore Magnes *et al.* (1961) demonstrated that low frequency stimulation of the area of the solitary tract nucleus induced widespread synchronization of the EEG that frequently outlasted the period of stimulation. Evidently this nuclear area *is* a hypnogenic structure. Corroborating evidence was offered by Bonvallet and collaborators (1961, 1962), who showed that arousal produced by reticular and nociceptive stimulation was more intense and more prolonged in cats in which discrete lesions had been placed in the cephalic part of the nucleus of the tractus solitarius.

In an attempt to clarify the intimate mechanisms involved, these authors suggested that there exists a (negative) feedback system operating between this nucleus and the reticular activating system which checks excessive arousal. Together with Bronzino (1968, 1971, see also Koella, 1970) we have reinvestigated this idea. We have been able to produce evidence that this negative feedback system indeed exists and further, that it is in all likelihood the neuronal mechanism through which serotonin exerts its "antiwaking" effect. For this study we made first the following assumptions: (1) The first component of this feedback loop is a facilitating (probably multisynaptic) pathway leading from the mesencephalic reticular formation (RF) to the nucleus of the solitary tract (NTS) and the amount of facilitatory information reaching NTS depends on the degree of arousal activity in the RF. (2) The NTS dispatches (again through multisynaptic pathways) inhibitory messages which eventually feed back upon the elements constituting the mesencephalic activating system. The amount of this inhibitory feedback depends upon the degree of activity in NTS. (3) NTS projects as a whole to both sides of the reticular formation. (4) The "gain" in NTS is variable in the sense that the ratio between outgoing reticulo-petal inhibitory information and the incoming reticulofugal facilitating infor-mation depends on additional inputs to NTS; signals reaching NTS through the sensory channels in the cranial nerves V, VII, IX and X as well as serotonin would constitute such "gain modulating" factors. (5) Finally, the assumption that this negative feedback loop carries information from RF to NTS and back to RF, led us to postulate that this information flow (if made to consist of more or less synchronized volleys) could be visualized by means of evoked potential techniques.

In decerebellated cats transected at the mesencephalo–diencephalic border we placed a longitudinal midsagittal cut through the lower brain stem extend-ing from the transection level down to the midpoint of the fourth ventricle, and separated, to avoid any possibility of "cross-talk," the two halves of the stem by means of a plastic sheet of appropriate size and shape. A bipolar stim-ulation electrode was placed in the right mesencephalic reticular formation and recording electrodes were introduced into the (left or right) NTS and the left RF respectively. Single electrical shocks applied to the right RF invariably were followed by evoked potentials in NTS as well as in the left RF, indicating information flow from the right RF to NTS and thence back to the left RF.

Placing cotton pellets soaked with Xylocaine on the floor of the fourth ven-tricle just over NTS, i.e., reduction of "gain" in this nucleus, invariably led to marked reduction of the evoked potentials not only in NTS but in the left RF as well. In turn, placing 5-HT-soaked small pellets over the areae postremae was followed in most cases by a distinct increase of the evoked potentials in NTS *and* in the left RF. Evidently serotonin leads to an increase in gain in NTS but, probably in contrast to the action of Xylocaine, does this indirectly, i.e., via action on 5-HT receptors in the area postrema and thence through neuronal pathways projecting into the NTS. Thus serotonin would increase the "antiwaking" activity of the RF-NTS-RF feedback system and in this way it would promote the onset of, and help to maintain, sleep.

This serotonergic antiwaking mechanism together with the directly acting serotonergic hypnotic mechanism of the raphe system could then be viewed as an example of a typical *reciprocal* control arrangement of the type we are used to seeing, for instance, in the motor sphere (activation of, viz., the flexors together with inhibition of the extensors) or in many areas of the autonomic system.

Discussion

Oswald: I think these are most beautiful and ingenious experiments but they raise questions about the universality and the specificity of the effects shown. In your presentation you referred to serotonin applied in the ventricle to produce sleep. Feldberg and Sherwood (1954) injected norepinephrine in the ventricle and also found sleep to occur. To what extent are these effects specific? Besides, all your work was done on cats and the cat is opposed to man in many ways. As I read the situation with regard to monoamines and sleep-mechanisms, by and large, humans and cats are quite different.

Koella: Serotonin is effective at much lower doses than anything else. It is an extraordinary substance as far as effectiveness is concerned. We used small doses. Feldberg and Myers (1964) injected serotonin and epinephrine into the third ventricle in doses about 10,000 to 100,000 times larger than we did. In answer to your second comment, I would say that I would love to do those experiments in humans but I need volunteers. I fully agree that the mechanisms may be different in different species. For instance, in humans we see an effect of PCPA on REM but very little on slow wave sleep. We have to be aware of those differences. At least, experiments in one species give us a look into various possible mechanisms. But I agree, this work ought to be repeated in higher animals.

Question: Do you have any information about the possible course of the pathway leaving the nucleus of the solitary tract?

Koella: It seems that the pathway from the nucleus of the solitary tract does not go through the raphe system, but is probably an entirely separate neuronal tract. Morest and Sutin (1961) have studied that question by stimulating the nucleus of the solitary tract and observing evoked potentials in the medial part of the midbrain reticular formation. We have repeated and extended that study and confirmed their data. We recorded evoked potentials in the midbrain reticular formation, but also in the midline thalamus.

Andersen: I like your scheme very much because we can start to attack it. The test would be to destroy the nucleus of the solitary tract and to see if the potentials disappear.

Koella: They disappear, indeed, if you apply Xylocaine on the floor of the fourth ventricle.

Oswald: Your work seems to point to the possibility of influencing sleep mechanisms from the general circulation. Could you comment further?

Koella: Halberg *et al.* (1967) have studied the circadian rhythm of blood serotonin in humans and found a high of serotonin level in the very early hours of the morning. So, in humans the level of serotonin is higher during the night than during the day. But maybe circulatory serotonin is of minor importance. On the contrary, intraventricular serotonin might play an important role as there are possibly serotoninergic endings very close to the ventricular surface. There is a good deal of serotonin in the pineal gland and one could speculate that serotonin is being discharged from the pineal gland through the recessus pinealis into the third and fourth ventricles where it could hit the area postrema and increase sleep.

Jouvet: I do not think there is 5-HT in the ventricles. It could be 5-HIAA. 5-HT is deaminated before it reaches the ventricles.

Koella: But Feldberg and Myers (1966) have shown that there is 5-HT in the ventricles in nanogram amounts.

Question: Is the level of serotonin affected in narcoleptic patients?

Koella: Dr. Dement can answer this question better.

Dement: Zarkoni and Barker sampled spinal fluid in narcoleptic patients and found that the level of 5-hydroxybutyric acid is normal. There is a suggestion that homovanylic acid might be excessive. But your question about narcolepsy is not really relevant because the primary disorder of narcolepsy is an abnormality of REM sleep and not of slow wave sleep. Thus you would not expect a serotonin abnormality.

CHAPTER ELEVEN

Somatic Reflex Activity during Sleep and Wakefulness[1]

MICHAEL H. CHASE

Except for slow postural adjustments, respiratory activity, and an occasional rapid twitch, while we sleep we do not move. The cessation of movement which accompanies the quiet and active phases of sleep is achieved, not by the withdrawal of facilitation, but by the advent of processes which actively inhibit somatic motor activity. Since these inhibitory processes are enhanced during the phase of active sleep, there results a reduction in motor activity when quiet sleep (QS) is compared with wakefulness (W) and when active sleep (AS) is compared with quiet sleep. The decrease in motor activity during sleep is dependent upon pre- and postsynaptic inhibitory processes. We know most about these inhibitory processes as they affect spinal somatic reflexes (monosynaptic and polysynaptic, extensor and flexor) which decrease in amplitude as the animal passes from wakefulness through quiet sleep into active sleep (Baldissera *et al.*, 1964; Beaudreau *et al.*, 1969; Gassel *et al.*, 1964b; Gassel and Pompeiano, 1965; Giaquinto *et al.*, 1963; Kubota *et al.*, 1965a; Pompeiano,

[1]This research was supported by a grant from the United States Public Health Service (MH 10083). Bibliographic assistance was received from the Brain Information Service, which is supported by the National Institute of Neurological Diseases and Stroke (Contract NIH NINDS 70–2063).

1967a,b). This reduction in amplitude reflects changes in the activity of gamma and alpha motor neurons as well as variations in the excitability of presynaptic sensory terminals. During quiet sleep there is depression of gamma motor neuron activity (Gassel and Pompeiano, 1965). During active sleep there is a further depression of gamma motor neurons as well as postsynaptic inhibition of alpha motor neurons (Gassel and Pompeiano, 1965; Morrison and Pompeiano, 1965a; Pompeiano, 1967a,b). Within the state of active sleep, during periods of rapid eye movements, there is presynaptic inhibition of the sensory terminals which are afferent to the alpha motor neuron pool (Gassel *et al.*, 1964b; Gassel and Pompeiano, 1965; Morrison and Pompeiano, 1965b; Pompeiano, 1967b.)

These changes in the activity of gamma and alpha motor neurons are principally due to variations in the discharge of descending spinal cord fibers of brain stem origin (Pompeiano, 1967b). The structures within the brain stem, the fibers which emanate from them, and their modulation of lower motor neuron and afferent terminal activity have been examined in detail (preceding references), reviewed extensively (Pompeiano, 1967a,b), and synopsized by the present author in other publications (Chase, 1970; 1972). However, a very brief description of the *spinal* somatic reflex and the factors which modulate its amplitude will be presented in order to provide a background for the major portion of this chapter, which deals with an examination of brain-stem somatic reflexes and an analysis of the variations in their amplitude which occur during sleep and wakefulness.

The monosynaptic reflex at the level of the spinal cord is composed of (1) muscle spindles and their gamma motor neuron innervation, (2) afferent fibers from the muscle spindles and their presynaptic terminals, and (3) alpha motor neurons whose fibers leave the cord to innervate somatic musculature. The degree of reflex contraction of somatic musculature is dependent upon the activity of muscle spindle afferents, their presynaptic terminals, and the membrane characteristics of alpha motor neurons. Under resting conditions, the active discharge of muscle spindle afferents is governed by the degree of contraction of the intrafusal muscle fibers which are innervated by gamma motor neurons. A consideration of the factors which modulate gamma motor neuron activity is therefore a logical beginning for this overview of the spinal cord monosynaptic reflex. Since no change in spinal cord reflex activity occurs during sleep and wakefulness when descending pathways to the spinal reflex arc are interrupted (Pompeiano, 1967b), their pattern of influence will be the prime consideration in this discussion.

Gamma motor neuron discharge is initiated by activity in a number of descending spinal pathways (Granit, 1955; Granit and Kaada, 1952) which arise from a variety of regions including the reticular formation, red nucleus, subthalamic nucleus and motor cortex; they course within the corresponding funiculi of the spinal cord. The gamma motor neurons which these fibers innervate directly or via interneurons influence the amplitude of the somatic reflex by modifying the discharge level of muscle spindle afferents (Granit, 1955; Granit and Kaada, 1952; Magoun and Rhines, 1946; Pompeiano, 1967b). Muscle spindle discharge is carried into the spinal cord to presynaptic terminals. Another opportunity occurs for descending suprasegmental fiber systems to modulate the somatic reflex by changing the reactivity of these terminals. The fibers which have been postulated to participate in the modulation of presynaptic terminal activity (specifically during sleep) course with the medial longitudinal bundles of the spinal cord and arise from the medial and descending vestibular nuclei (Morrison and Pompeiano, 1965b; Pompeiano, 1967b; Pompeiano and Morrison, 1966). The effect of their activity is to reduce postsynaptic discharge. It may be possible that their *pattern of effect* is also excitatory; however, only the reduction in postsynaptic activity, which occurs as the result of presynaptic inhibition, has been examined in detail (Pompeiano, 1967a,b; Wall, 1958). Suprasegmental modulation may also affect reflex contraction by changing the characteristics of the alpha motor neuron membrane. Descending fibers may either increase or decrease its excitability (Morrison and Pompeiano, 1965a,d). It has been postulated that the decrease in alpha motor neuron excitability which is specifically linked to the sleep states occurs as the result of activity within the inhibitory (medial) regions of the brain-stem reticular formation; the fibers which emanate from these areas course within the ventral half of the lateral funiculi of the spinal cord (Gassel et al., 1965; Giaquinto et al., 1964; Morrison and Pompeiano, 1965a; Pompeiano, 1967a,b). Those fibers which increase its excitability (during sleep) course within pyramidal *and* extrapyramidal spinal cord tracts (Morrison and Pompeiano, 1965c,d; Niemer and Magoun, 1947).

In summary, if one starts with the level of excitability of the reflex during resting wakefulness as a base line, there is a decrease in responsiveness during quiet sleep. This decrease is due to a reduction in the excitability of gamma motor neurons. During active sleep there is a further decrease in the excitability of gamma motor neurons as well as postsynaptic depression of alpha motor neurons. During the periods of rapid eye movements of active sleep there exist, in addition to the ongoing depression of alpha and gamma motor neuron excitability, presynaptic inhibition of the afferent terminals of the reflex arc. The myoclonic twitches which occur during active sleep are present principally during the periods of rapid eye movements and are the result of the activity of fibers descending from the brain stem which course within the dorsolateral funiculi of the spinal cord (which includes the corticospinal and rubrospinal tracts (Gassel et al., 1965; Pompeiano, 1967a,b). Thus, during rapid eye movement periods of active sleep there is an increased preponderance of inhibition, both pre- and postsynaptic, as well as the concurrent excitation postsynaptically of alpha motor neurons (which briefly overrides the ongoing inhibitory processes). Both myoclonic twitches and rapid eye movements are abolished by bilateral vestibular lesions (Gassel *et al.*, 1964a; Morrison and Pompeiano, 1966; Pompeiano, 1967a,b).

This survey of the factors which modulate the spinal cord monosynaptic reflex during sleep and wakefulness also applies to the spinal cord polysynaptic reflex, with the exception that between the afferent terminal and the efferent motor neuron there lie interneurons whose excitability may also be changed by segmental or suprasegmental influences. It is generally assumed that the same suprasegmental structures and patterns of effect which are responsible for state-dependent monosynaptic reflex activity are also responsible for the modulation of polysynaptic reflexes (Pompeiano, 1967a,b).

We do not know whether the suprasegmental structures which influence spinal cord somatic reflexes during sleep and wakefulness exert a similar pattern of activity upon brain-stem somatic reflexes, for there have been no studies to elucidate the mechanisms of brain stem somatic reflex modulation. Only the variations in brain-stem reflex *amplitude* during these states have been examined in detail. Of the two reflexes which have been studied, one is a monosynaptic reflex—the masseteric reflex—the structure and function of which is similar to spinal cord reflexes, and the other is a polysynaptic reflex— the digastric reflex—the structure and function of which is different from either the brain-stem monosynaptic reflex or spinal cord reflexes.

I. Data

A. The Monosynaptic Masseteric Reflex

The excitation of proprioceptive endings located within the masseter muscle initiates jaw closure which occurs by synaptic organization located entirely within the brain stem (Hugelin and Bonvallet, 1957; Szentagothai, 1948). Activity is carried into the brain stem over fibers whose cell bodies lie within the mesencephalic nucleus of the fifth nerve (Hugelin and Bonvallet, 1957; Szentagothai, 1948). Fibers from these sensory cells connect monosynaptically with neurons in the motor nucleus of the fifth nerve. Excitation of these motor neurons leads to contraction of the masseter muscle. The masseteric reflex may also be induced electrically by direct excitation of the sensory cells which comprise the mesencephalic nucleus of the fifth nerve (Hugelin and Bonvallet, 1957). A monosynaptic reflex response results which may be monitored by recording the electromyographic activity of the masseter muscle (Chase *et al.*, 1968). It is this electrically induced monosynaptic reflex which was utilized in the investigations reported in this chapter (Fig. 11.1). An abbreviated description of the surgical procedures for establishing this reflex in the freely moving

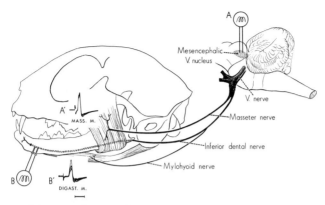

Fig. 11.1. Adult cat: Reflex stimulation and recording paradigm. Masseteric reflex: An electrical pulse delivered to the mesencephalic nucleus of the fifth nerve (A) excites cells whose fibers originate in proprioceptors within the masseter muscle. Discharge from these sensory cells induce, monosynaptically, activity in the motor nucleus of the fifth nerve and contraction of the masseter muscle (A′), resulting in jaw closing. Digastric reflex: Stimulation of the inferior alveolar nerve (B), as it runs within the mandibular canal, yields polysynaptic excitation of cells in the motor fifth nucleus, resulting in contraction of the anterior belly of the digastric muscle (B′) and jaw opening. Calibration line: 10 msec and 200 μV. [From Chase, 1972]

kitten and adult cat and the recording procedures for monitoring its response is presented. A more complete description of these procedures may be found in the following reports: Chase, 1971b; Chase and McGinty, 1970a; Chase *et al.*, 1968.

The electrically induced brain-stem monosynaptic masseteric reflex is ideally suited as an experimental tool with which to investigate brain-stem reflex activity in the freely moving animal during sleep and wakefulness. A stable pattern of response is achieved for long periods by delivering electrical stimulation to the mesencephalic nucleus of the fifth nerve via electrodes which are permanently placed within the brain (Fig. 11.1). This technique affords little opportunity for the effectiveness of stimulation to change over time, as it normally would with electrodes placed around peripheral nerves where movement of the animal, tissue reaction, or injury to the nerve may lead to changes in response.

The reflex was monitored by placing wire loops within the substance of the masseter muscle (Fig. 11.1). These recording electrodes were stable with respect to the amplitude of the recorded response over periods exceeding 3 months. Moreover, if the recording wires broke at any point between their insertion into the muscle or the recording plug, they were easily mended without changing their configuration within the muscle parenchyma. In order to monitor the reflex response on an ink-writing polygraph, it was necessary to lengthen the recorded response to allow the polygraphic pen time to follow. This lengthening process was achieved by a simple capacitor and time-expanding circuit, which, when combined with a window circuit, permitted the polygraphic analysis of individual waves of the electromyographic potential. The electrical activity generated by the cerebral cortex, eye movements, and the neck musculature was also recorded polygraphically. Thus, it was possible to maintain an on-line analysis over long periods of time and to correlate changes in the state of the animal with changes in reflex amplitude.

After recovery from the surgical procedures (approximately 3 days for kittens and 2 weeks for adult cats), the animals were placed in an environmental chamber, a reflex induced at a rate of either 0.5 per second or 1 per second, and an analysis made of its amplitude changes during consecutive cycles of sleep and wakefulness. Following an analysis of the reflex amplitude as the animal passed from wakefulness to quiet to active sleep, a more detailed investigation was carried out to examine those variations in response which occurred during specific periods within these states.

1. The Adult Cat

In the adult, freely moving cat, the mean amplitude of the masseteric reflex was largest during wakefulness, smallest during active sleep, and of an intermediate value during quiet sleep (Fig. 11.2). These determinations, however, did not reflect many of the dynamic changes which occurred within each state. It was therefore important to examine intrastate fluctuations which were time-locked to variations both in central neural patterns of activity and in the animal's behavior. During wakefulness, analyses thus far have included discriminations of amplitude variations which were linked to periods (1) when the cat was immobile or mobile, and periods (2) which consisted of no eye movements, few eye movements, or many eye movements. In general, the amplitude of the masseteric reflex was positively correlated with the degree of activity (Fig. 11.2). When the animal was quiet and immobile, the reflex was small; it increased in amplitude as the animal moved or appeared in a hyper-excited state. The masseteric reflex was positively correlated in its amplitude with the frequency or density of eye movements (Fig. 11.3). Against a background of wakefulness, periods of rapid eye movements were correlated with a relatively increased amplitude of response, while periods which were comprised of few eye movements were correlated with a reduced response (Fig. 11.3). The amplitude of the reflex was extremely variable during those episodes when the animal was actively moving his jaw (Chase and McGinty, 1970a). In summary, the largest amplitude responses occurred during wakefulness; they decreased in size during quiet sleep, and were minimal during active sleep (Fig. 11.2). This pattern was the exact opposite from that observed in the kitten, as will be described in the following section.

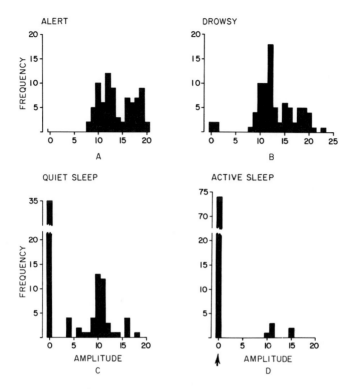

Fig. 11.2. Frequency histograms of the amplitude of 80 consecutive masseteric reflex responses. These potentials were obtained during the (A) alert, (B) drowsy, (C) quiet sleep, and (D) active sleep states. The amplitudes of the motor responses were plotted on an arbitrary scale as a function of the frequency of their occurrence. High amplitude potentials were reduced and then almost totally abolished as the animal progressed from wakefulness, through drowsiness and quiet sleep, into active sleep. [From Chase *et al.*, 1968]

2. The Neonatal Kitten

When one places neonatal kittens (that is, those less than 2 weeks of age) into an experimental chamber and records masseteric reflex activity, one is immediately struck by its very low amplitude at the beginning of the session, when the kitten is aroused. Indeed, the more aroused the kitten, the smaller the amplitude of the reflex response (Fig. 11.4). It was only when the animal began to calm down and assumed a position of rest that a response followed each stimulus (Fig. 11.4). The response grew in amplitude and consistency as the kitten entered the quiet sleep state (Fig. 11.4). During the active sleep state the amplitude of the reflex became large and was consistently present; i.e., the reflex response occurred following each stimulation of the mesencephalic

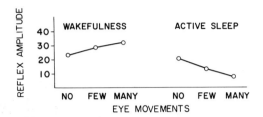

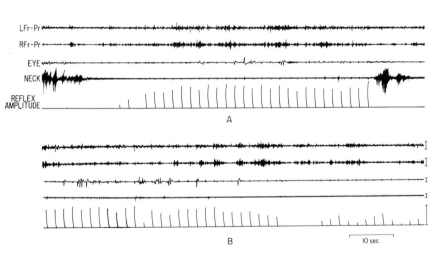

Fig. 11.3. This figure depicts the amplitude changes of the masseteric reflex during the eye movement and no-eye movement periods which accompany wakefulness and active sleep. The amplitude of the reflex was plotted on an arbitrary but relative scale. During wakefulness in conjunction with an increase in the frequency of eye movements the masseteric reflex was augmented. During active sleep, during periods of rapid eye movements, the reflex was maximally depressed. Thus, as the density of eye movements increased during wakefulness, the masseteric reflex increased in amplitude. As the density of eye movements increased during active sleep, the masseteric reflex amplitude decreased. [In collaboration with Dr. Margaret Babb]

nucleus of the fifth nerve (Fig. 11.4). Thus, its general pattern of reactivity was distinct from that which was observed in the adult cat (Figs. 11.5, 11.6).

An examination of the amplitude of the masseteric reflex during periods of

Fig. 11.4. Relation of reflex amplitude to abrupt changes in state. In the young (10-day-old) kitten, changes in state were accompanied by rapid variations in reflex amplitude. In A, note the correspondence between the increase in reflex amplitude during active sleep and its decrease during arousal. Occasionally, the kitten would pass from active sleep directly to quiet sleep (B); the reflex amplitude followed closely this change of state. Masseteric reflex; 3 V, 0.5 msec, 0.5/sec. Calibration: EEG, EOG, EMG, 50 uV. reflex, 500 uV. For this and subsequent figures the following abbreviations for the cortical recording sites were employed: LFr-Pr, left frontal to left parietal; RFr-Pr, right frontal to right parietal; Trans-Fr, transfrontal. [From Chase, 1972]

many eye movements, few eye movements, and no eye movements was undertaken during wakefulness and active sleep. The periods of eye movements during active sleep varied little from the control periods (which consisted of contiguous periods of no eye movements) until the kitten was about 2 weeks of age, at which time the amplitude occasionally decreased during eye movement episodes (Fig. 11.5). By about 6 weeks of age very striking reductions occurred in conjunction with the rapid eye movements of active sleep as reported for the adult cat (Fig. 11.5). In summary, as the kitten (2 weeks of age or younger) became more alert the amplitude of the masseteric reflex decreased. As the kitten moved into quiet sleep from wakefulness the amplitude increased and as the kitten moved from the quiet sleep state into the active sleep state there was a further increase in the response. Thus, the general pattern observed in kittens which were less than 2 weeks old was exactly the opposite from that observed during similar states in the adult cat (Fig. 11.6).

B. THE POLYSYNAPTIC DIGASTRIC REFLEX

We can ask whether the responses of the masseteric reflex are similar to the variations in other reflexes which are organized at the level of the brain stem. The answer is a negative one, for the amplitude changes of its antagonist, the digastric reflex, follow a dissimilar pattern. The structure of the digastric reflex

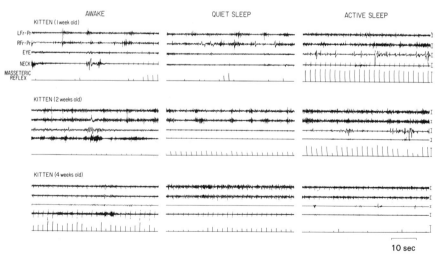

Fig. 11.5. Masseteric reflex modulation in the 1, 2, and 4-week-old kitten. This reflex was of greatest amplitude during active sleep in 1 and 2-week-old kittens. By 4 weeks of age the mean amplitude of the reflex was largest during the awake state and smallest during active sleep. Note the lack of a clearly differentiable state-dependent EEG pattern in the 1-week-old kitten. Masseteric reflex: 3 V, 0.5 msec, 0.5/sec. Calibration: EEG, EOG, EMG, 50 uV; reflex, 500 uV. [From Chase, 1971b]

is different not only from the masseteric reflex but also from all spinal cord reflexes in that it lacks muscle spindles; therefore, it lacks a gamma motor neuron system (see Discussion). The method of induction of this reflex is also unique, i.e., via fibers from receptors located in the periodontal area or

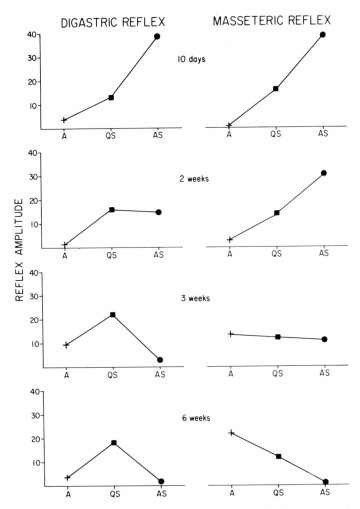

Fig. 11.6. The mean amplitudes of 100 consecutively induced reflex responses (evoked at the rate of 0.5/sec) are plotted in this figure on an arbitrary but relative scale for each animal in each age group. The adult pattern for the digastric reflex appeared to be achieved by a gradual reduction in amplitude during active sleep and an increase during quiet sleep. As the kitten grew older this reflex remained relatively reduced during the awake state. The pattern of masseteric reflex activity during wakefulness and active sleep in the first two postnatal weeks was the opposite from that which occurred at 4 weeks of age, when the responses were similar to those reported in the mature cat. [From Chase, 1971b]

by excitation of fibers coursing in the dental nerve (Fig. 11.1). In any event, the reflex does not reflect the excitation of muscle stretch receptors, as is the case for the masseteric reflex. The following sections consist of a description of the amplitude changes of the digastric reflex in the adult cat and neonatal kitten. A detailed description of the method of establishing and recording this reflex in the freely moving animal may be found in Chase, 1970, and 1971b.

1. The Adult Cat

The digastric reflex in the adult cat exhibited state-dependent amplitude variations which were distinct from those observed for its antagonist, the masseteric reflex. During wakefulness, the amplitude of the digastric reflex was less than that occurring during quiet sleep (Figs. 11.7, 11.8). When the animal was very alert, there was a further decrease in amplitude. During the quiet sleep state, just prior to the transition to active sleep, an increase in the amplitude of this reflex occurred (Figs. 11.7, 11.8). As with the masseteric reflex, the digastric reflex exhibited its smallest amplitude during *active sleep* (Figs. 11.7, 11.8), especially during rapid eye movements. During the rapid eye movements which accompanied wakefulness, there was also a reduction in amplitude. The control periods consisted of active sleep and wakefulness without rapid eye movements. Thus, the amplitude variations of the digastric reflex which were similar to those of the masseteric reflex appeared to be circumscribed to

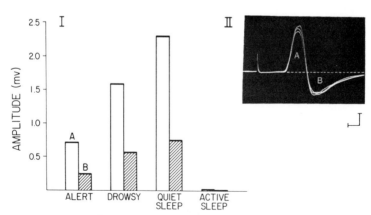

Fig. 11.7. Digastric reflex responses during states of sleep and wakefulness in the adult cat: Mean amplitude of 50 consecutive responses. Each wave of the reflex (II: A, B) was measured separately as the extent of its excursion from the base-line level (II: dotted line). As the animal changed state the amplitude of both waves varied in parallel fashion (I: A, B). An increase in amplitude occurred when the drowsy state was compared with the alert state (actually quiet alert) and when quiet sleep was compared with the drowsy state. During active sleep the reflex response decreased below the level obtained during the quiet alert state. Inferior dental nerve: 1.5 V, 0.1 msec, 1/sec. Calibration (II): 2 msec and 200 uV. [From Chase, 1970]

260   *Michael H. Chase*

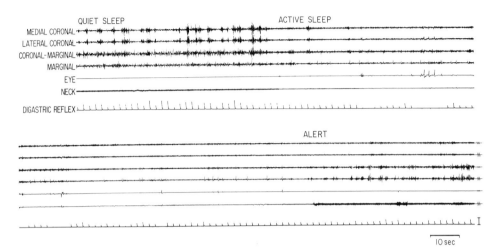

Fig. 11.8. Digastric reflex during sleep and wakefulness in the adult cat: On-line record of the EEG, EOG, EMG, and reflex response. In the initial part of this continuous record the animal was in the quiet sleep state. Since the reflex was evoked with a supraliminal stimulus, it was present throughout most of the active sleep episode, except during single eye movements or bursts of EOG activity. The alert pattern which followed active sleep was not accompanied by any obvious change in reflex amplitude due, most probably, to the fact that the animal was not aroused or actively moving (note synchronization in marginal leads). With this level of reflex excitation the only striking change in reflex amplitude occurred as (1) facilitation during quiet sleep, (2) suppression during the eye movements of active sleep, and (3) suppression during arousal. Inferior dental nerve: 1.6 V, 0.1 msec, 1/sec. Calibration: EEG, EOG, EMG, 50 uV; digastric reflex, 1.5 mV. [From Chase, 1970]

those variations which occurred during active sleep. On a continuum, the amplitude of the digastric reflex was largest during quiet sleep, smaller during wakefulness, and smallest during active sleep or very alert behavior.

2. The Neonatal Kitten

In kittens less than 2 weeks of age the amplitude of the digastric reflex was largest during the active sleep state (Figs. 11.6, 11.9). The reflex response was smaller during quiet sleep and smallest during wakefulness (Figs. 11.6, 11.9). Thus, on a continuum, as the neonatal kitten emerged into quiet sleep from wakefulness there was an increase in response (Fig. 11.6). As he passed into active sleep from quiet sleep there was a further increase. These variations in response *are the same* as those which were observed for the masseteric reflex in neonatal kittens (Figs. 11.5, 11.6, 11.9). It was not until approximately 2–3 weeks after birth that there occurred the divergent adult reflex patterns (Figs. 11.5, 11.9).

As in the adult, the digastric reflex in the kitten was reduced in amplitude during the rapid eye movements which accompanied wakefulness (Fig. 11.9).

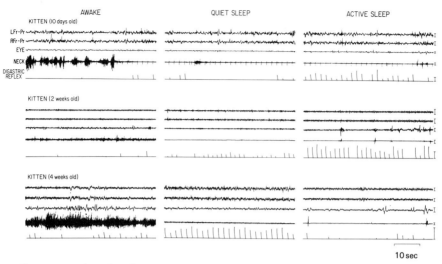

Fig. 11.9. Digastric reflex modulation in the 10-day, 2 and 4-week-old kitten. The mean amplitude of both waves of the digastric reflex fluctuated in parallel during sleep and wakefulness. The records shown in this figure represent the amplitude of the initial component of the reflex response which was reduced in all age groups during the awake state compared with quiet sleep. In 10-day and 2-week-old kittens it was largest during active sleep, whereas it was greatest during quiet sleep in the 4-week-old animal. By 3 to 4 weeks of age the adult pattern of modulation was present. Digastric reflex; 6 V, 0.75 msec (10 days); 5 V, 1 msec (2 weeks); 2 V, 0.5 msec (4 weeks); 0.5/sec. Calibration: EEG, EOG, EMG, 50 uV; reflex, 500 uV. [From Chase, 1971b]

During active sleep in kittens less than 2 weeks old there was very little variation in amplitude during the rapid eye movements which accompanied active sleep (Fig. 11.9). In summary then, the digastric reflex in the neonatal kitten during wakefulness reacted in much the same manner as it did in the adult cat. During quiet sleep in both the neonatal kitten and the adult cat there was an increase in amplitude above that which occurred during wakefulness. However, in the neonatal kitten during active sleep the amplitude of the digastric reflex increased over that which occurred during quiet sleep; whereas in the adult cat its size was minimal during active sleep. Thus, during active sleep, in the neonatal kitten, the amplitude of the digastric reflex was largest while in the adult cat its amplitude was smallest.

II. Discussion

There appears to be no special problem attached to the descriptive and functional analysis of spinal cord somatic reflex activity during sleep and wakefulness (Baldiserra *et al.*, 1964, 1966a; Gassel *et al.*, 1964b; Gassel and Pompeiano, 1965; Giaquinto *et al.*, 1963; Kubota *et al.*, 1965a). Essentially the level of reactivity is greatest during *wakefulness*, specifically during those periods of time when the animal is required to move his somatic musculature or to maintain antigravity or postural functions. During *quiet sleep* the reduction in amplitude in all likelihood reflects and maintains the quiescent nature of this state. During *active sleep* there is a further reduction in the amplitude of response, perhaps in order to preserve the "sleep state" at a time when most areas of the brain, including motor systems, are extremely active. During the rapid eye movements of active sleep, presynaptic inhibition of afferent terminals overrides, to some degree, the direct facilitatory discharge which impinges on the alpha motor neurons which lead to muscular twitches. If one assumes that quiet and active sleep subserve specific functions, without defining them, then the preceding pattern of spinal cord somatic reflex activity appears to be appropriate for the maintenance of these states.

The bases for brain-stem reflex variations during sleep and wakefulness are not as apparent. Specifically, the digastric reflex appears to be distinct with respect to its pattern of reactivity. This divergent pattern of response may be based upon its unique function and/or structure.

The *functional significance* of the digastric reflex has been discussed in a previous article (Chase, 1970). Since it is not involved in postural functions, as are spinal cord reflexes, its function may emerge only during quiet sleep when its amplitude is greatest. During the quiet sleep state there is a possible protective mechanism subserved by the maintenance of the mouth in an open position or by the facilitation of those factors which would tend to initiate jaw opening as an alternative airway to the nasal passage under conditions of respiratory distress. During active sleep it is possible that this respiratory function is overridden or is of less importance owing to the reciprocal inhibition of antagonists. When other brain-stem reflexes which are involved in similar mechanisms have been analyzed during sleep and wakefulness we will be able to extend our hypotheses of the state-dependent functions of this reflex. For example, if respiratory reflexes show an increased response during the quiet sleep state we can, with more assurance, assume that the increase in amplitude of the digastric reflex reflects a state-dependent respiratory process.

The digastric reflex is related to a variety of other functions, including those concerned with mastication and protection of the buccal structures (Dumont, 1964; Hoffman and Tonnies, 1948; Kidokoro *et al.*, 1968; Kubota *et al.*, 1965a; Lubinska, 1932; Sherrington, 1917). In addition, the afferent limb of the digastric reflex is thought to be involved in the evaluation of the quality and texture of food within the buccal cavity (Wyrwicka and Chase, 1969). In this context, it has been proposed that sensory endings from the periodontal receptors are critical in the maintenance of normal patterns of food consumption. Therefore, sensory information may be conveyed to the central nervous system during wakefulness which is independent of reflex activity but which may nevertheless induce it. Since the inferior dental nerve conveys information which does not originate in the digastric muscle, it is possible that digastric reflex activity is but an incidental response to the excitation of sensory afferents of buccal–pharyngeal origin.

The *structural* feature which is different in the digastric reflex from other reflexes which have been studied is the absence of muscle spindles (Baum, 1900; Hosokawa, 1961; Kidokoro *et al.*, 1968; Smith and Marcarian, 1967; Szenta-gothai, 1949). This lack of muscle spindles precludes the presence of gamma motor neurons. We know that variations in somatic reflex activity, at least with respect to spinal cord reflexes, are in large part dependent upon the modu-lation of gamma motor neurons. We may therefore, by virtue of subtracting their influence, hypothesize as to the reactivity of a reflex in which this system is not present. To a large measure such hypothetical variations in reflex activity occur for the digastric reflex. If there were no activation of gamma motor neurons—which are absent from the digastric reflex—one might expect a decrease in its amplitude during wakefulness due to "reciprocal inhibition" by the masseteric reflex. Additionally, in conjunction with electroencephalo-graphic desynchronization, spinal cord reflexes are facilitated by supraspinal activation of gamma motor neurons (Buchwald and Eldred, 1961; Euler and Söderberg, 1956; Gassel and Pompeiano, 1965; Hongo *et al.*, 1963). We assume that the increase in the amplitude of the masseteric reflex is partially due to gamma motor neuron activation. The increased digastric reflex amplitude during quiet sleep may represent its truer "base-line" level, when there is no suprasegmental inhibition or activation; or, as suggested in the discussion of its functions, there may be facilitation of its response which is specific to this state.

At the present time it is impossible to generate substantive hypotheses to explain brain-stem reflex modulation since we do not know the neurophysio-logical bases for the variations in amplitude which occur as state-dependent phenomena. Rather, our best bet is simply to stipulate those factors which might contribute to digastric depression during wakefulness, facilitation during quiet sleep, and enhanced depression during active sleep and to a decrease in masseteric reflex amplitude during quiet and active sleep. The possible combinations of inhibition, disinhibition, facilitation, defacilitation of postsynaptic and/or presynaptic origin negate, a priori, realistic neuro-physiological models to explain functional changes in reflex amplitude. In lieu of additional experiments it is best at the present simply to accept the variations in reflex amplitude as a "given," and from there (1) carry on further examinations of the factors which modulate these reflexes and (2) use them as known physiological variables for the study of other central neural pro-cesses.

The state-dependent variations in spinal somatic reflex amplitude have been used to examine the central nervous system sites which modulate their activity (see introductory remarks for references). No studies have been carried out which would indicate whether the same or different central nervous system (CNS) structures regulate brain-stem reflexes in either the adult cat or developing kitten. Theoretically it is not difficult to determine the responsible CNS structures. In most instances these studies consist of the stimulation of a specific area of the CNS and an examination of the somatic reflex response. Subsequent studies are carried out to determine whether a given effect is accomplished by presynaptic or postsynaptic processes. Central nervous system lesions are also used to determine the influence of a given structure on spontaneous reflex variations; lesions are expected to complement the results of stimulation. Since a great many areas of the CNS are capable of influencing motor processes either directly or indirectly, a panorama of their potential to modify somatic reflexes would be expected to clarify their inter-relationships and the role which they play in state-dependent phenomena. According to this scheme, if we take the masseteric reflex as a prototype, the following areas of the CNS have been shown to exert an influence upon its

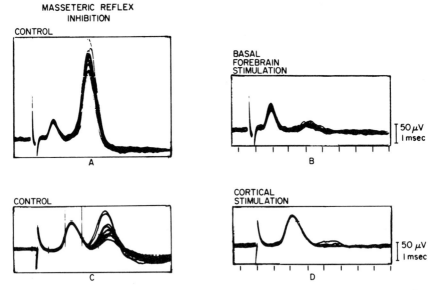

Fig. 11.10. The control masseteric reflex is illustrated in A and C. Following the artefact, the antidromic volley is followed by the reflex volley (recorded from the masseteric nerve). In B, which shows basal forebrain stimulation, almost complete inhibition of the reflex response is observed during stimulation of the ipsilateral preoptic area, while D shows an even more pronounced effect during stimulation of the ipsilateral orbital gyrus. [From Clemente *et al.*, 1966]

activity: orbital cortex (Fig. 11.10) (Chase, 1971a; Chase and McGinty, 1970a), motor cortex (Chase, 1971a; Sauerland *et al.*, 1967), mesencephalic and bulbar reticular formations (Dumont, 1964; Hugelin, 1961), and the basal forebrain (Fig. 11.10) (Clemente *et al.*, 1966). These areas of the CNS, as well as vagal afferent activity (Fig. 11.11) (Chase *et al.*, 1970a,b), appear to exhibit a common pattern of influence. In conjunction with excitation of each of these areas (with the exception of the reticular formation) the masseteric reflex is profoundly depressed. This depression of masseteric reflex activity may be used as a tool with which to investigate state-dependent patterns of central neural control. Thus far only the orbital cortex has been examined in this manner (Figs. 11.12, 11.13) (Chase and McGinty, 1970a,b). Its potential for masseteric reflex inhibition predominates during wakefulness (Figs. 11.12, 11.13). There is a decrease in effect during quiet sleep which reaches minimal levels during active sleep (Figs. 11.12, 11.13). Thus, the conclusion is drawn that one should look to wakefulness when examining the motor functions of the orbital cortex. By analyzing the CNS in this fashion it may be possible to gain a comprehensive

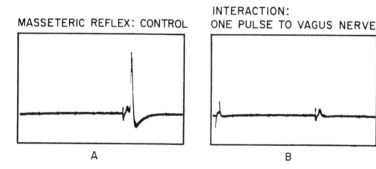

MASSETERIC REFLEX: CONTROL

INTERACTION:
ONE PULSE TO VAGUS NERVE

A

B

INTERACTION:
THREE PULSES TO VAGUS NERVE

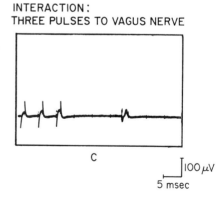

C

$100 \mu V$

5 msec

Fig. 11.11. Inhibition of the masseteric monosynaptic reflex by afferent vagal stimulation (three superimposed traces). In A, the control reflex was elicited by stimulation of the mesencephalic nucleus of the fifth nerve. The reflex was completely abolished when preceded by either single (B) or multiple (C) vagal pulses. The antidromic potential persisted unchanged. Mesencephalic Vth nucleus: 4 V, 0.2 msec, 1/sec; Vagus: 10 V, 1 msec. [From Chase and Nakamura, 1968]

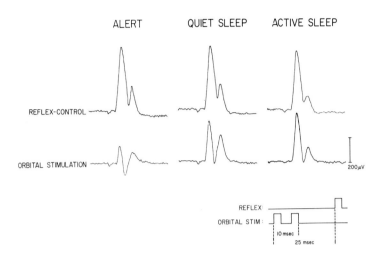

Fig. 11.12. Orbital cortically induced changes in the masseteric reflex during sleep and wakefulness. Each trace is the average of 15 responses. The control reflex was maximally induced, therefore little change in amplitude was noted during the different states. Inhibition by orbital stimulation was most evident during the alert state and least during active sleep. Orbital cortex: 9 V, 0.75 msec; Mesencephalic Vth nucleus: 6 V, 0.8 msec. [From Chase and McGinty, 1970b]

picture of its state-dependent functions not only during the general states of wakefulness, quiet sleep, and active sleep, but also during specific substates. For example, during wakefulness, there are easily recognized patterns of activity such as eating, drinking, copulating, etc. Additionally, there are other substates more subtle, such as those involving internal inhibition, drive, expectancy, etc. Undoubtedly, there are neural systems whose activity predominates only during circumscribed states of behavior.

By extending these investigations to the neonatal animal, it may be possible to gain an appreciation of the fashion and time when specific areas of the CNS begin to exert their function. For example, it is possible and probable that areas of the CNS which affect somatic activity do so during wakefulness at a different point in development than they do during the sleep states. Given that the orbital cortex exerts its motor functions primarily during wakefulness, and given that the developing animal spends a majority of its time in sleep, it would be fruitless to investigate the orbital cortical function for masseteric reflex modulation during the sleep state in the developing kitten. It would be during wakefulness that one would expect to determine that point in time when the orbital cortex begins to function in the control of somatic reflex activity. For other orbital cortical functions different patterns may emerge. Thus, in

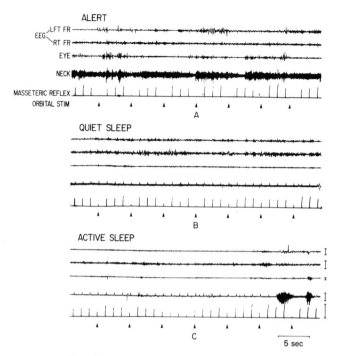

Fig. 11.13. By recording the masseteric reflex on a polygraph, along with the EEG, EOG, and EMG, variations in the effectiveness of cortically induced inhibition of this reflex during sleep and waking states could be examined. The masseteric reflex was evoked at a rate of 1/sec; orbital stimulation (indicated by arrowheads) preceded every fourth reflex by 15 msec. When the animal was in the alert state the degree of inhibition was greatest; it decreased during quiet sleep and was least during active sleep. Orbital cortex: 8 V, 1 msec, 4 pulses (500 pulses/sec); Mesencephalic Vth nucleus: 5 V, 1 msec. Calibration: EEG, EOG, EMG, 50 uV; masseteric reflex, 500 uV. [From Chase and McGinty, 1970b]

order to obtain a comprehensive analysis of the central neural modulation of behavior it is essential to carry out developmental-dependent and state-dependent analyses of activity. Only by this kind of investigation can we hope to extend our knowledge of the dynamic processes of the central nervous system which occur not only during wakefulness, but also during sleep.

ADULT HUMAN SLEEP STATES

CHAPTER TWELVE

An Introduction to Sleep[1]

WILLIAM C. DEMENT
MERRILL M. MITLER

The purpose of this paper is essentially pedagogic. We will try to lay some groundwork for understanding the articles that follow and to explicate a few of the "principles" of sleep research, at least as we view them at Stanford University.

For the most part, we will be presenting descriptions and definitions of sleep phenomena and some details of the organization of sleep. The material will be presented roughly in an historical context and the reader will discern, in order, three major themes. First, sleep and wakefulness may be thought of as cyclic fluctuations in behavior throughout the day. Second, organisms partition their existence among three entirely separate and unique "states." Third, sleep research can profit from a "process" view of the states of existence, such that each state is considered as a collection of processes. Adopting such a viewpoint will allow each process to be analytically studied.

[1]Preparation of this manuscript was supported by National Institute of Mental Health Grant MH 13860, National Institute of Health Grant NS 10727, National Aeronautics and Space Administration Grant NGR 05–020–168. WCD is supported by Career Development Award MH 5804 and MMM is supported by NIH Grant MH 8304.

Sleep and wakefulness are essentially functions of the whole organism vastly extended in the temporal dimension. Scientific observation is ordinarily either cross-sectional or longitudinal, but the very essence of most sleep research is that it is simultaneously longitudinal and cross-sectional.

In many fields, undue concentration upon mechanism and function often occurs somewhat prematurely and tends to undermine the necessary attempt at overall careful open-eyed observation without preconceptions. When pure description is no longer a goal, certain dramatic transients are easily overlooked among the myriad variables that constitute the behavior of the whole organism in time. Perhaps the best example of this general principle is in sleep research itself. There were innumerable experimental studies on the mechanisms of sleep before the true nature of mammalian sleep was fully comprehended—that is, before the existence of REM sleep was known. It is a mystery to us, given the methods in use, how REM sleep was so long overlooked. One explanation, as we have implied above, may lie in the fact that descriptive work generally holds second-class citizenship *vis-a-vis* experimental work.

The identification of REM sleep was solely a descriptive process. It is clear, we think, that every approach has its appropriate and most timely application; our advocacy of pure observation is only intended to underscore the fact that description is not entirely finished, in spite of spectacular developments in the theoretical–experimental areas.

Another way of looking at these considerations refers back to the cross-sectional versus longitudinal aspects of sleep. Historically, there was a strong tendency (which still persists in little enclaves) to view sleep as a single totally uniform state. From such a viewpoint, investigators attempted to describe the entirety of sleep by single nighttime observations of individual variables. A great many interpretations were made on this basis. For example, Pietrusky (1922) published a "definitive" study of eye position during sleep in human subjects. He made *single* observations on 300 individuals. From these data he concluded that the characteristic stationary resting position of the eyes during sleep was in divergence. In addition, this conclusion may have been "predisposed" in the sense that Pietrusky saw divergence during sleep as an inevitable consequence of predominant ocular convergence during wakefulness. By nightfall, he reasoned, the more fatigued internal recti could not maintain the midposition against a slight tonic pull of the less fatigued lateral recti. We now know that the eyeballs *do not* maintain a single characteristic resting position during sleep. Actually, much of Pietrusky's data could have been duplicated by making observations on one individual at 300 different points in a single night. Any position in which we might find the eyeball is simply one of the relatively brief pauses separating the countless episodes of slow and rapid motility (Dement, 1964).

Thus, any description of sleep must take the temporal dimension into account. In this sense, sleep is something like a river—basically the same, yet different at every point depending upon the shape of its bank, the size of projecting boulders, the presence or absence of tributaries, the traffic upon it, the rate of flow, and so forth.

I. Early Work: The EEG and the ARAS

The somnolent state has occupied the attention of laboratory scientists for more than a hundred years. During this time the one thing which, more than any other, stimulated work in this area was the development of electro-encephalography (EEG). Thus, an instrument was available which permitted continuous observation of the electrical activity of the brain during sleep without disturbing the sleeper.

One of the first things to become obvious to Berger (1930) after his discovery of the presence of brain waves in humans was their consistent change when passing from wakefulness to sleep or vice versa. As is well known, an exciting series of papers in the late 1930s emanating from the Loomis group at Harvard (Loomis et al., 1937; Davis et al., 1938, 1939) and from the University of Chicago (Blake, 1937; Blake and Gerard, 1937; Blake et al., 1939) presented relatively detailed descriptions of the various EEG patterns during sleep in humans. These investigators did not fall into the trap of oversimplifying their observations. Although they did use sampling procedures, they nonetheless recognized and reported dramatic differences in sleep EEG patterns depending upon the time of night and the distance from the onset of sleep.

A general conception developed in the 1930s and 1940s that the EEG waves represented a kind of integrated display at the scalp level of envelopes of unit discharge. Accordingly, it was felt that the important parameter in sleep and arousal was EEG synchrony, stipulating an inverse relationship between frequency and amplitude. It was very logical, then, that neurons would be discharging slowly and synchronously in deep sleep.

The work of Magoun and his colleagues greatly strengthened this formulation (Moruzzi and Magoun, 1949; Lindsley et al., 1949, 1950). Cortical activation was equated with arousal; both were thought to be specifically related to fast frequencies and low amplitudes (desynchronization) in the EEG. The level of cortical activation was assumed, in turn, to depend upon the amount of activity in a hypothetical ascending extralemniscal system in the brain stem. This system was called the ascending reticular activating system (ARAS). Thus, the whole continuum of sleep and arousal was presumed to be controlled by an essentially unitary mechanism residing in the brain-stem core.

In addition, the ARAS was found to receive collaterals from all the main sensory pathways. Accordingly, its activity reflected the amount of stimulation impinging upon the organism. Furthermore, by interposing this system between external stimulation and the cerebral cortex, one could account for a certain amount of independence from immediate sensory stimulation in terms of amplifying and modulating functions performed by the ARAS. This formulation was so beautiful and seemed so amenable to experimental manipulation in laboratory animals that it was reified before all the descriptive facts were available.

The above conception did allow for variation in the "depth" of sleep. Thus, the bigger and slower the EEG waves, the deeper the sleep. This was also consistent with the notion that cortical units were discharging slowly and synchronously, in contrast to their presumed patterns in response to the evocations of wakefulness. Figure 12.1 depicts this vertical continuum of sleep and wakefulness.

Several studies were also done which presented evidence supporting a relationship between EEG patterns and arousal threshold (Blake and Gerard, 1937; Simon and Emmons, 1956; Coleman *et al.*, 1959). Here again, the relationship was reified before all the evidence was gathered. For example, in their otherwise superb *Atlas of Electroencephalography*, the Gibbs (1950) eschewed numbers or letters to name the EEG stages of sleep, preferring instead a nomenclature based on depth of sleep.

Figure 12.2 presents examples of some EEG patterns seen during human

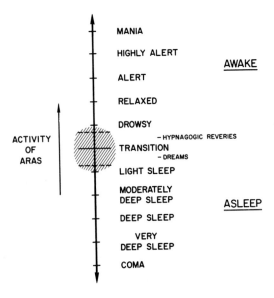

Fig. 12.1. This figure graphically presents the relationship between activity of the ascending reticular activating system (ARAS) and points along a phenomenological continuum of arousal.

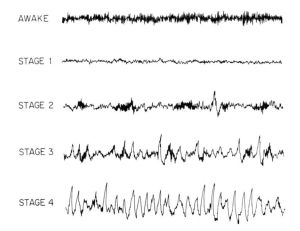

Fig. 12.2.   These five tracings represent typical EEG patterns of wakefulness and sleep stages 1 through 4.

sleep and will serve to make the point that the current classifications are not very different from the major descriptive categories set forth by the Loomis group.

As is well known, this group originally used letter designations: the letter "A" designated waking alpha rhythm; "B" through "E" corresponded roughly to EEG stages 1 through 4.

II. REM Sleep and the Temporal Course of Events

In spite of the clear knowledge that EEG patterns during sleep were not uniform, a concern with the temporal course of events did not develop until Aserinsky and Kleitman (1953) observed the occurrence of rapid binocularly synchronous eye movements during sleep in human adults. This, together with the additional observation that dream recall was high when eye movements were present radically altered the situation: the temporal course of events actually became the focus of attention. Intense interest in the temporal location and physiological concomitants of the rapid eye movement dream periods led to absolutely continuous monitoring over many hours instead of sampling techniques. As suggested earlier, the EEG was the perfect instrument because it enabled the continuous monitoring not only of brain wave patterns, but of eye movements as well. A dependable instrument, one of the first, was available in Kleitman's laboratory, and a period of intense observation began. This observation was aimed at a detailed, minute-by-minute description of the 8-hr nocturnal sleep period in man (Dement and Kleitman, 1957).

We have never fully understood why the so-called Dement–Kleitman classification of sleep stages utilizing numbers became so popular; we have always felt that it was a matter of the utmost triviality whether numbers or letters were used. We suspect the reason was simply that the Dement–Kleitman classification was the first relatively precise description of brain wave patterns during sleep. We made fairly specific statements of frequency, amplitude, and wave forms which enabled one to decide whether a pattern was or was not stage 1, stage 2, stage 3, or stage 4. In addition, these stage definitions enabled us to deal with the unprecedented mass of data which had been accumulated from multiple all-night sleep recordings before computers.

After looking at many nights of EEG records, it was apparent that all sleep epochs would indeed fit comfortably into these four levels. More significant, it was obvious that the four stages seemed to alternate in a kind of cyclic fashion. With the bursts of rapid eye movements as a guidepost, distinctly repetitive sequences of change were clearly visualized. The further understanding of the relationship between rapid eye movement periods and dreaming led to the first longitudinal generalization about the nature of sleep, the so-called basic rest activity cycle (BRAC) (Dement and Wolpert, 1958; Kleitman, 1963).

It was assumed that the characteristic all-night EEG changes represented a cyclic alternation in depth of sleep. It was further assumed that central nervous system activity at the peak of the cycle (signaled by the appearance of low voltage, relatively fast EEG patterns) was sufficient to support the psychological experience of dreaming. This psychological activity, in turn, was presumed to be responsible for other manifestations occurring at the peak of the cycle, namely, the rapid eye movements and certain other physiological events, such as respiratory and cardiovascular changes. At the time (1958), it seemed obvious that the only aspect of the rapid eye movement (REM) period which might lend it special importance for the human organism was its seemingly unique association with dream activity. Although interesting quantitative data were compiled on lengths and locations of REM and stage 4 periods, there was no concept of two kinds of sleep.

III. Two States of Sleep

Several very important observations led to drastic modification in the above formulation. The first was the finding that rapid eye movement periods also occurred in the laboratory cat (Dement, 1958). This finding greatly increased the opportunity for experimental work. In the next year, Jouvet and Michel

(1959) made one of the most outstanding observations in the history of sleep research. Every precedent favored closer scrutiny of the brain and diminished scrutiny of peripheral events, yet Jouvet and Michel had the temerity to observe the electrical activity of the muscles. They noticed a remarkable occurrence which none before had seen. Everyone had assumed that electromyographic (EMG) activity would more or less parallel depth of sleep and level of EEG activation. Jouvet and Michel found that the EMG was quite active during slow wave periods, but when EEG activation with rapid eye movements appeared, EMG activity was totally suppressed! Berger (1961) confirmed this finding in man. Thus, there was for the first time a strong suspicion that sleep was not a unitary state.

Finally, Jouvet and his colleagues (Jouvet et al., 1959; Jouvet and Michel, 1960) discovered a very unique electrical activity in the pons of the cat during REM sleep. They initially referred to this activity as "spindles," but later recognized it as bursts or clusters of individual monophasic sharp waves, or spikes. Brooks and Bizzi (1963) found the same activity in the lateral geniculate nuclei, and Mouret et al., (1963) completed the picture by describing these waves in the visual cortex. Even in human scalp recordings, it has been possible to identify certain unique features in the EEG of REM sleep. Schwartz (1962) was the first to see bursts of peculiar waves that had escaped the notice of everyone else. These waves were related to rapid eye movements and have come to be known as "sawtooth" waves. Thus, it became clear that some very unique phenomena were part of the spontaneous electrical activity of the brain during REM sleep, in addition to nonspecific arousal (Dement, 1958) or hyperarousal (Shimazono et al., 1960).

In an almost explosive way, sleep researchers realized that sleep was two processes. It is difficult to overemphasize the revolutionary nature of this shift of viewpoint. It was totally against the personal experience of sleep and was a complete departure from all previous thinking about sleep. I believe that Oswald (1962) was the first to actually state this radical new notion in print, but I think that Jouvet probably deserves the most credit because of the impact of his epochal paper (Jouvet, 1962b) which appeared later in the year. This paper summarized a tremendous amount of anatomical, physiological, and behavioral work, and clearly established the brain stem origins of REM sleep. Thus, it was recognized that the REM period was one kind of sleep and that all the rest, albeit encompassing several very different EEG patterns, was another kind of sleep.

Two kinds of sleep—what does this mean? From a taxonomic point of view, it means simply that there are two periods of sleep which, though outwardly very similar in terms of recumbency, quiescence, increased response threshold, etc., are totally dissimilar when observed more closely. Indeed, as we all know and as has been demonstrated repeatedly, nearly every physiological variable observed longitudinally during sleep shows markedly contrasting behavior as a function of the two kinds of sleep.

Nonetheless, it is apparent that some confusion still exists. Therefore, we wish to define very clearly the difference between *state* and *stage*. The term *state* usually refers to a condition in which something exists that is qualitatively different from other possible conditions in which it may exist. A specific condition or *state* is usually recognized by the necessary presence of one or more attributes that are essentially absent at other times. For example, when H_2O exists in the frozen state, it possesses attributes of solidity and rigidity that are present at no other time. In complex living organisms, the taxonomic problem of defining states becomes, to some extent, a matter of judgment and consensus. As a rule, a single variable will not suffice to define a state; a cluster of attributes whose simultaneous and repeated occurrence is highly unique must be present. It is commonly accepted that there are two, and only two *states* of sleep. They are called REM and NREM sleep and appear to be present in nearly all mammals.

The word *stage* usually refers to a relatively precise, but arbitrary subdivision in the course of a continuously progressing quantitative change. Thus, H_2O in the liquid state between 0° and 10° C could be called stage 1, from 10° to 20° could be called stage 2, and so on. It is obvious that almost any number of *stages* could be defined arbitrarily within a state. In the case of the sleeping human, only four stages defined by the EEG have been commonly accepted as subdivisions of NREM sleep. There are *no* commonly accepted subdivisions of REM sleep. This is not to say that other possibilities have not been proposed.

Stage designations, as opposed to state, become a part of discipline and its language only when they have functional significance and/or outstanding usefulness. The putative functional significance of the NREM EEG stages is that they represent levels in a NREM continuum of depth-of-sleep. These stages also show quantitative changes in several clinical conditions. It may be assumed that no stage subdivision of REM sleep has been widely accepted because a clear-cut functional significance does not exist, or has not yet been conclusively shown to exist. Certain divisions of REM sleep have been used from time to time to facilitate an experimental approach. Most frequently, such a division is used for the study of the correlation between a REM sleep-associated variable and some aspect of dreaming. For example, epochs of REM sleep have been differentially classified according to the absolute frequency of individual eye movement potentials, heart rate changes, respiratory changes, and so forth.

The realization that two entirely independent states of being alternated during the period of bodily quiescence (sleep) gave rise to two major concerns. The first concern was with the separate mechanisms of the two states, exemplified by the work of the Lyon group. This work led to the early biochemical proposal of Jouvet that NREM sleep might be dependent upon serotonergic neurons, while REM sleep might involve catecholaminergic elements (Jouvet, 1969a).

The second concern initiated by the concept of two states of sleep reflected on the age-old problem of the function of sleep. If one could distinguish two kinds of sleep, it followed that these two kinds of sleep might perform two totally different functions. Thus, it was necessary to repudiate the total sleep deprivation studies as confounding the effects of the loss of both REM and NREM sleep. It was felt that functional clarity could come only as a result of selective sleep deprivation.

The first such study involved the selective deprivation of REM sleep. The early experiments (Dement, 1960, 1965) were rather successful in eliciting the postdeprivation REM rebound, which seemed to suggest a "need" for REM sleep. In addition, there was a feeling that the rebound served a quantitative makeup function. While clarification of the specific role of REM sleep in the biological economy of the mammalian organism has remained controversial (Dement, 1969; Dement, in press; Ferguson and Dement, 1968), the mere fact that one could conceive of a possible "need" for a certain amount of REM sleep led to an augmented concern with quantification of sleep states and stages. Parenthetically, there was also a notion that stage 4 might have some unique functional significance and it was also subjected to quantitative manipulation.

Accordingly, great consternation developed when Monroe first presented the results of his study of inter-rater reliability in the scoring of sleep stages (Monroe, 1969). To wit, he found that the numbers (minutes of stage 4, REM, etc.) everyone had been presenting as experimental data did not have a generally reliable meaning. Monroe had distributed copies of exactly the same all-night sleep recording to a number of laboratories, and the results showed significantly different values for the sleep states and stages among the laboratories.

Primarily as a result of this debacle, the UCLA Brain Information Service sponsored a specific project to develop a standard manual for the scoring of human sleep stages. Under the chairmanship of Rechtschaffen and Kales, a committee was formed to set forth absolutely precise definitions of the sleep states and stages so that anyone, at least in theory, should get identical results scoring human adult sleep records. This manual has been completed (Rechtschaffen and Kales, 1968) and Monroe has set about checking its effect on inter-rater scoring reliability.

The *Standard Manual* not only details definitions of the sleep stages, but illustrates standard techniques and procedures for human sleep recording as well. Instructions are included for recording the three chief modalities used in sleep research, EEG, EOG, and EMG. Ample figures are presented in the manual for illustrating all the criteria and special rules for scoring sleep stages. To give a general idea of the thoroughness of the manual, we should like to abstract some of the sleep stage definitions:

> *Stage 1:* This stage is defined by a relatively low voltage, mixed frequency EEG with a prominence of activity in the 2–7 Hz range. The faster frequencies are mostly of lower voltage than the 2–7 Hz activity. Stage 1 occurs most often in the transition from wakefulness to the other sleep stages or following body movements during sleep. During nocturnal sleep, stage 1 tends to be relatively short, ranging from about 1 to 7 min. The highest voltage, 2–7 Hz activity (about 50 to 75 μV), tends to occur in irregularly spaced bursts mostly during the latter portions of the stage. Also during the latter portions of the stage vertex sharp waves may appear ... (whose) amplitude is occasionally as high as 200 μV ... stage 1 requires an absolute absence of clearly defined K-complexes and sleep spindles ... stage 1 ... is characterized by the presence of slow eye movements. . . . Rapid eye movements are absent. Tonic EMG levels are usually below those of relaxed wakefulness. . . . When the amount of the record characterized by alpha activity combined with low voltage activity drops to less than 5% of the epoch and is replaced by relatively low voltage, mixed frequency activity, the epoch is scored as stage 1 [see Fig. 12.3].
>
> *Stage 2:* This stage [see Fig. 12.4] is defined by the presence of sleep spindles and/or K complexes and the absence of sufficient high amplitude, slow activity to define the presence of stages 3 and 4. . . . The presence of a sleep spindle should not be defined unless it is of at least 0.5 sec duration. . . . K-complexes are defined as EEG wave forms having a well-delineated negative sharp wave which is immediately followed by a positive component. The total duration of the complex should exceed 0.5 sec. Waves of 12–14 Hz may or may not constitute a part of the complex ... [Rechtschaffen and Kales, 1968, p. 6].

The beauty of this manual is that it enables everyone to say that "this epoch

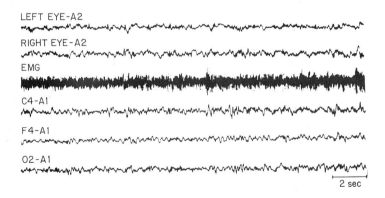

LEFT EYE-A2

RIGHT EYE-A2

EMG

C4-A1

F4-A1

O2-A1

2 sec

Fig. 12.3. Stage 1 sleep (reading down: left and right electrooculogram; electromyogram; and central, frontal, and occipital electroencephalogram). [After Rechtshaffen and Kales, 1968]

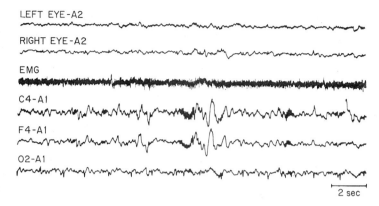

Fig. 12.4. Stage 2 sleep (reading down: left and right electrooculogram; electromyogram; and central, frontal, and occipital electroencephalogram). [After Rechtshaffen and Kales, 1968]

is REM sleep, this epoch is stage 2, this epoch is stage 4, this epoch is wakefulness," and so on.

There are many implications underlying what become arbitrary decisions about stages, but such peripheral problems usually develop when temporal quantification is involved. Thus, it is true that an epoch containing eye movements and sleep spindles both may be scored stage 2, but it is obviously true that this epoch is not pure stage 2. If transitions in sleep, and we will say more about this later, can occur at rates greater than once every 30 sec, then it is obvious that the scoring is not ultimately precise.

A similar scoring manual has recently been published (Anders *et al.*, 1971) for the scoring of sleep stages in infants. This manual was more difficult to prepare because, as will be seen later in this conference, the criteria and the actual descriptive phenomenology of sleep in newborn infants is much more complicated than in human adults.

Investigators have worked on similar standardization in other animals but very little progress has been made. Ursin (1968) has proposed a two-stage division for NREM sleep in cats. Adey *et al.* (1962) have described sleep stages in the chimpanzee and Weitzman *et al.* (1965) have described sleep stages and sleep cycles in the monkey, but precise criteria have not been widely accepted. Kales *et al.*, 1967c) and Kahn and his colleagues (1970) have described sleep in the elderly and it is clear that there are differences, particularly in that the stage 4 criteria would not apply in the elderly. Whether these problems will be solved in the same way that they have been solved in the past, or whether new ways of processing these kinds of data will simply take over and obviate the need in this area remains to be seen.

In addition to the move toward quantification, another great push in the last decade or so, which may become known as the first "golden age of sleep re-search," was a far-reaching developmental description (e.g., Anders *et al.*, 1971; Bowe-Anders *et al.*, 1972; Jouvet-Mounier *et al.*, 1970; Parmelee *et al.*, 1961; Roffwarg *et al.*, 1964, 1966) and phylogenetic description (e.g., Allison and Van Twyver, 1970; Dement, 1958; Kripke *et al.*, 1968; Reite *et al.*, 1965).

Although development of the concept of two kinds of sleep was a major advance, it was inevitably carried too far. In some way, the notion of two kinds of sleep was transmogrified so that these states became things in their own right. People began to assume, *a priori*, that what was true for one state would not be true for the other. Thus, as an example, if serotonin were the neuro-transmitter for NREM sleep, it could play no role in REM sleep. Jouvet has recognized this error in proposing that serotonin plays a priming role for the onset of REM sleep. It is almost as if people regarded a car that is moving and the same car standing still as two entirely different and unrelated entities.

In addition to influencing biochemical approaches, this notion of mutual exclusiveness definitely colored the functional approach. Thus, because the phenomenological aspects of REM and NREM sleep seemed so divergent, we felt that their functions ought to be equally divergent. The kind of mythology grew up where we assumed the selective loss of NREM sleep would lead to sleepiness, whereas the selective loss of REM sleep would lead to excitation. Because sleep loss in total sleep deprivation is around 75% NREM sleep, we assumed the overt consequences of total sleep loss primarily reflected the loss of NREM sleep. We further assumed that REM sleep loss contributed some excitation and thus diluted the effect of sleep deprivation. According to this notion, if an animal had 50% NREM and 50% REM sleep, sleep deprivation will have no effect. And if an animal had only NREM sleep, it would be more vulnerable to the depressing effects of total sleep loss than an animal that had both kinds of sleep. An attempt to test this notion was made by sleep depriving chickens. We observed that chickens did succumb to sleep loss very quickly. However, such a finding was probably more the result of anatomical considera-tions (i.e., chickens, having only two feet, are just not able to remain active as long as most mammals that have four feet). At any rate, we would like to mention a few findings that gave us pause in this regard. There is some evidence that sleep is, after all, on some level, a unitary process in opposition to wake-fulness. We would like to mention two things: one is an unpublished study by Naitoh and Johnson who totally sleep-deprived subjects for two full days and then deprived them selectively of REM or NREM stage 4 during the recovery period. They found that regardless of the procedure the recovery function proceeded at the same rate, probably being dependent only on total amount of sleep time. Second is the casual but very startling observation that the sleepiness of a narcoleptic patient, which is in no way distinguishable from the drowsiness of someone who has suffered prolonged sleep loss, can be reversed if he has 20 min of pure REM sleep. In other words, there is no cortical synchronization, no slow waves, just the furious activity of REM sleep. Yet, the sleepiness is reversed.

We are not mentioning these things to suggest that the old theorists who felt that REM and NREM were really manifestations of a unitary process were right, but merely to suggest that there is more to the problem than we think. There may be a great many things going on, some of which are common to both of the defined states of sleep and some of which are not.

IV. The Process View

This leads quite logically to a discussion of what we are calling a "process view" of sleep. The meaning of this will become apparent as we discuss these things, but essentially we are talking about the concept that sleep is really the outward manifestation of a number of processes that are going on independently, simultaneously, in combination, at different times, with different relationships, and so on. The beginning of this concept, or way of thinking about sleep, could probably be dated to the Lyon conference in 1963 and more specifically to the discussion by Professor Moruzzi in which he said it would be a very good idea to distinguish between phasic (short lasting) and tonic (long lasting) activity. This led to the notion that there were at least two things about REM sleep that might be dealt with more or less independently. Certainly, the mere fact that PGO spikes occurred prior to the defined onset of the REM period indicated that what was true for one state could be true, at least in a transition period, for the other. All of this led up to our next topic and a newer point of view. We would like now to discuss the independent processes in the states of sleep. We will start with REM sleep because it is in some ways the most interesting of the behavioral states.

Full-blown REM sleep is defined when we can note the simultaneous occurrence of at least three distinct processes. Perhaps the most essential and characteristic process of REM sleep is an actively induced tonic nonreciprocal motor inhibition. The most widely used and convenient indicator of this inhibitory process is a continuous recording of the electromyogram, or EMG. The EMG suppression is highly correlated with the onset of REM sleep (see Fig. 12.5) and with other indicators of active motor inhibition, for example, electrically induced reflex suppression in humans (Hodes and Dement, 1964) and a number of measures as studied by Pompeiano and his associates (see Pompeiano, 1965, 1970). According to Pompeiano, during REM sleep there is a tonic hyperpolarization of alpha motor neurons, and if the cataplectic attack in narcoleptic patients is representative of the effectiveness of this inhibitory process (Dement and Rechtschaffen, 1968), REM sleep is a time of profound motor paralysis, in which tendon reflexes cannot be elicited and in

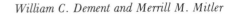

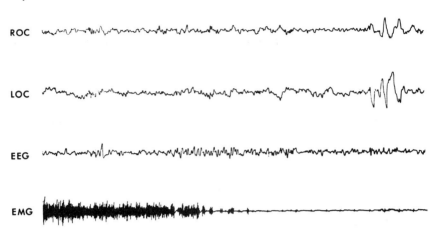

Fig. 12.5. Representative onset of REM sleep (ROC and LOC, right and left outer canthus; EEG, electroencephalogram; EMG, electromyogram of digastric muscles). Note the abrupt diminution of EMG activity associated with a flattening of the EEG and the large rapid conjugate eye movements.

which voluntary movement is totally impossible. In cats, the presence of motor paralysis is also confirmed by an extreme flaccidity. The mechanism of this inhibition is relatively unclear. Inhibitory pathways descend from the brain stem to the spinal cord in the dorsal fasciculi. There is evidence that the locus coeruleus is involved (Jouvet and Delorme, 1965) and, in some way, the lumbar spinal cord (Morrison and Bowker, 1972). This kind of inhibition, from a behavioral and global point of view, can be produced by an implantation of cholinomimetic drugs into the pontine reticular formation (George *et al.*, 1964) or by electrical stimulation of areas such as the orbital cortex (Sauerland *et al.*, 1967) and the ventromedial medulla (Magoun and Rhines, 1946) in the lightly anesthetized cat. Those of us who work with this phenomenon assume that the medullary inhibitory area of Magoun and Rhines is some sort of final common pathway.

The second process is CNS arousal. It is a well-known fact that in many respects the brain in REM sleep appears to be aroused or awake. We must, therefore, postulate some sort of nonspecific arousal process as a system that operates more or less tonically during REM periods. It is a matter of great puzzlement whether the observed CNS arousal is true wakefulness or a totally different process which merely resembles wakefulness in terms of most of the nonspecific measures of CNS activity levels such as brain temperature, EEG activation, cerebral blood flow, and so forth. Certain differences between wakefulness and REM sleep could, of course, be quantitative. Thus, atropine might block EEG activation during waking behavior but not during REM sleep at one dose, but would block EEG activation in both states at a higher dose. Early studies suggested different pathways by showing that lesions in the reticular formation brought about prolonged EEG synchronization in wakefulness, yet, when REM periods occurred, normal EEG activation was seen. Recent behavioral observations in narcoleptics lead us to feel that perhaps REM arousal is truly the same arousal process as in wakefulness. That is, the awake brain in the narcoleptic appears to be gradually preempted by internal hallucinatory activity, but that at some point, the narcoleptic on the verge of full-blown REM sleep is clearly awake in terms of the usual definitions of wakefulness.

The third, and most interesting process which is so highly characteristic of REM sleep is called phasic activity. The exact definition of phasic activity is still somewhat up in the air; the underlying neurophysiology is far from clear. Different people will think of different things when the term is used. In its most global definition, phasic activity refers to short-lasting events. The exact interval beyond which this definition would not apply has not been specified nor would it be practically useful to do so. Generally we are thinking of phenomena lasting for a second or less. These events may, of course, occur in bursts. The most important aspect of this phasic activity derives from the assumption that phasic activity is generated exclusively from *within* the brain. What are some examples of phasic activity? The first activity to be described, of course, was the rapid jerk of the eyeballs. Such eye movements occur in bursts or singly and in all directions and sizes of arc. This activity was discovered in man and subsequently in the cat and numerous other animals. Other things we can mention are muscle twitches (Baldridge *et al.*, 1965), sudden changes in pupil diameter (Berlucchi *et al.*, 1964a), sharp fluctuations in penile tumescence (Fisher *et al.*, 1965), cardiovascular irregularities (Baust and Bohnert, 1969; Gassel *et al.*, 1964c), phasic middle ear contractions (Baust *et al.*, 1964; Dewson *et al.*, 1965), and finally the unique bursts of high amplitude biphasic sharp waves in the electrical recordings from the pons, ocular motor nuclei, lateral geniculate nuclei, and visual cortices of the cat (the PGO wave) (Mikiten *et al.*, 1961; Jouvet and Michel, 1959; Mouret *et al.*, 1963; Brooks, 1967). Many people have speculated that these PGO waves are the primary phasic event in that they in some way trigger eye movements, middle ear muscle contractions, and so on. Certainly, if there were a generator for PGO waves, this generator might stimulate many areas of the brain where a potential change resembling a PGO wave could not be recorded. This is suggested by unit studies which show phasic bursts of firing in almost every area of the brain without exception which seem to be correlated fairly well with PGO waves. Thus, it is important to know whether or not every other phasic event is uniformly linked in time to the occurrence of PGO waves. Another problem is whether or not the PGO wave is unique to REM sleep since there are waves in the lateral geniculate which appear to be merely a response to eye movements in the waking state. Currently there is a controversy as to whether these eye movement potentials have the same anatomical substrate as the REM PGO wave. At the present time, clear relationships have been described in the cat between PGO waves and eye movements, twitches, and other phasic phenomena. It is also clear that PGO waves appear to lead the defined onset of the REM period by a minute or more. It is important to emphasize here that there is little cross-species data to affirm (1) the apparent "pacemaker" properties of the feline PGO wave *vis-a-vis* other phasic events and (2) the generality of the distribution of the feline PGO wave in sleep. Nevertheless, we all assume that there is some phasic generator in all the many mammalian and avian species who have REM sleep characterized by other phasic events such as muscle twitches and eye movements. The desire to look at this activity in association with dreaming in humans has led to a search for some sort of PGO analog in humans. There are three important candidates. The first is the phasic integrated muscle potential (PIP) described by Rechtschaffen *et al.* (1972a), who observed that discharge in the eye muscle was always associated with PGO waves in the cat and decided to look at this activity in the human. Second, the phasic EMG suppression described by Pivik and Dement (1970), which is apparently analogous to the phasic inhibition described by Pompeiano (1970), can be seen only during NREM sleep in humans because it is observed against the tonically active EMG background. It has been confirmed by H-reflex studies that such phasic inhibition is short lasting but generalized. Third, there are EEG events which may be related to phasic activity. The sawtooth waves of REM sleep could be human cortical or scalp derivations of phasic electrical activity, and the so-called K-complex, seen more frequently in NREM sleep, may represent a kind of response to some spontaneously occurring internal event.

What about NREM sleep? Most people think of NREM sleep as slow waves and spindles in the EEG and further feel that these imply a kind of deactivation of the brain. However, we might ask the question, what is the essential difference between being awake and being asleep? As far as we can determine, the salient feature of wakefulness is the environmental engagement of the organism. He sees, hears, and responds to the world around him. The onset of sleep, which seems to be the onset of NREM sleep in most humans, entails the cessation of the above processes. There is a moment somewhere in the transition from wakefulness to sleep where the organism essentially, though not entirely, stops perceiving his environment. This is not, we hasten to add, the moment at which slow waves and spindles appear. Therefore, the significance of spindles and slow waves in the EEG may not be crucial, convenient though they may be as "signs" of slow wave sleep.

It is important to be aware of the fact that many characteristics that we call correlates of NREM sleep or sleep in general are not necessary correlates.

Most of them, such as lower blood pressure, lower heart rate, and lower body temperature can be achieved by prolonged recumbancy and relaxation or by prolonged meditation. Thus, at some point the additional development of frank sleep entails no further change in these variables.

The moment of sleep (i.e., the cessation of perception) is apparently quite abrupt. While there may be important predisposing changes leading up to it, and consequences of its occurrence leading away from it, the point of sleep onset itself seems relatively easy to determine within a second or two. For example, suppose we ask an individual to sit with his eyes taped open and to make a motor response when a light flash (S^d) is presented. At some point he will not respond to the S^d. The moment of sleep is best defined as the point of perceptual disengagement (i.e., failure to respond to the S^d). Immediately after such a failure the EEG patterns may still show waking patterns, such as alpha rhythm. Thus we could conceivably abolish slow waves and spindles without abolishing the process of perceptual disengagement. Accordingly, we must acknowledge that it is not clear if slow waves and spindles are processes which really begin at the point of response inhibition and only build up enough to appear in the EEG a few minutes later, or are entirely separate and perhaps redundant processes. But until proven otherwise, we must think of slow waves and spindles as meaningful although often belated signs of a central inhibitory state. However, aside from the kind of behavioral study we have mentioned, even the more sophisticated neurophysiological techniques, such as unit activity studies, have not shown changes in firing patterns that are commensurate with the vast functional differences among states. It may be, however, that such studies compare unit activity at the onset of sleep (i.e., after perceptual changes but before the conventional signs such as slow waves and spindles) with the sleep stage a few minutes later when slow waves and spindles have appeared. At the present time, the best sign of the moment of sleep appears to be the breakdown of visual fixation and the appearance of slow eye movements. According to other investigators, pupillary myosis in dim light may also be such a precise sign, the implication being that pupillary myosis precedes slow waves and spindles as do slow eye movements and perceptual disengagement. Thus, we may conclude that there may be at least two independent processes in NREM sleep, the control of cortical rhythms being one and the higher processing of sensory input being the other.

V. Dissociative Aspects of Sleep and Wakefulness: Implications for the Process View of the Sleep States

At this time, the significance of this discussion must be clarified. We can take any phenomenon and conceptually divide it into "independent processes," but the real test is whether these processes can be experimentally dissociated from one another on a temporal basis. This is crucial to both the whole issue of whether states are really different things and whether processes are really independent.

The best place to start this discussion is in the area of phasic activity. Phasic activity, as exemplified by the PGO spike, always shows some dissociation from REM sleep. From over 2000 REM periods distributed among various sleep episodes of perhaps 20 to 30 cats in our laboratory, we failed to find, in normal intact cats, a single instance where REM sleep (as defined by EEG activation closely followed by EMG suppression and eye movements) ever occurred before at least a few PGO waves (usually 10–30 waves) had preceded. Thus, the first event to appear of the three we have discussed is phasic activity. Generally, it appears for about 30 sec as single PGO waves. In addition, phasic activity in the form of PGO waves is far more distributed throughout slow wave sleep than most people realize. Although absolutely characteristic of REM periods in the cat, it is also true that phasic activity in the form of PGO waves may be present in more than 50% of the total amount of NREM sleep, at least in certain cats. In addition, intervals of NREM sleep in the cat in which there are absolutely no PGO waves at all are relatively brief, for the most part no longer than 2 or 3 min. Discharge rate of PGO spikes during REM period varies from cat to cat, ranging from about 40 per minute to more than 100. The discharge rate during epochs of NREM sleep are highly variable, although well below the rates seen during REM periods. The total number of PGO spikes per day in the cat has been estimated to vary between 10,000 and 20,000. Approximately 15% of this total typically occurs in NREM sleep as defined by slow waves and spindles in the EEG and the presence of tonic electrical activity in the neck muscles. Most of the other phasic activities tend to be less prominent in NREM sleep but the truth of the matter is that we have not looked at them closely. Thus, there may be occasional rapid eye movements in NREM sleep, occasional fluctuations in heart rate, penile tumescence, and so on, but we have simply not emphasized these findings. In other areas there is no question that phasic activity is widely distributed in NREM sleep. Rechtschaffen has reported a plentiful and almost continual discharge of PIPs in NREM sleep (Rechtschaffen and Chernick, 1972). Dement and Pivik (1970) have reported the same for EMG suppressions (see Fig. 12.6).

Finally, K-complexes, if they represent phasic activity, also are distributed throughout NREM sleep. Thus, there is this normal dissociation. If we look at the EMG suppression, we find that it, too, can precede the onset of the REM period, often by a minute or more. In one of the early studies of long-term REM sleep deprivation, we observed that the gap between EMG suppression and EEG activation (NREM stage 2 to REM stage 1) underwent a steady enlargement. If motor inhibition were shifted to the waking state, it

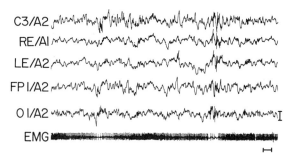

Fig. 12.6. Three examples of phasic EMG suppression during sleep in the human (derivations reading downward: central electroencephalogram; right and left electrooculogram; frontal electroencephalogram; occipital electroencephalogram; and electromyogram. Calibrations: 1 sec and 100 μV).

would be cataplexy. This had never been accomplished experimentally by REM sleep deprivation, although it is seen consistently in narcoleptic patients. Penile tumescence, which appears to be a consistent concomitant of REM periods in humans and monkeys, has been reported to occur in NREM sleep in humans if REM sleep is prevented from occurring. Surgical dissociations have been accomplished: for example, the locus coeruleus preparation of Jouvet and Delorme (1965) and the lesions of the brain stem which permit waking behavior in the presence of slow waves and spindles in the EEG. Perhaps the most striking dissociations of these so-called state manifestations can be produced by neuropharmacologic manifestations. The classical finding in this vein is described in a report by Wikler (1952) on the effects of high doses of atropine in dogs. These animals showed waking behavior simultaneous with clear-cut NREM sleep patterns in the EEG (slow waves and spindles). One of the most interesting and striking dissociations in cats was accomplished by the administration of compounds which caused a marked reduction in the level of serotonin in the brain, notably PCPA and reserpine (Ferguson *et al.*, 1969b; Dement *et al.*, 1972a; Delorme *et al.*, 1965). In the former case adequate treatment was associated with a spectacular occurrence of PGO waves during what otherwise appears to be a normal waking state. By treating PGO waves as independent processes in PCPA or REM deprivation preparations, which allow PGO activity to be studied under conditions resistant to nonspecific experimental influences, some advances have been made in understanding the PGO waves' biochemical mechanisms. For example, looking at PGO waves alone, there is plentiful evidence to suggest that serotonin is an inhibitory regulator of this activity and that, in some way, the PGO wave is cholinergic in nature. It is clear that in certain doses, atropine will suppress PCPA-induced waking PGO waves (Jacobs *et al.*, 1972), but although atropine can block normal PGO waves in REM sleep, it will not block REM sleep *per se* (Henriksen *et al.*, 1972).

VI. Microepochs: A Closer Look at
the Temporal Process in Sleep

One of the major reasons for assuming that the states of sleep are very stable continuous phenomena, at least in adults, has been the arbitrary decision involved in the size of the epoch that will be scored. Thus, if we must call a 30-sec epoch wakefulness, or sleep, or REM sleep, we may overlook as many as three or four clear-cut changes of state within this epoch. Along this line we also overlook in NREM sleep scoring the occurrence of phasic events, such as PIPs, K-complexes, EMG suppressions, an occasional eye movement, and the like. Out of curiosity to know a little more about this, we decided to look at sleep stages in the cat to the nearest 3 sec; in other words, we adopted a 3-sec scoring epoch (Ferguson et al., 1960a). The appropriate criteria were set up and then every 3-sec epoch throughout a 24-hr recording period was scored. This meant scoring 28,800 epochs per day. Figure 12.7 presents some examples of the fact that brief state transitions do occur. We felt that their behavioral significance was just as great as when behavioral states are scored by conventional methods. In other words, a cat could apparently be soundly asleep, wake up, look around, and apparently be soundly asleep again within only a few seconds. When we examined distributions of un-interrupted intervals of wakefulness scored to the nearest 3 sec, and the un-interrupted intervals of NREM sleep scored to the nearest 3 sec, we found the vast majority of such intervals were very short, on the order of 1–2 min.

Thus, it should be clear that sleep, wakefulness, REM sleep, and phasic events are far more dynamic than we have ever imagined or been willing to face. This is particularly relevant when considering experimental attempts to extirpate states as in sleep deprivation and REM deprivation. For example, after an excessively long period of wakefulness, microsleeps begin to occur. As the potency of sleep systems increases, these microsleeps become much more frequent and perhaps they finally reach a point during which we assume that the subject is awake but is getting considerable amounts of sleep in microparcels. In other words, the sleep process begins to intrude upon wake-fulness. The same thing may happen in REM deprivation where REM pro-cesses begin to intrude upon slow wave sleep and upon wakefulness (e.g., more PGO waves in slow wave sleep). A crude analogy for this process would be the damming up of a stream. Eventually the water begins to overflow the banks in many little rivulets.

VII. The Failure of Total and Selective Deprivation
to Elucidate Functional Consequences

Given all of the preceding discussion about independent processes, dyna-mism dissociations, and so forth, it is immediately obvious that deprivation

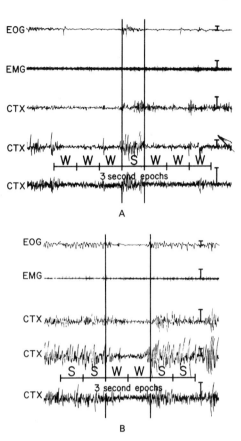

Fig. 12.7. Polygraph tracings of sleep and wakefulness in the cat (EOG, electro-oculogram; EMG, electromyogram from the dorsal neck muscles; CTX, various derivations from the cerebral cortex; calibration: 100 μV). Note the rapid change from slow wave sleep (S) to wakefulness (W). B. Depicts a reverse case. Scoring in 3-sec epochs will resolve such transitions.

of states, analogous to the extirpation of a cerebellum, a kidney, or the prevention of food intake, is just not a valid approach. What does it mean to waken an organism at the precise point where EEG activation occurs if he has already had a minute of PGO waves and a minute of EMG suppression? What does it mean if he has had EEG activation but EMG suppression has not yet occurred? What if he has a few seconds of slow waves and spindles in the EEG? It seems apparent that at some point an equilibrium is reached, and indeed, most of the deprivation studies, whether they be total or partial, show this. Figure 12.8 illustrates by showing that further effects of selective REM sleep deprivation cannot be attained beyond 20 to 30 days of deprivation. The more one attempts to deprive REM sleep, the more effective REM processes must become; inevitably, an equilibrium point is always attained.

A final consequence which we feel deserves discussion because it will undoubtedly come up on the remainder of this conference, is the question of the phasic generator. There are three possibilities. First, there may be one phasic

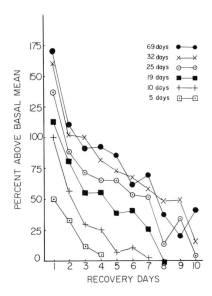

Legend:
69 days ●——●
32 days ×——×
25 days ⊙——⊙
19 days ■——■
10 days +——+
5 days ▱——▱

Fig. 12.8. Percent of REM sleep above base line means as a function of days after REM deprivation. The curves summarize the recovery of six cats after undergoing individual periods of REM deprivation ranging from 5 to 69 days in duration. Note that after 25 days of REM deprivation the recovery curves all share the same general shape and acceleration.

generator whose discharge is accurately indicated by PGO waves, middle ear muscle contractions and other phasic events more or less independently and not all simultaneously. There is some evidence in favor of this possibility. For example, middle ear muscle contractions apparently do not always co-incide with PGO waves (Roffwarg, personal communication). Third, there may be many phasic generators which may discharge synchronously or not, depending upon many other factors. To decide among these possibilities would involve gathering extensive data on the temporal distribution of many phasic events and determining the conditional probabilities of detecting each phasic event for all combinations of the remaining phasic events. Even this approach involves the dubiously appropriate assumption that the time of experimental detection of each event's occurrence is negligibly different from that of the actual necessary and sufficient neurophysiological processes under-lying each phasic event studied.

VIII. The Psychological Side of Sleep

The emphasis of this conference is on physiology and biochemistry, but we cannot totally ignore the psychological side of the coin. Therefore, we would like to say few words about dreaming.

Clearly, the associations of REM sleep with dreaming has preoccupied the attention of many sleep researchers, at least in the United States. The under-standing of dreaming, particularly the physiological substrate, presupposes an adequate conceptualization of the two kinds of sleep. Notions such as "what is true for one state cannot be true for another" may be counterproductive. Consequently, the process view has stimulated a great deal of renewed activity in this area. When REM sleep was first discovered and it was shown that a high incidence of vivid detailed dream recall could be obtained 80% of the time when subjects were wakened during REM periods. It was quickly assumed that REM sleep and dreaming were essentially synonymous. Since REM sleep was so different from NREM sleep, we more or less tacitly assumed NREM sleep was a kind of psychological vacuum. Many psychodynamic studies were attempted using REM sleep as the measure of dreaming, and seeing whether or not dreaming would increase or decrease in a variety of situations. The concept of exclusivity was quickly challenged by Foulkes (1962) who got reports of dreaming and dream content from awakenings in NREM sleep with a fairly high incidence. Previous studies which found 5% to 10% NREM recall were discarded as normal variability. Since Foulkes's study, and a number of others, the existence of NREM dreaming has been widely accepted and has left those concerned with the problem of the dream's physiological substrate in something of a dilemma. Associated difficulties include adequate definitions of dreaming, adequate ways of scoring the subject's report when he is awakened, allowing for memory lapses, confusion, and time of night. When all is said and done, what most people would call vivid dreaming is reported approximately 80% of the time across all subjects and across all arousals from the middle of REM periods. Something like 20% to 30% may be reported from all NREM arousals across subjects and across nights. However, investigators have pointed out that there is much more subject-to-subject variability in NREM recall than in REM recall. If REM sleep *per se* is not the best correlate of dream recall, or of dreaming, then what is? The process view of sleep has been most helpful in making progress on this issue. One promising process approach is the PIP awakening technique of Rechtschaffen's group (Rechtschaffen *et al.*, 1972a,b; Watsonn, 1972).

IX. New Directions in Sleep Research

At this point it is appropriate to look at new trends in sleep research. Obviously we expect continued advances from the laboratories of Michel Jouvet in the biochemical and anatomical mechanisms of sleep. We would like to mention possible trends in better description. Such new directions will come from increasing the intensity with which we observe sleep processes.

The first area is data processing. As the scope of our observations extends in time, among species, and into odd locations, like the moon, the sky lab, and perhaps Mars, it becomes necessary to process more and more data.

Further, in addition to the classical measurement of EEG, EOG, and EMG, we have become much more interested in recording other variables when possible. In the human this includes blood pressure, cardiac functions, and respiration. In animals additional variables include primarily unit data, biochemical data by push-pull cannulae, and reflex facilitation. The most important thing is use of the computer in a manner analogous to the human scorer. Systems have been developed by Itil (1969, 1970), by the Florida group (Smith et al., 1971; Smith and Karacan, 1971), and by others (Johnson *et al.*, 1969) that will perform this task. To date, while computers perform much more rapidly, they are not really able to match the accuracy of human scorers. However, one implication is that the standards, presumably more consistent, which are used in computer scoring, will in some way shape our future concepts of sleep. The computer may also be used to look at other events in the sleep period in ways analogous to that which obviated the drudgery of looking at evoked potentials. There are now programs for counting K-complexes, eye movements, and PGO spikes. Advanced techniques of pattern recognition, masking techniques and so forth may apply in recognizing patterns of discharge, phasic activity units, and other electrophysiological phenomena. We have just begun to utilize advanced methods of data processing in this area, but we expect great advances in the future. This may also include fairly radical departures in looking at the data. An example of this is the Stanford Slowgram (Sinha *et al.*, 1972) and a similar approach developed by Johnson *et al.* (1969) in terms of delta cycles. The point is that instead of looking at the amount of stage 4 we measure the decay in amplitude, the rate of rise, and so on. All of this can be done almost totally by a computer at the end of the night and written out. Figure 12.9 illustrates a Stanford Slowgram.

A second area which will unquestionably be of greater importance in the ensuing years is the area of circadian rhythms and their relation to functional problems of sleep (Aschoff, 1969; Halberg, 1953). At the present time, almost nothing is known about these interactions except that sleep is favored at certain phases of the circadian oscillation. A recent study in our laboratory (Dement *et al.*, 1972b) suggests that circadian programming of sleep stages may override the conventional contingency point of view wherein REM sleep can only occur after a certain amount of slow wave sleep. In this study, one subject lived on a 90-min cycle (30 min sleep and 60 min of wakefulness) for 6 days. The limited sleep period obviated the normal occurrence of REM sleep. Yet, although the subject obtained approximately 5 hr of sleep per 24 hr, REM sleep occurred during 16 of the sleep periods. In fact, many sleep onset REM periods were seen. It is interesting to note that this simple alteration of scheduling produced sleep onset REM periods quite easily as opposed to the heroic methods of REM sleep deprivation or pharmacological manipulation utilized in the past. We do not know what happens to sleep sequencing when phase relationships are

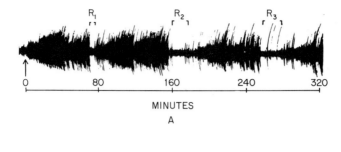

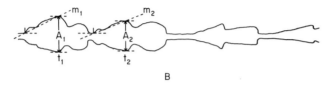

Fig. 12.9. A. Cortical electroencephalogram of a human male recorded on a compressed time scale during a night's sleep. R_1, R_2 and R_3 are REM sleep periods. B. Diagrammatic representation of sleep electroencephalogram. m_1 and m_2 are rates of approaching maximum EEG amplitude cycles 1 and 2 respectively. A_1 and A_2 are midpoints of the maximum amplitude plateau in that particular cycle. [After Sinha et al., 1972]

radically altered or when the organism is free-running. It is quite possible to interpret many of the sleep deprivation effects in terms of phase alterations. To further underscore the importance of circadian rhythms, we should note that if we assume that sleep–wakefulness is biochemically controlled, we will have to explain eventually why there are large circadian changes in level and turnover of biogenic amines, but very small changes in these variables as a function of state (Sinha et al., 1973).

Finally, there is going to be a great increase of activity in the area of sleep pathology. Even though sophisticated sleep research has been pursued for approximately 10 years or more, our knowledge about the so-called primary sleep pathologies is still in its infancy. An example of this is the notion of insomnia. Even today, we retain a monolithic concept of insomnia that reduced sleep is the primary symptom. Yet there are many complications. It is known from Jouvet's work that almost total insomnia can occur as a result of certain brain lesions (see Jouvet, 1969a,b). Kales et al. (1969) has well described drug dependency insomnia, the insomnia caused by the chronic use of sleeping pills. There is our surprising finding that many clinical patients with profound insomnia, as defined by history, turn out to sleep more than most people (Dement et al., in press); and finally, we have recently described an entirely new syndrome, the insomnia–sleep apnea syndrome, as a result of merely looking more intensively at our patients (Guilleminault *et al.*, in press). What other ailments are lurking under the rubric of disturbed sleep? In the area of hypersomnia, Mouret and his co-workers (1972) have recently described a totally new syndrome, which he calls the nonwakefulness syndrome. Mouret has also pointed out that there are at least two kinds of narcolepsy based on 24 hr sleep recordings.

These are only a few of the many areas in which we expect sleep research to be even more active in the future. Indeed, it is almost time for the area to be viewed as a discipline with specialized training, clinical practioners, and so on.

In conclusion, we cannot help mentioning that in our years of work, we have continually been asked if sleep research is sort of "petering out". Sometimes we think it may be, but on reflection, we realize that sleep research is branching into many new areas. Sleep research continues to accelerate and exciting new findings continue to pour from the laboratory. As the remainder of this book will show, challenging problems face us and lure us on. We hope that research can make progress on what continue to be the greatest mysteries: Why does REM sleep exist? Why does NREM sleep exist? Do we really need sleep, and if so, how much do we need? These questions may turn out to be pseudoproblems, but whatever the outcomes may be, we are sure they would be great surprises if we could see them now from our present vantage point.

ACKNOWLEDGMENTS

We wish to thank Mary Carskadon, Steve Henriksen, Barry Jacobs, and Terry Pivik for their assistance in manuscript preparation and allowing us to summarize some of their research findings.

CHAPTER THIRTEEN

Pharmacology of Sleep

IAN OSWALD

The techniques of human sleep research that have evolved in recent years have opened up a new area of pharmacological study. Illustrations have been forthcoming of how the brain changes slowly in the course of weeks under the influence of a drug and how it recovers slowly during the weeks after a drug has stopped. It cannot yet be said that each class of CNS drugs has a characteristic profile of action on sleep variables but there are indications of that kind: For example, the monoamine oxidase inhibitors (MAOIs) may slightly increase paradoxical sleep, or bring it on early when first administered, but when given repeatedly in adequate dose will, after some days, cause complete abolition of the signs of paradoxical sleep. Likewise, the benzodiazepine hypnotics appear to differ from most other hypnotics in that they suppress stages 3 and 4 sleep.

I. Rebounds of Paradoxical Sleep

A great many drugs reduce the proportion of sleep spent as paradoxical sleep. After repeated consumption of such drugs and then withdrawal, there is a rebound increase above normal that tends to persist. Return to base line occurs slowly in the course of about 2 months. The rebound cannot be considered as a simple compensation for the lost paradoxical sleep. It is much larger than is found after depriving subjects of paradoxical sleep by selective awakenings and commonly reaches 150–200% of the loss (Oswald, 1969).

One common feature of rebound of paradoxical sleep after drug withdrawal is seen in the delay or latency between first falling asleep and the first episode of paradoxical sleep of the night. In about 98% of instances normal young subjects have a delay or latency exceeding 45 min. After drug withdrawal it may be zero, or may just be a few minutes. Latencies shorter than 45 min may persist for as much as 2 months.

In Fig. 13.1 is shown the general pattern of the time course of effects on paradoxical sleep caused by the common hypnotic drugs. The very existence of a rebound makes it at once obvious that the classical drug trial requires rethinking. Very commonly, such trials have included a brief period on placebo, a brief period on drug A, a brief period on placebo again, a brief period on drug B, and variations on this order. The placebo period that follows the administration of either drug A or drug B is likely to be abnormal in a direction opposite to the drug effects, merely because the drug had previously been given. Furthermore, the patients in such trials have usually been on other hypnotics previously. Ideally they would have to be withdrawn from all other drugs about 2 months before a trial started.

The time taken for the rebound curve of Fig. 13.1 to reach its peak appears to

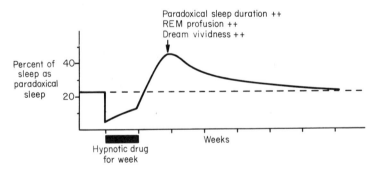

Fig. 13.1. When a hypnotic, such as amylobarbitone sodium, 400 mg, is given, sleep is altered and, among other things, the proportion spent as paradoxical sleep is reduced. Continued administration is associated with a reduced effect, as one manifestation of tolerance brought about by neuronal modifications. These modifications persist after the drug is withdrawn and cause rebound abnormalities opposite in kind to those initially caused by the drug. The inevitable but slow turnover of neuronal protein is believed to underly the gradual elimination after withdrawal of the drug-instituted neuronal modifications, but this takes several weeks. The number of days between stopping the drug and the peak of the rebound reflects the time taken for the drug to leave the brain.

depend upon the time taken to eliminate the drug from the brain. Consequently, it depends upon the nature of the drug and upon the dose that had been taken. After withdrawing small quantities of sodium amylobarbitone, about 2 days may elapse to reach the peak (Oswald and Priest, 1965). After a very large dose of phenobarbitone that takes 3 weeks to disappear from the blood stream, the rebound takes 3 weeks to reach its peak (Haider and Oswald, 1970). After heroin, where the urinary products of the drug may take 10 days to disappear, the rebound peak is similarly delayed (Lewis *et al.*, 1970).

The degree to which an hypnotic drug will lead to a curve like that shown in Fig. 13.1 depends upon the nature of the drug and the dose. The larger the dose, the more likely such an effect is to appear. In the case of 150 mg methaqualone, there may be no discernible effect on the paradoxical sleep percentage, but paradoxical sleep may nevertheless be altered, as manifested by a decrease in the profusion of rapid eye movements (Rechtschaffen *et al.*, 1970).

II. Tricyclic Antidepressants

Many other drugs besides hypnotics will cause an effect on paradoxical sleep similar to that seen in Fig. 13.1, for example, many of the tricyclic antidepressant drugs. The most powerful among these appears to be chlorimipramine, but imipramine and desipramine appear very similar and all three cause a rebound lasting about 1 month (Dunleavy *et al.*, 1972). On the other hand, trimipramine, a widely used antidepressant, has no such effects, which would appear to indicate that there is no direct correlation between antidepressant effect and suppression of REM sleep, contrary to certain theories that have been put forward. The effect on paradoxical sleep of tricyclic drugs such as imipramine diminishes during continued administration. By way of contrast, imipramine, chlorimipramine, and desipramine cause increased intrasleep restlessness, as manifested by an increased frequency of shifts to stage 1 sleep or wakefulness from any other stage of sleep per unit time. The latter effect of the drugs *does not diminish* with the passage of a month and there is *no rebound* when the drugs cease. Doxepin, which is widely held to have some daytime sedative properties, appears to reduce intrasleep restlessness (Dunleavy *et al.*, 1972).

One may note that chlorimipramine is the most potent of all these antidepressant drugs in increasing the serotonin (5-HT) "available" to receptors. The fact that it makes sleep much more restless assorts oddly with the claims that have been made that serotonin is a sleep-inducing agent. Desipramine is much more potent in increasing the noradrenaline available to receptors, whereas imipramine is the more potent of the two in increasing the available serotonin. It is therefore interesting that these two drugs appear to have

identical effects upon paradoxical sleep (Dunleavy *et al.*, 1972), suggesting that
the available norepinephrine and serotonin have nothing to do with the suppression of REM sleep.

A wide variety of drugs and a wide variety of other conditions causing organic
impairment of the brain reduce paradoxical sleep percentages. As Hartmann
has aptly said, it is a "fragile" condition. Very few drugs will increase paradoxical sleep, but among these are reserpine (Hartmann, 1966), possibly LSD
(Muzio *et al.*, 1966), L-tryptophan in narcoleptic patients (Evans and Oswald,
1966), and 5-hydroxytryptohan in man (Wyatt *et al.*, 1971a) and rabbits
(Tabushi and Himwich, 1970). The effects on sleep of drugs that may interfere
with brain amines seem to vary greatly according to the species studied.

III. Need for Chronic Studies

When one conducts pharmacological studies using sleep as a tool, one learns
through bitter experience how important it is to conduct chronic studies. The
initial effects of monoamine oxidase inhibitors may be to increase paradoxical
sleep, and the same has been seen with a small dose of chlorpromazine (Evans
and Lewis, 1969) and also debrisoquine (Dunleavy *et al.*, 1972). If one conducts
an acute study, using only a single night, one can easily get a misleading
answer. Most striking are the MAOIs. Phenelzine given in a daily dose
of 90 mg can abolish all signs of paradoxical sleep after about 5 days, but
if it is only given in a dosage of 60 mg daily it may take about 3 weeks before
the signs of paradoxical sleep are abolished. In the first week there may be
no discernible effect upon that particular variable.

IV. Other Types of Drug Effects

The preceding discussion has concentrated upon paradoxical sleep and in
the early years of drug studies of this kind it was paradoxical sleep that was
seen to be so very sensitive to drugs. However, we should not forget that the
EEG rhythms themselves may be changed by drugs. Tricyclic antidepressants,
for example, can cause enhancement of the sleep spindles (Lewis and Oswald,
1969), while many hypnotics, including the barbiturates and some of the
benzodiazepines, cause enhanced fast activity at about 18 Hz, most easily seen
during stage 1 or during paradoxical sleep. Stages 3 and 4 sleep are also much
affected by some drugs and just as one may have to wait for many weeks for
recovery in paradoxical sleep, so one may have to wait for weeks after stages
3 and 4 have been suppressed by a single large dose of hypnotic drug (Haider
and Oswald, 1970). When one has seen how many weeks are needed for recovery of human sleep after a single large dose of a hypnotic, one cannot but

wish that similar studies had been conducted with rats. It appears to have been common to implant electrodes after a single large dose of a barbiturate and then commence studies of sleep a few days later. If the human studies are any guide, base line measures at such a time could be totally misleading.

Rebounds of paradoxical sleep are well known, but other variables can also show rebound after drug withdrawal. An example is phenelzine (Akindele *et al.*, 1969), withdrawal of which can cause increased intrasleep restlessness (just the opposite of what would be expected if it were a "stimulant" drug, as pharmacologists sometimes have loosely classed it). More commonly, rebounds of increased intrasleep restlessness are seen following the withdrawal of hypnotics, whether after a long-continued modest dose or after a single massive dose (Haider and Oswald, 1970).

One can also see negative rebounds (Oswald, 1970). The drug fenfluramine causes increased intrasleep restlessness and when it is withdrawn there is sometimes a rebound inertia, as Fig. 13.2 illustrates. Likewise, the same drug can cause a rebound of stages 3 and 4 sleep (Lewis *et al.*, 1971). In the case of a drug that is fairly quickly metabolized, there may be an *intranight* rebound, in which, for example, paradoxical sleep is suppressed at the beginning of the night but increases to well above normal values in the later part of the night. The overall effect may be to mislead one into thinking the drug does not have any action on paradoxical sleep and it is always important to study the effect

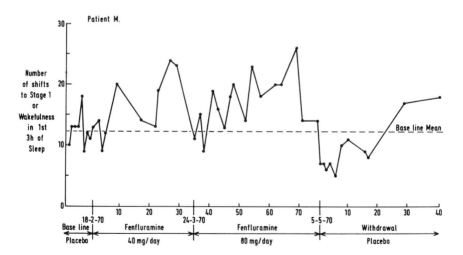

Fig. 13.2. Increase of intrasleep restlessness above the base line mean during fenfluramine intake and a fall below base line in the week after withdrawal of the drug. Among the 45 recorded nights the lowest values are on the five that immediately follow withdrawal.

of the drug upon the intranight distribution of sleep variables (e.g., Oswald, 1970).

V. Behavioral Correlates

When one reflects upon the very great increase of research into brain function and particularly sleep in the past 20 years, one has to recognize that the money has been made available because grant-giving bodies have hoped that in the long run clinical benefits would ensue. It is therefore important that research should relate if possible to the clinical scene. One may, for example, try and measure behavior concomitantly with the measurements of brain variables while drugs are being administered over a period of weeks. There is some evidence, for example, that in those depressed patients who respond to phenelzine there is a relation in time between the delay to the abolition of paradoxical sleep sign and the delay to mood improvement (Akindele *et al.*, 1969; Wyatt *et al.*, 1971b).

Equally, one may look for behavioral correlates of the rebound. After fenfluramine has been administered for some months, there is a rebound of paradoxical sleep when the drug is withdrawn and the rebound curve reaches its peak at 4 days after withdrawal. Self-ratings of mood conducted throughout the same time indicate that depression of mood may appear when this amphetamine derivative is withdrawn and may be at its worst about 4 days after drug withdrawal. In the case of the same appetite-reducing drug, we have also seen evidence of an appetite rebound (Oswald *et al.*, 1971).

In conclusion, we may say that sleep research offers techniques for looking at the human brain with clinical doses of drugs. By observing the long time course of events, one may gain some insight into basic brain mechanisms and be led to psychophysiological correlations. Finally, I must again emphasize that the effects of drugs on the sleeping brain depend upon the species, the dose, and the time since first administration, and must emphasize once more the importance of conducting chronic studies if one is not to obtain misleading results.

Discussion

Question: Might the REM effect, the rebound effect, be due to a protein?
Oswald: When you keep a human or an animal selectively deprived of paradoxical sleep by waking them, and when they later show a rebound, I cannot think of anything else that something is building up. We know that

some withdrawal effects can be prevented by concurrent administration of protein synthesis inhibitors at the same time as the drug. Something changes in the brain. So the brain must be producing something that acts against the drugs. If the brain has been changed by continuous administration of the drug what can we learn from the long rebound period? For instance, heroin has a rebound period of $2\frac{1}{2}$ months. If we look for what brain constituents have a life span of that order, we realise the brain proteins do.

Question: If you had a drug that was eliminated in a short period of time, and the REM rebound was 50% more than the initial REM time, you would expect the half-life elimination to be equivalent to a drug that had a rebound also of 50% more. Or would you expect the half-lives to be the same?

Oswald: We have to be careful about what half-life we are talking about. If the rebound curve goes up to a peak very quickly, then the half-life is very short.

Question: What is the effect of occasional intake of hypnotics on the rebound effect? What is the dose one has to take in order to see that long rebound effect that you describe?

Oswald: Just one night is enough in order to have a very little rebound but usually drugs are taken by people for a long time.

Question: Do you know something about sedatives which produce sleep with normal proportions of REM and slow wave sleep?

Oswald: Practically all drugs do in small doses, for instance, it has been stated that Dalmane at low dosage does not change the proportions of REM and slow wave sleep though it does at high dosage. Rechtschaffen (Rechtschaffen *et al.*, 1970) and his group have done counts of eye movements per unit time. They found a decrease in intensity of REMs even when the duration remained the same after methaqualone. They measured not only the duration of paradoxical sleep but also its intensity and there was a rebound in duration at withdrawal.

Question: Could you relate some of your data on drugs with what is known about the action of serotonin and noradrenaline? For instance, the tricyclic antidepressants are said to interfere with noradrenaline. Dr. Jouvet has shown in this conference that in the absence of noradrenaline, the amphetamine effect is modified. What is the effect on slow wave sleep of drugs of the amphetamine class that lower serotonin, for instance, metamphetamine?

Oswald: Actually nobody knows how barbiturates affect behavior and induce sleep. The tricyclic drugs are said to alter the brain amine functions, not only epinephrine but also serotonin. I showed you some slides of effects of desipramine and imipramine. There is nothing to choose between them in their effects. Desipramine is particularly potent in blocking the uptake of noradrenaline whereas imipramine acts more upon 5-HT uptake. Chlorimipramine is very potent in reducing paradoxical sleep and is the most potent of all in blocking the uptake of 5-HT. Chlorimipramine makes people restless although it is said to make more serotonin available.

Question: (1) Some patients claim not to recall any dream when you put them on antidepressive drugs such as 10 or 15 mg of amytryptiline, which is a low dose. They usually say that in the beginning they recall more dreams. (2) Do you have any idea about the type of sleep and of REM and the amount of REM in epileptic children and adults who are on phenobarbitone for years?

Oswald: I agree completely with you on the first question. We had one woman who had been for several months on amytryptiline, 200 mg daily, and who had normal percentages of REMs and claimed to dream a lot. We have no experience of epileptics with phenobarbitone.

Question: Would you say that all the monoamine oxidase inhibitors would have the same effect on REM sleep of patients? What is their dosage and time?

Oswald: At low dosage the drugs do not have any effect and it is only after continuing a large dose that REM sleep drops to zero.

Question: Antibiotics are said to act upon protein synthesis. Do you know about antibiotic effect in REM sleep?

Oswald: There is some evidence that antibiotics, including penicillin, do increase paradoxical sleep in the first two REM periods of the night.

Question: Concerning the effect of drugs on sleep, your main criterion was REM sleep. The difficulties to characterize REM sleep are known. Can you specify the hierarchy of your criteria concerning REM sleep?

Oswald: Well, the criteria are not that loose. Experienced observers have a high interrater reliability.

Question: In relation to that question, is there any drug that dramatically changes the form of REM sleep?

Oswald: The illustrations that I showed you were based not only on REM sleep but also on intrasleep restlessness, shifts to stage 1, stages 3 and 4, rebound of stages 3 and 4, recovery of stages 3 and 4, and total sleep duration. With some monoamine oxidase inhibitors, for instance chlorimipramine, when REM sleep disappears there are at first a few periods of eye movements but the muscle tone is retained. Muscle tone is actually very high and this is a deviant feature of REM sleep. You get the same with chlorimipramine.

Question: We studied the effects of amphetamine in cats. During the administration period there is a slight increase of REM sleep, but we didn't see any changes during the recovery period. With the chronic suppression of paradoxical sleep, whatever the preparation is, could you draw a curve of the rapid eye-movement intensity? What are the different types of intensity changes that you see?

Oswald: We have not worked with cats. But in patients, there is an increased profusion of eye movements during the rebound period, whereas there is a decreased profusion of eye movements during the barbiturate administration period.

Question: (1) Is it possible to classify drugs according to your criteria which might be helpful in formulating a new drug in animal experimentation? (2) In your self-rating mood scale, do controlled people not have cyclic changes in their mood?

Oswald: I would hesitate to draw conclusions from my human data relevant to animal work, e.g. benzodiazepines, used in humans as hypnotics, make cats more active. Your second question: in our data people served as their own controls. The ratings are variable from subject to subject but you should take each subject as his own control.

Metcalf: What about people who are exposed to heavy doses of anticholinesterase agents e.g. industrial workers. All these people have chronically prolonged REM sleep.

Oswald: Those were maybe patients in the withdrawal periods? Are you saying that it is a consequence of the drug being present?

Metcalf: No, it is a consequence of *past* exposure to such compounds. Another question: Dr. Dement asked you whether there is a dissociation among some of the criteria that you use for judging the presence of REM sleep. That is among the combined patterned criteria of EEG, EMG, and EOG. I am wondering if you do a microanalysis of your sleep data, that there may be intermittent dissociation of EEG, EMG, and EOG which later falls into an entrainment. REM sleep shows a constellation of physiological patterns. We have seen people in the recovery period having lots of alpha in the EEG, a low EMG, eye movements, and irregular respiration. So they fulfill some but not all the criteria of paradoxical sleep.

CHAPTER FOURTEEN

General Discussion: Significance of Sleep Signs and Their Use in the Classifications of Sleep Stages

Dement: There is some ambiguity in the term, "sleep sign." It could mean a physiological event or property that is used to define the presence of sleep, or it could be anything that takes place in sleep. In the former instance, it should probably be called a primary sleep sign, and in the latter, a secondary sleep sign. I would include as primary sleep signs those changes in the EEG, the EMG, and the EOG that define whether or not any particular 30-sec epoch should be classified as NREM sleep, REM sleep, or wakefulness.

Secondary sleep signs can confirm what the primary sleep signs show, or can be more crucial if great precision is desired. For example, some people contend that a change in respiration is the most precise indicator of the exact moment of the sleep onset. An interesting secondary sign of the presence of REM sleep is the penile erection. However, when REM sleep is eliminated, the penile erection takes place in NREM sleep.

One has to understand a great deal to make the correct interpretation of a sleep sign. One might say that the failure to respond is a sign of sleep. Obviously, this is not always true and could, in some instances, indicate a very high level of arousal and concentration. The primary signs in the EEG, EOG, are certainly the most important, and will be the focus of our interest throughout this meeting.

Albe-Fessard: In one of the cases that you discussed, Dr. Oswald, you claimed that there was no REM sleep at all. What was the test you were using for deciding that: the EMG, the ocular movements, or the cortical activity, or the three at the same time?

Oswald: I said that there was an abolition of the signs of PS. I didn't say that PS disappeared because all we have are the signs. Maybe there are others inside the scalp that we cannot obtain. The criteria of PS are the low-voltage EEG, sometimes with sawtooth waves, frequencies within the range of 4–6 (occasionally others), rapid eye movements, and loss of muscle tone. If you give monoamine oxidase inhibitors, the percentage of PS that conforms to those criteria drops. However for some nights, you get a few minutes when you have some rapid eye movements, and every now and then low voltage EEG, but you have a lot of muscle tone. Since it does not meet the criteria of PS, we do not call it PS.

Albe-Fessard: All right! But you still had some ocular movements!

Dement: Occasionally, the experimenter will find cases which the rules do not cover. Although the answer is more obvious, the same question might be asked about a *cerveau isolé* preparation which shows EMG suppression together with spindles and slow waves in the neocortex. We once recorded all-night sleep in a patient with psychomotor epilepsy who appeared to fall asleep in a more or less normal fashion, but whose EEG tracings all through the night showed nothing but spike and wave seizure activity. Nonetheless, there were periods of EMG suppression which were accompanied by irregular respiration, some rapid eye movements, and in one instance, we detected penile tumescence. When EMG suppression was not present, he snored and the respiration was more regular. In the morning, the EEG normalized and the patient behaved as if he had had a good night's sleep. We decided to call the periods of EMG suppression REM periods; we decided to call the rest of the behaviorally quiescent time NREM sleep. At the very least, we can assume that EEG changes are not a necessary component for the continued manifestation of the 90-min sleep cycle. Labeling the specific stages is another problem and is essentially a matter of the experimenter's judgment.

Question: What is the effect of REM sleep deprivation? In relation to what Dr. Oswald has shown and what Dr. Dement has said before, it is not clear whether it is harmful or not.

Dement: I believe that I can give you a reasonably clear answer. The Stanford group has probably done more work with selective sleep deprivation than anyone else in the world. Rapid eye movement sleep deprivation, as carried out by instrumental techniques (nondrug), does not appear to be immediately harmful to either human or animal. You have asked this question in the summer of 1971. I arrived at the above conclusion in the summer of 1965. I would like to quote from a paper that was given at the end of this year

(Dement *et al.*, 1967). "The REM state does not appear to be absolutely necessary to maintain life in the adult animal. In other words, prolonged deprivation
is not lethal. In fact, some sort of equilibrium appears to be reached at around
30 days of deprivation." In terms of the ways in which REM sleep deprivation
is likely to occur in nature, I do not think that it has any clinical relevance. On
the other hand, there is a great deal of relevance to drug-induced REM sleep
suppression in terms of the consequences of subsequent withdrawal."

As I have tried to point out elsewhere (Dement, 1972), we can no longer
regard instrumental REM sleep deprivation as a critical manipulation because
we know that the processes whose simultaneous occurrences define the REM
period can occur independently in a REM sleep-deprived animal. An example
of this is the fact that more PGO spikes occur in NREM sleep in an animal
that is undergoing REM deprivation than in a normal animal.

Twelve years ago when we began experiments with selective sleep deprivation, our knowledge of sleep was relatively primitive; our thinking about REM
sleep was psychoanalytically biased and metaphorical. We thought of REM
sleep as a thing and we used the metaphor of pressure when describing the
deprivation rebound phenomenon and the tendency for REM period onsets to
become more frequent during the deprivation procedure, almost as if a pressure was building up. In 1963, we tried to REM deprive some human volunteers
until we saw serious consequences. In these three individuals, the problem was
not so much the appearance of a serious consequence, but the difficulty in continuing the REM sleep suppression while maintaining a normal amount of
NREM sleep. In the case of cats, we were able to selectively deprive them of
REM sleep more or less without limit. I suspect that we could have done it for
years, if we had had the energy. In 1964 and 1965, we deprived cats of REM
sleep for more than 2 months and, again there were no apparent serious consequences for the cats. Obviously, there are many subtleties involved in this
problem, but it is quite clear that the original speculations about dreaming in
order to stay sane and so forth, for which I do not claim credit, turned out to
be unjustified. I don't know why this idea has persisted with such tenacity.
I would like to go on to another point, however, which is that the selective
deprivation of REM periods does affect the central nervous system (CNS).
Some sort of change occurs so that the animal is in what we often call a REM
deprived state. The effect of REM sleep deprivation is apparent in the following
ways:

1. *Changes in sleep.* Parenthetically, in the figure that Dr. Oswald displayed
to illustrate instrumental REM sleep deprivation as compared to drug-
induced REM sleep deprivation, the REM rebound was relatively small. As
a matter of fact, if the instrumental deprivation is greatly prolonged, the
rebound is a good deal larger than this illustration would suggest. At any
rate, the organization of sleep states changes to favor REM sleep, and in

addition, REM sleep may become spectacularly more intense. This intensity is more apparent in the frequency of rapid eye movements in cats and in the intensity of the muscular twitching. In both animals and in humans, we have succeeded in dramatically changing the usual sequence in going from wakefulness to sleep. In other words, we have succeeded in producing sleep onset REM periods which may have some relevance to narcolepsy. There is absolutely no information that bears directly upon the mechanism of the postdeprivation REM sleep rebound. Arabinda Sinha and Jack Barchas at Stanford University have done some preliminary work with cycloheximide which suggests that protein synthesis may be involved. The changes in monoamine turnover demonstrated by others probably only represent a nonspecific biochemical sign of an overall enhancement in CNS activity, or perhaps, of the activating effect of nonspecific stress.

2. *Changes in CNS excitability.* We have done a number of studies which clearly demonstrated that a specific effect of selective REM sleep deprivation was an enhancement of CNS excitability measured in several ways. These findings have been confirmed in other laboratories. The most recent study concerned a change in evoked potentials in human subjects deprived of REM sleep for only two consecutive nights (Koppel *et al.*, 1972). We have long assumed that these changes would have clinical relevance for seizure activity. Recently this speculation was confirmed (Bergonzi *et al.*, 1970, 1971).

3. *Changes in pharmacological response.* An animal that has been REM deprived for a long time will not respond to many drugs in the same way as before deprivation. I will give two examples. The first is a drastically different response of REM-deprived rats and control rats to exactly the same dose and dose schedule of amphetamine (Ferguson and Dement, 1969). Second, there is a dramtic change in the response of a REM-deprived cat to parachlorophenylalanine. In effect, the REM-deprived animal appears to be immune to this very potent metabolic inhibitor.

4. *Changes in behavior.* The interpretation of the behavioral changes is somewhat controversial, but I feel we have been quite consistent. Indeed, we are willing to generalize and say that selective REM sleep deprivation has a drive-enhancing effect in terms of observations of intensification of sexual behavior, aggressive behavior, and eating behavior.

Koella: There is evidence that there is a good deal of mentation going on in non-REM sleep. Have there been any studies, indicating that if you REM deprive man, you would get compensation, so that you would have more non-REM-mentation? In a sense, would you have a transfer from the REM that you have deprived into NREM sleep?

Dement: The kind of study you are suggesting would be very difficult to carry out although it would be very interesting. The reason for the difficulty would be simply that REM-deprived subjects have very poor dream recall, probably as a result of the partial sleep loss that is always experienced by subjects undergoing instrumental REM sleep deprivation. At any rate, in subjects whom we have deprived of REM sleep for five or more consecutive nights, we have found that awakenings from the greatly prolonged and intensified REM periods of the first recovery nights produced essentially zero recall. The same problem exists if you try to elicit NREM recall in REM-deprived subjects. We do not feel that it is reasonable to assume that REM deprivation leads to a cessation of dreaming; therefore, we prefer to assume that the difficulty is due to an interference with recall. As I said earlier, there is definitely an increase in the number of PGO spikes in NREM sleep during REM deprivation. Other investigators have shown similar results. For example, during REM sleep deprivation, human subjects will have penile erections during NREM sleep periods. The whole concept of selective REM sleep deprivation needs careful evaluation. I have recently discussed this problem at length (Dement, 1972).

Question: Following REM-deprivation in rabbits and cats, there is a lowering of seizure threshold electrically induced. Convertely, following convulsion what kind of sleep change do you see?

Dement: There seems to be an increase of non-REM sleep and a decrease of REM sleep. There is almost a reciprocal interaction of convulsion and REM sleep in the cat. If the cat is convulsed every day, REM sleep time will drop and then will not rebound. If the cat is deprived of REM sleep for a few days and then convulsed, the subsequent rebound will be greatly attenuated. I suspect that some neurochemical changes also affect the REM sleep in this situation.

Question: Isn't it evident that during the REM period, there could be other output than neurological signs activities, for example, endocrine activation?

Koella: You probably have heard about the more recent reports about growth hormone output mostly during NREM sleep. So it would be a negative aspect.

Question: It has been mentioned that the occurrence of the REM stage in chickens correlates very strongly with the imprinting process and that the final connections of this may take place during REM sleep. Phylogenetically mammals and humans have much more information to process than in a simple imprinting process. If you look at the amount of REM sleep in relation to how much learning the organism has to do in the phylogenetic scale, may we associate REM sleep with the very simplest basic kinds of learning and information processing?

Dement: There have been many studies in which people looked for changes in memory and learning processes as a function of REM sleep deprivation. The findings are not terribly impressive. I do not believe that anyone has succeeded in harmlessly eliminating REM sleep in a baby duck or chicken. Therefore, I cannot answer your question. The major interest has been in possible correlations between amount of REM sleep and optimal time of the imprinting process. I would remind you that it is very difficult to deprive a newborn organism of anything, let alone REM sleep.

Question: We might get into theories which relate the stages or signs of sleep to waking function. Should the notion that REM sleep simply reveals something that is also present during wakfulness not be considered?

Dement: I think that this is a very interesting possibility. Years ago we speculated, somewhat naively to be sure, that the intensity of PGO spikes in REM sleep and /or the overall predominance of REM sleep would give an indication of the waking motivational state of the cat. We felt that there was some sort of equivalence between REM sleep and/or PGO spikes and instinctual energy. In some cats who were very aggressive, very fierce, very sexual, we felt that we could demonstrate a high level of PGO spikes. Actually, we have not proved this one way or another. We do know, however, that a clear-cut two-way reciprocity between REM sleep and drive-oriented behavior has not been demonstrated. For example, Steve Henriksen in our laboratory put male cats on a 12–12 hr sleep and wakefulness schedule. He compared the amount of REM sleep in the 12-hr sleep period during a time when the cat was just walking on a treadmill with a period when he spent his 12 waking hours in the company of several estrous females. We expected that the excess of "drive discharge" during wakefulness would lower REM sleep time. It did not. Somewhat more realistic explorations have been done by other investigators, primarily in the area of oculomotor function. There is some evidence of a relationship between waking eye movements and sleeping eye movements. In summary, however, we must admit that your question merely highlights our vast and continuing ignorance about the function of REM sleep.

Question: I was wondering whether in any population there are individuals who require much less sleep than others. I think there are individuals who require only 2 or 3 hr of sleep every night and I was wondering whether their signs of REM-sleep and slow wave sleep are different and what are the conditions?

Dement: The most remarkable study of such individuals was carried out by Oswald (Jones and Oswald, 1968). Presumably these subjects had been doing this all their lives. I would like to take this opportunity to get more details from Dr. Oswald. Were these gentlemen fully alert during the 21 plus hours that they were not sleeping? If they had rated themselves according to the Stanford Sleepiness Scale every 15 min around the clock (except when they were asleep, of course), would they have consistently shown low ratings (1 = feeling active and vital; alert; wide awake)? Were you absolutely sure they did not fall asleep at other times? Did they ever get very sleepy at any other time? Do you feel that the 7-day period of your study was a sufficient sample?

Oswald: These were two men who slept regularly less than 3 hr. They have done this for years and were both extremely active people. They had the same percentage of PS as normal people, 23%. Of course, the absolute amount was rather small. They had a great deal in absolute terms of stage 3 and 4 and were especially short in stage 2. They were unpaid volunteers, a sort of middle-class professional type. I couldn't follow them around all day but I could only rely on what their wives said and what they said. I had no reason to disbelieve it and the pattern that they showed in sleep was consistent over the period that we studied it. It could not be regarded as compatible with people taking amphetamine or people getting more and more sleep deprived. We know that if you have a nap at 9 o'clock or 10 o'clock in the evening and then wake up, you are short of stages 3 and 4 thereafter, whereas they went into stages 3 and 4 and then woke up at 5 or 5.30.

Question: Would it be conceivable that wakefulness has different stages too, and not only the two stages that we usually distinguish: arousal and normal wakefulness? Perhaps with modern techniques, maybe telemetry, one could record people around the clock and make fine distinctions of wakefulness! Maybe we could see that people who stay awake for 21 hr are differently awake than we are.

Dement: That is a very good point. I don't think that it would be easy, however, to distinguish EEG stages during wakefulness that would correlate highly with variations in the subjective feeling of sleepiness. Nonetheless, there is a wide range in subjective level of arousal during what we call wakefulness. The Stanford Sleepiness Scale (SSS) is a 7-point rating scale which allows us to look at these variations during the waking state. More recently, the SSS has been cross-validated against performance tests of the Wilkinson type (Hoddes *et al.*, in press).

Albe-Fessard: Concerning animals during wakefulness, the observation of the organization of spiking in different areas shows that wakefulness is a highly nonstationary state. People who studied units in several thalamic locations have shown that wakefulness is a nonhomogeneous state whereas slow wave sleep and PS are homogeneous.

Dement: Subjectively, people can distinguish seven stages of wakefulness with some reliability.

Question: Yawning? Has it anything to do with sleep at all?

Dement: It is a social communication.

Schlag: I am disturbed by the great number of possible exceptions that you have to accept in dealing with the concept of REM sleep. A concept is made up of a number of attributes. When I see an apple, I recognize it as an apple because it has attributes A,B.C. . . If one is missing, I may still decide that the object is an apple because the missing attribute is unimportant. Which attributes are essential and which are secondary to identify REM sleep? If we cannot answer this question, maybe it would be preferable to get rid of the concept of REM sleep and adopt a different categorization in terms of the component signs.

Dement: To begin with, I fell reasonably certain that the concept of an apple is much clearer than the concept of REM sleep. If we could show that REM sleep existed in the apple, then we would have a comparable problem. As I have said many times, however, REM sleep is a confluence of many events and we have not completely sorted them out in terms of which are primary and which are secondary, which are necessary in some way for the concept of the state and which are not, etc. Quite honestly, I think we are almost at the point of a paradigmatic crisis with regard to REM sleep and what to do with it.

Purpura: You were very careful indeed in indicating those signs that you call PS. Could all these signs be absent and the pontomesencephalic area still ticking away in a very cyclic fashion? If you really want to go that way, I think you will get into very serious problems. Is it conceivable to you that there is still the phenomena of this ticking away of the fundamental process which cannot be seen?

Oswald: Yes, I think that those activities are locked in the brain. You can get rid of the signs of PS as far as eye movements and muscle tone are concerned but still see every $1\frac{1}{2}$ hr changes in the EEG.

Purpura: There is a fundamental issue here which I would like to have some discussion about. Suppose one could do the theoretical experiment of recording from a single raphe neuron and a neuron of the locus coeruleus region in a paralyzed anencephalic monster. Let us also assume that the metabolic activities of these neurons were similar. Now is it your view, Dr. Oswald, that under these conditions these neurons would still exhibit a clocklike alternation in phasic and tonic activities?

Oswald: No, but the clock would still be there. The neurons must have been changed by drugs or a rebound would not occur.

Purpura: There are several examples in the literature of neurons that exhibit rhythmical clocklike increases in activity in isolation. What I want to know is whether there are cells in the raphe, reticular, or locus coeruleus regions which might be so classified as autorhythmically active elements with a built-in clockmechanism. The possibility exists of removing small portions of neural tissue from these regions in fetal animals and transferring them to tissue cultures. Do you think it would be worthwhile to see if such elements in tissue culture would generate rhythmical activities?

Oswald: Dr. Purpura, I would like to ask you first how you would conceptualize the rebound. If you gave a drug for a couple of weeks, stopped it, and then got signs of PS much increased in duration and intensity and gradually recovery to normal over a period of about 2 months, how would you, in your way, conceptualize this sort of thing happening?

Purpura: You are dealing with a time scale that is very difficult for neurophysiologists to handle. Consequently I cannot give you an answer. We know that it is possible to completely block synaptic activity in growing neural tissue cultures without affecting the morphological maturation of neurons and synapses. Such elements as are blocked could show an enhanced activity following removal of drugs. It is not necessary to postulate synthesis of new protein to account for the changing responsiveness of the synaptic organizations.

Oswald: I do not know why you are thinking in terms of synapses. What is wrong with the rest of the cell?

Purpura: I believe the major job of a neuron is to maintain its synaptic functions and to modify these in accordance with changing requirements of the neuron and its synaptic relations.

Oswald: No, it is the time scale we must come back to. I don't see why you think only of synapses.

Purpura: Because I do not think of synaptic functions just in terms of a few milliseconds. You know, I have the feeling that things are changing quite a bit all the time and I think we don't have the best techniques to see these changes.

Dement: Can cells interact in terms of a depletion or excess of transmitter in terminals independent of number of impulses?

Purpura: They certainly can.

Metcalf: May I introduce a quite different question: What is the present state of electro-sleep or electro-anesthesia?

Dement: There is absolutely no standardization in what is called the electro-sleep technique. This applies to frequency, voltage, and wave form. As it is currently used, the actual stimulation is administered during the day. It is then claimed to have some mysterious ameliorative effect on a variety of human conditions such as hypertension, neurosis, insomnia, migraine, premenstrual tension, and so forth. There is a great need for a nondrug method of treating true insomniacs. If this technique really helped insomniacs it would be very useful. However, we do not have the slightest idea about the possibility of harmful effects as a result of daily passage of electric current through the head. There is one thing about which I am very certain: there is no evidence whatsoever that these currents have a direct and specific sleep-inducing effect.

Question: What about transcendental meditation?

Dement: In terms of the notion of states of existence, we might consider transcendental meditation. Transcendental meditation has been called the fourth state of existence, along with REM sleep, NREM sleep, and wakefulness. Dr. Keith Wallace of Harvard University has studied the physiological concomitants of meditation. He has made a point of the prominence of a hypersynchronous frontal alpha rhythm. Interestingly enough, many of the things he describes are characteristic of the onset of sleep, or the moment of transition between wakefulness and sleep. One variable that was not studied by Wallace was eye motility. If transcendental meditation were accompanied by slow rolling eye movements, I would be convinced that, rather than a separate state, it is merely a prolongation of the moment of sleep onset, i.e., early NREM stage 1. The technique of meditation, which includes the repeating of the mantra and an erect body position, may actually serve to prevent a further progression into the sleep state, or to prolong a kind of sitting on the fence.

All of this underscores the fact that defining a state is a complex process. Another way of deciding about transcendental meditation might be in terms of its relationship to the so-called sleep need. If transcendental meditation is indeed sleep onset, it ought to take care of the sleep need as if it were so many minutes of frank sleep. On the other hand, perhaps it is naive to assume that the deprivation of a state can only be relieved by the occurrence of that state.

This leads to a corollary argument that since there are two kinds of sleep, there should be two kinds of sleepiness. This, however, does not appear to be the case in that we cannot distinguish two kinds of sleepiness in narcoleptics, and it is very clear that the sleepy feeling they experience is relieved by 15 min of NREM sleep, *and* is equally relieved by a sleep onset REM period (only REM sleep) of 15 min duration. Perhaps the overall sleep need is related to metabolic processes in the peripheral organs about which we know nothing at the present time. The feeling of a sleep need may also be related to circadian rhythm processes.

Question: Might sleep have an adaptive function?

Dement: As I suggested in my presentation earlier, perhaps REM sleep is nothing more than the confluence of three individual processes, namely, nonreciprocal motor inhibition, cortical activation, and phasic activity. Since each of these processes can and does occur independently, we cannot easily assess their importance to the organism by considering only those periods when they occur simultaneously. Maybe motor inhibition as indicated by EMG suppression is the only important part of REM sleep. Then it is surely just as important when it occurs during what we now call NREM sleep, i.e., in association with slow waves and spindles. Maybe phasic activity is the most important aspect of REM sleep. In terms of this possibility, we should certainly not be misled by the fact that rapid eye movements do not occur in NREM sleep. PGO spikes certainly do occur in NREM sleep without eye movements. In addition, PGO spikes can be augmented by a certain level of barbiturate narcosis. In the human, we are accustomed to the action of barbiturate which is a marked reduction of eye movements within REM periods. We must face the fact that we do not know what is the critical feature of REM sleep, if any.

CHAPTER FIFTEEN

Clinical Disorders in Man and Animal Model Experiments

WILLIAM C. DEMENT
JAIME VILLABLANCA

Dement: There is no widely accepted and therefore "official" nomenclature of sleep disorders. At the present time, at the Stanford University Sleep Disorders Clinic, we classify sleep disturbances into three major categories: primary, secondary, and interactive. In the secondary disorders, the sleep disturbance is considered to be a direct consequence of some other pathological condition. A prosaic example would be an abscessed tooth with nocturnal pain. Various psychiatric illnesses are often associated with sleep disturbances of varying degrees of severity.

In the case of the interactive disorders, the disease manifestations, while clearly of independent origin, are nonetheless related to sleep stages or the prolongation of the recumbent position. Examples are sleep-related seizure discharges, nocturnal angina, and peptic ulcer. In the latter instance, the Kales group has shown that the rate of gastric acid secretion is greatly elevated during REM periods.

We group the primary sleep disorders into three categories. First the dyssomnias. In this category we include those problems where we know or infer the presence of some impairment or imbalance of the neuroanatomical and/or the neurochemical mechanisms that regulate and control sleep and wakefulness. Second are the syndromes of drug dependency. From the point of view of frequency, these are easily the most important. The third category we call the syndromes of inadequate sleep: In some way that we do not completely understand, the entire sleep–wakefulness cycle is not working properly. There is sleepiness during the day and sleeplessness at night. When both are present we call it insomnia; when only sleepiness during the day is present, we call it hypersomnia.

There are three kinds of dys-somnias: REM-type, NREM-type, and generalized. Narcolepsy is a dys-somnia involving REM sleep. This illness is a highly specific symptom cluster whose pathophysiology is clearly related to REM sleep mechanisms. The narcoleptic patient complains of inappropriate sleep episodes or "attacks" during the day *and* brief episodes of muscular weakness or paralysis, usually triggered by strong emotion, commonly laughter and anger. The latter episodes are known collectively as cataplexy. During cataplectic seizures, there is no impairment of waking consciousness. As far as we know, generalized, nonreciprocal motor inhibition is a normal process that occurs in everyone, every night during REM periods. In narcoleptics, this normal REM component is dissociated from REM periods and appears in wakefulness. Occasionally, the cataplectic episode continues and develops into a full-blown REM period.

The diagnosis of narcolepsy can be made by asking one question: Do you have attacks of muscular weakness or paralysis that seem to be caused by strong emotions such as laughter or anger? In every patient who answers "yes" to this question, we expect to see a highly characteristic and totally abnormal sleep response in clinical laboratory testing. *During a daytime diagnostic sleep recording, these patients go directly from wakefulness into REM sleep. In other words, they have sleep onset REM periods.* This is illustrated in Fig. 15.1. Normals never do this. Neither do patients who complain of sleepiness or fatigue during the day, but *do not* have cataplexy.

Two other complaints that narcoleptics may have are sleep paralysis and hypnagogic hallucinations. Sleep paralysis is seen when the patient suddenly realizes that he is paralyzed just as he is about to fall asleep. Almost every time a narcoleptic begins to fall asleep, indeed before sleep has actually started, motor inhibition occurs. We must assume that the complaint of sleep paralysis depends upon the patient noticing that he is paralyzed. We assume that he will not notice if he does not attempt to move, but the inhibition will simply continue into a full-blown sleep onset REM period. Remember, motor inhibition is *not* a property of NREM sleep, and therefore, is not an attribute of the sleep onset in normals or patients with other kinds of sleep problems.

Narcolepsy tends to be familial, which strongly implicates a genetic component. It usually begins at puberty and continues for the remainder of the patient's natural life.

Finally, narcoleptics do not necessarily sleep more than normals. The problem is more in the timing of both full-blown and partial REM attacks than in

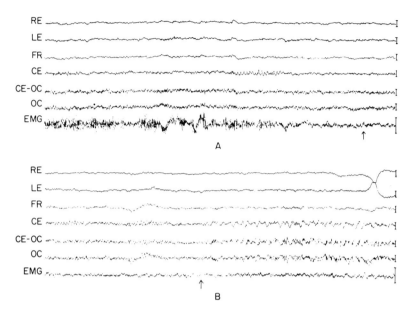

Fig. 15.1. Sleep-onset REM episode with zero latency. Tracings A and B are continuous. At the beginning of A, the patient is awake and the EEG is unchanged from that seen at the start of the recording session 4 min earlier. However, a transient EMG suppression is seen almost immediately, and at the arrow, the EMG is suppressed completely, although the EEG patterns still resemble those seen during full wakefulness. The sleep onset REM episode starts (by definition) at the point where a discernible change is evident in the EEG (second arrow); in this case, the change is the appearance of sawtooth waves. At the extreme right of B, the first rapid eye movement potential is seen. RE, right outer canthus; LE, left outer canthus; FR, frontal; CE, central; OC, occipital; EMG, submental (chin). All derivations monopolar to ears unless otherwise indicated. Calibration: 50 μV. Paper speed: 15 mm/sec. [Reprinted with permission of the author from Dement *et al.*, 1966. The nature of the narcoleptic sleep attack, *Neurology* **16**, No. 1, 18–33. Copyright The New York Times Media Company Inc.]

the total amount of sleep. Many of the facts in textbooks and in the literature are confounded by the fact that one label, narcolepsy, has been applied to any vague or undocumented complaint of sleepiness. Our findings are based on information obtained exclusively from patients who present the syndrome of sleepiness during the day, cataplexy, and sleep onset REM periods.

Treatment of narcolepsy should include education about the nature of the illness. When daytime sleepiness is the most prominent feature, low doses of methylphenidate or amphetamine may be prescribed. When cataplexy is the most prominent feature, tricyclic antidepressants are indicated. Twenty-five milligrams (or slightly more) of imipramine three times a day will immediately relieve these episodes. We sometimes use Ritalin and imipramine in combination.

The NREM dys-somnias are all behavioral episodes that take place or start in NREM sleep. Their differences are essentially quantitative variations in complexity and intensity. The least complicated behavioral episode involves only the simple act of emptying the bladder. It is called enuresis. The most complex and intense behavior is the night terror syndrome (*pavor nocturnus*). In between is sleep walking. There are several things that these episodes have in common. According to Kales and others (Jacobson and Kales, 1967), they usually begin in stages 3 and 4 early in the night when the sleeper is presumably too deeply asleep to be able to achieve normal alertness. Too, an instigating stimulus is presumably present. This stimulus can be either internal or external. Characteristic attacks can be easily elicited in the laboratory merely by attempting to arouse the patient. In addition, according to Broughton (1968), there is also a specific impairment of arousal processes in these patients. He bases this contention on data from auditory evoked potentials. He finds that auditory evoked potentials characterizing normal alertness do not immediately appear after such individuals are aroused from sleep, whereas they appear immediately in normal subjects.

The NREM dys-somnias tend to be familial; in other words, sleep walking runs in families. We have one patient in our clinic whose entire family sleep walks—father, mother, aunts and uncles, and siblings. He recounted to us a possibly apochryphal story of a family reunion at Christmas in which he awoke and found himself with the entire family in his grandfather's dining room.

Sleep apnea is the name we apply to a condition which occurs in both REM sleep and NREM sleep. Accordingly, it is classified as a generalized dys-somnia. It seems, as I am saying this, that many physicians are unaware of the ramifications of this condition, or even of its existence. The syndrome of sleep apnea is characterized by completely normal respiratory function in the waking state. However, there is a functional impairment of the respiratory center in the brain such that when deprived of the activating or energizing influences of wakefulness, the respiratory center ceases to function. In other words, whenever the patient falls asleep, he stops breathing. Apnea often has two phases. The first is called central apnea and refers to the apparent cessation of activity in the respiratory center and the consequent immobility of the diaphragm and of the intercostal muscles. This phase lasts for about 15 to 30 sec, during which time oxygen saturation of the blood falls and the carbon dioxide tension rises. At some point, this change in blood gases apparently stimulates the respiratory center, and respiratory effort begins. However, ventilation does not occur because the patient has become functionally obstructed. When respiratory effort begins, the patient enters what is called the obstructive phase of the sleep apnea. The obstruction is due to a collapse of the posterior nasopharynx due to muscle atonia. Thus, although respiratory effort begins and increases, the patient cannot move air through his airway. Finally, after about a minute of apnea, the patient wakes up, tone returns to the pharyngeal muscles, the patient takes a series of cacophonous, choking respirations, the blood gases normalize, and as a rule, the patient returns to sleep and the cycle is repeated.

It appears that most patients will have complete sleep apnea, that is, they will never breathe when they are asleep. Other patients, however, have apnea, or periodic respiration such as I have described, only during a portion of their sleep. When apnea during sleep is complete, the patient will wake up every 30–60 sec and thus can have as many as 500 arousals during a single night of "sleep." Small wonder that some patients are sleepy during the day. In point of fact, however, we do not know whether the sleepiness is directly related to the impairment of the respiratory center, and indeed is an analogous impairment of the arousal system, or whether it is a consequence of the many brief arousals during the night. What is amazing about these patients is that they are never really conscious of it. Sometimes they are conscious of the unusual respiratory effort when they wake up, but they still do not suspect that they stop breathing during sleep.

A patient with sleep apnea typically presents one of two complaints. Either he complains of falling asleep during the day or he complains of insomnia. Patients who complain of sleepiness during the day and who state that they spend a normal or greater than normal amount of time in bed at night sleeping have been, in the past, labeled as hypersomnia. When the respiratory problem was discovered, the condition was called hypersomnia with periodic respiration. We prefer to refer to it as sleep apnea, hypersomnia type. We must assume that such patients habituate to their many arousals and cease to be aware of them. When recorded in the sleep lab, and when all of the arousals, however brief, are carefully subtracted from the total sleep time, sleep is rarely excessive.

Recently, my colleague in the Stanford University Sleep Disorders Clinic, Dr. Christian Guilleminault, discovered sleep apnea in a patient complaining of insomnia. This is a very important discovery. In the first place, it establishes the more general prevalence of this disorder, and it means that many such patients may exist among the millions who complain of insomnia. We must assume, in such patients, that they do not habituate to the arousals, and further, that they may not return immediately to sleep. Finally, we should mention that we have seen sleep apnea coexisting with narcolepsy in two patients. Figure 15.2 is a sleep tracing from a patient showing the periodic breathing characteristic of this illness.

Question: What happens to patients with bilateral chordotomy? When they fall asleep, they must stop breathing and they almost consciously have to restart breathing.

Dement: Yes, this would be a sort of iatrogenic alveolar hypoventilation

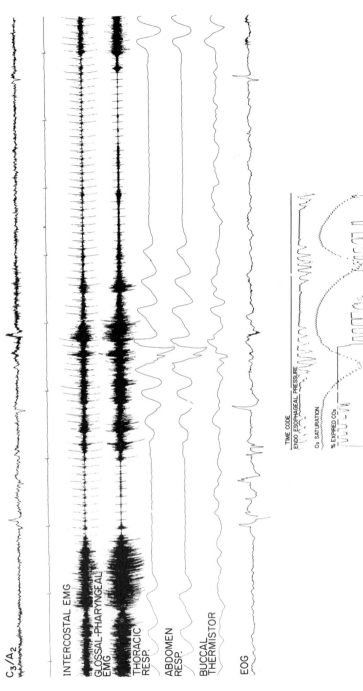

Fig. 15.2. Two concurrent 1-min records of two apneic periods. Upper tracings show muscle activity drops in intercostal and glossal-pharyngeal muscles. The apneas are of the so-called "central type." From the lower tracings it can be seen that endo-esophageal pressure does not increase when respiration resumes. There is only a short delay between initiation of diaphragmatic movements (endo-esophageal record) and expiration through nostrils (percent expired CO_2). This delay is due to the resultant anatomic and physiologic dead space. Oxygen saturation is recorded through an ear oxymeter which is recalibrated several times during the night by sampling blood gases.

C$_3$/A$_2$

INTERCOSTAL EMG

GLOSSAL-PHARYNGEAL EMG

THORACIC RESP.

ABDOMEN RESP.

BUCCAL THERMISTOR

EOG

TIME CODE

ENDO ESOPHAGEAL PRESSURE

O$_2$ SATURATION

% EXPIRED CO$_2$

syndrome. When individuals who have sleep apnea and complain of sleepiness during the day are also obese, this subtype has been called the Pickwickian syndrome. However, in the original description, the obesity was thought to be causal, and the somnolence was thought to be due to hypercapnea. This is not correct.

With regard to the drug dependency syndromes, we distinguish an insomniac type and a hypersomniac type. Whenever a patient complains of insomnia and gives a history of taking sleeping pills, our tentative diagnosis is always hypnotic dependency or drug dependency insomnia. Current understanding of this syndrome is due largely to the work of Dr. Anthony Kales and his colleagues. Drug dependency insomnia is a syndrome of disturbed sleep that is *caused* by sleeping pills. We know this because when patients are withdrawn from sleep medication, most typically barbiturates, their sleep disorders disappear. What we say in discussing this problem will apply to virtually all sleep medications. Thus, glutethimide is no different in this respect from sodium amytol. These principles will include the antihistaminic sedatives and, as Kales and his group have recently shown, they will also apply to across-the-counter medications such as Sominex and Nytol (Kales *et al.*, 1971).

The concept of drug dependency can be illustrated as follows: If you take a normal subject and give him 200 mg of a barbiturate at bedtime, his sleep time will increase. REM sleep time will be reduced. If we give the same dose every night at bedtime, very quickly, within a week or two, the increase in sleep time will disappear and, indeed, the total sleep time may actually be less than the base line value, even though the patient is taking barbiturate every night. At this point, the dose can be increased and the same cycle of events will be repeated. As the subject takes more and more barbiturate, he becomes more and more dependent. By this I mean that if he attempts to sleep without any drug, he will not sleep at all or his sleep will be tremendously disturbed. In addition, if he does sleep, he will suffer from a very pronounced REM sleep rebound in which large amounts of very intense REM sleep will occur. These intense REM periods are often accompanied by horrible nightmares. According to Kales, some patients would rather take the drug than experience these terrible dreams. Thus a normal subject can be converted into a patient who, although he may be taking thousands of milligrams of barbiturate every night, nontheless has insomnia. With one or two exceptions, all sleeping pills will always cause or worsen insomnia.

In real life, this cycle of dependency and increased hypnotic intake is often begun at the time of some transient situational episode during which the patient has difficulty sleeping. Sleeping pills are prescribed and the vicious cycle is underway. The all-night sleep patterns of patients who are taking large doses of barbiturates show no stages 3 or 4, very little REM sleep, many arousals, and some reduction in total sleep time. The diagnosis of uncomplicated drug dependency insomnia must remain tentative until the withdrawal is complete.

Analeptic dependency, or drug dependency hypersomnia, is diagnosed whenever a patient complains of falling asleep during the day, is sleeping well at night most of the time, and is being treated or takes analeptic medication such as amphetamine, phenmetrazine, and methylphenidate during the day. Drug dependency hypersomnia is essentially the mirror image of drug dependency insomnia. If the patient uses the medications chronically, he is likely to develop a tolerance which leads to an increasing dose and finally, the patient will fall asleep, or "crash" during the day in the presence of very high doses of these drugs. In such instances, the episodes of sleep during the day are always NREM sleep.

At the Stanford Sleep Disorders Clinic, we classify patients who complain about their sleep and do not have other disorders, under the syndromes of inadequate sleep. The reason for this title will become apparent. At any rate, in order to make the tentative diagnosis of idiopathic insomnia, we require that two conditions be fulfilled. The first is that the patient give some history of disturbed sleep at night. We get this information from standard sleep diary forms in which the patient keeps very close track of his sleep time over the course of a week. Generally, the mean nightly sleep times derived from such a diary are somewhat longer than the patient's original estimate. Second, we require some evidence that the patient's sense of well-being during the day is impaired in some way and that he attributes this to the disturbed sleep at night. This is generally done by means of the Stanford Sleepiness Scale which we have developed in our clinic.

At the present time, we insist that every patient who complains of insomnia undergo all-night sleep recordings to accurately assess total sleep time and organization of sleep states and stages. We generally record from two to four successive nights of *ad lib.* sleep in the laboratory. At the same time we can add a night or two with an hypnotic to evaluate its effectiveness in that particular patient.

Figure 15.3 presents the data on mean nightly sleep times from the first 26 patients we recorded in this manner. As you can see, the total sleep times distributed themselves more or less evenly from 4 to more than 8 hr. There is no particular relationship to age of the patient, although nearly all were middle-aged or older. Every patient showed values of 6 hr or less on the sleep diaries; thus it is clear that in this group the complaint of insomnia does not correlate with the total sleep time. We are not sure what this means in terms of defining insomnia, but it is clear that this complaint is not necessarily the result of abnormally short sleep.

A diagnosis of idiopathic hypersomnia is made when a patient complains of sleepiness during the day, does not use analeptic medication, and gives a

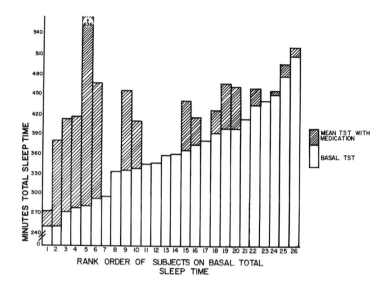

Fig. 15.3. Total sleep time for 26 presumed insomniacs from several experimental treatment studies. Subjects 1, 2, 3, 10, 15, 19, 25, and 26 were from the flurazepam studies; subjects 4, 6, 18, and 20 were from the doxepin studies; subjects 8, 12, 13, 17, 21, and 23 were control "insomniacs"; numbers 5, 9, 16, 22, and 24 were patients recorded on base line and flurazepam. Numbers 7, 11, and 14 were patients recorded only on base line. Unshaded areas represent the mean total sleep times of from 2 to 4 base line nights. Shaded areas represent the mean total sleep times of from 2 to 14 nights on medication.

history of normal sleep at night. The complaints are evaluated in the same manner as they are for insomniacs. The number of patients we have seen in our clinic in whom we have made this diagnosis is relatively small. At the present time, we insist on recording their sleep, but because they sleep during the day, or at least they say they do and they claim that they have long periods of sleep during the night, we must have 24 hr a day for several days, and this is a very difficult and costly procedure. However, it is clear that these patients do not necessarily have markedly excessive sleep time. Rechtschaffen and Roth recorded five patients for two nights each and found a mean sleep time slightly in excess of 8 hr. We have also studied five such patients and have found a mean sleep time of about 8½ hr. None of the patients had impressively long sleep times. All gave abnormally high (sleepy) ratings on the Stanford Sleepiness Scale during the day. In some patients there is clearly a need for a great deal of sleep, and if this is not allowed, they present marked symptoms of sleep loss and are unable to perform. This has been called sleep-drunkenness by Roth in Czechoslovakia. Again, it is clear that the definition is not exclusively an abnormally large amount of sleep.

There is something wrong with the sleep of the insomniac and he experiences it as a nocturnal disturbance; there is something wrong with the sleep–wakefulness rhythm of the hypersomniac, and he focuses on sleepiness during the day. At the present time there are no facts that can tell us what is wrong with these patients. However, our working hypothesis is that the difficulties will lie in an area of biological function called circadian oscillation.

We feel that chemotherapy for the complaint of insomnia is only indicated when the patient shows less than 6 to $6\frac{1}{2}$ hr of sleep as an average of several laboratory all-night recordings. The reason for this is that when hypnotics are administered to patients who complain of insomnia and sleep *more* than this, there is no significant change in their time. In other words, the drug does nothing. When chemotherapy is indicated, only an effective medication should be used. For our standards of hypnotic effectiveness, we are again indebted to Dr. Anthony Kales who has pioneered the development of hypnotic evaluation. His standard effectiveness protocol involves the recording of four base line nights in an insomniac, 2 weeks of administration of the hypnotic compound at bedtime, of which the first three nights and the last three nights are recorded in the laboratory, and finally immediately the first four withdrawal nights are recorded. In order to be judged effective, the compound must increase sleep time during the first three treatment nights, and the last three must be no different than the first three. Finally, there should be no significant suppression of REM sleep on any of the treatment nights nor an excessive rebound on recovery nights. Obviously barbiturates show a marked difference between the first three treatment nights and the last three treatment nights. The only compound that we are thoroughly familiar with which fulfills these effectiveness criteria is flurazepam. The dose is ideally 15 mg or 30 mg at bedtime. Other possibilities involve psychotherapy, relaxation therapy, and certain other physical approaches.

In the case of idiopathic hypersomnia the only treatments available are analeptic medications which we use only in the desperation because of their likelihood of eventually worsening the condition.

Purpura: What happens in REM in Parkinsonian patients?

Dement: Nothing. The tremor usually disappears at the onset of sleep. As far as I know, it does not return during REM periods.

Minard: The REM onset sleep that you show will not trigger our REM detector. It was not a slow eye movement but it was yet not fast enough. I wonder if you have nonambiguous cases of REM-sleep attack?

Dement: The answer to that is an emphatic yes. To be sure, some sleep onset REM periods have eye movements that appear a little "sluggish." However, we have seen many daytime sleep onset REM periods, or REM "attacks," in which the eye movements were very fast, if anything, faster than waking saccadic eye movements.

Minard: You find with REM deprivation that the characteristics tend to appear during NREM. It has been suggested by Rosalind Cartwright that waking activities can compensate for REM deprivation. It is possible that these people who are hyposomniac can somehow manage to accomplish during wakefulness things that REM accomplishes for the rest of us.

Dement: I do not think that is a very promising hypothesis for patients with true insomnia because it implies a successful alternative. True insomniacs feel much better when their insomnia is alleviated. In individuals who do not complain of sleepiness during the day (i.e., normals), but who have relatively low sleep times like Jones and Oswald's subjects, there might be some possibility that their waking activities are in some way compensating for REM sleep and that total sleep time is in some way a function of the "need" for REM sleep. However, such an hypothesis is difficult to prove. It is sort of like trying to prove the existence of the unconscious mind. I will say that normal hyposomniac subjects that we have studied do not have the very active fantasy life which I believe Rosalind Cartwright associates with a compensatory function.

Petre-Quadens: Endocrine steroid dysfunctions have been mentioned in narcoleptics. Could you comment on that?

Dement: We have not seen endocrine dysfunction in any of our narcoleptic patients. In some cases, we searched very carefully for such a dysfunction. I would like to remind you of our definition of narcolepsy. We must have cataplexy and sleep onset REM periods. We feel that sleep onset REM periods do not occur in patients without cataplexy. Sleep "attacks" alone, which are usually NREM sleep, do not qualify. We have seen one or two cases of endocrine dysfunction associated with hypersomnia.

Oswald: According to the literature a lot of narcoleptics become fat. In addition, fat people have hardly any growth hormone. There are lots of similarities between these patients and the Pickwickian syndrome.

Dement: As I indicated earlier, we have seen sleep apnea in patients with absolutely unambiguous narcolepsy. Dr. Guilleminault is studying these patients. There are three and, at least two are definitely not obese. We feel that the Pickwickian syndrome is a subgroup of the sleep apnea condition. Many Pickwickians will continue to be apneic even when they lose weight. Others will improve. Obviously, there are many fat people who have neither sleep apnea nor daytime somnolence.

Freemon: I know a family in which three persons have sleep attacks during the day and two others have sleep walking.

Dement: That is very interesting. Sours (1963) has also reported many cases where narcolepsy and schizophrenia coexist in families.

Purpura: Ries has done a lot of work with catecholamines and norepinephrine in the spinal cord in relation to phasic activities, and circadian rhythms. I do not think he knows where they came from but there are at least three pathways that have been described. The general area is the pontine reticular system mostly. I do not know how much is raphe but he certainly described this change along with bursts of sham rage. So there is a powerful input to the cord. But the same pathway seems to be the one which controls the reflex inhibition of motorneurons.

Petre-Quadens: Maybe this would be a good time to ask Dr. Villablanca to present his Jacksonian viewpoint on sleep.

Villablanca: The idea of a "sleep center," which has enjoyed considerable popularity for a long period in the history of sleep research, appears to be losing ground today. This is mainly because a multiplicity of structures along the entire neuraxis have been demonstrated to be involved in the control of sleep processes.

The hypothesis that the thalamus acts as the "head ganglion" in the coordination of all other brain areas concerned with sleep (Koella, 1967) seems more tenable. However, since only a difference in degree exists between this viewpoint and the traditional "sleep center" concept, one could argue that other CNS areas also deserve the title of "head gaglion" of sleep, i.e., the pontine-mesencephalic core, the basal forebrain area, or the hypothalamus.

It seems to me that a more realistic integrative view of sleep regulatory mechanisms be based on the model proposed by H. J. Jackson (1932) for the general functional organization of the CNS. Since Jackson's theory implies that different structures along the neuraxis contribute specific features to a given CNS function, it is unnecessary to invoke the concept of a "sleep center" when applying the theory to the physiology of sleep. The coordination of the different structures underlying sleep, only apparently missing in this conception, would result from the integrative nature inherent to all brain activities (Sherrington, 1906).

The origin of this concept as applied to sleep stems mainly from the results of lesion experiments (in which we have been involved for over 12 years) but also draws support from results obtained by other research methods such as electrical stimulation of the brain (see Parmeggiani, 1968). Those lesion experiments have demonstrated that the deterioration of sleep increases as the lesion progresses from the "highest" to the "lowest" brain levels (similar to the "dissolution" of other CNS functions, such as motor activity following such lesions). Thus, for instance, there is parallelism between the markedly curtailed behavioral manifestations of sleep and the "lowest level" motor functions, such as stereotype walking, in the chronic mesencephalic cat (Bard and Macht, 1958; Villablanca, 1966a). The demonstration in the classic *cerveau isolé* of the cat (in the chronic condition) that the forebrain has intrinsic capabilities for displaying an alternation between desynchronized and synchronized bioelectrical activities (Batsel, 1960; Villablanca, 1962) and some of their correlative sleep–wakefulness behavioral manifestations (Villablanca, 1965, 1966b; Zernicki *et al.*, 1967) is also relevant in terms of a Jacksonian viewpoint.

The main data which suggest that after brain lesions the deterioration of sleep follows a Jacksonian pattern are the following. In the neodecorticate animal, several "highest level" features of sleep as well as wakefulness are lost. Kleitman and Camille (1932) showed that in decorticate dogs the nycthemeral periodicity is lost, with the animals turning into "polyphasic sleep" creatures. In the cat, in which there is a clear sleep–wakefulness cycle (Sterman *et al.*, 1965; Ursin, 1970) but not a nycthemeral periodicity, there is a loss of the cyclic sleep–waking activity after a lesion in the basal forebrain area (Lucas and Sterman, 1971) or after complete neodecortication (see Chapter 4 in this volume). Whether or not a rostral brain area is specialized in this control—as claimed by Lucas and Sterman (1971) for the rostral preoptic area—has not been decided as yet. At any rate, the cyclic nature of sleep appears to depend on cortical or, at least, rostral brain mechanisms. In this context, it should be pointed out that in the chronic *cerveau isolé* periods of electrocortical synchronization and its behavioral concomitants also follow a cyclical pattern (Villablanca, 1965, 1966a). Furthermore, some behavioral manifestations which could be considered as "social" and "voluntary" factors associated with the action of going to sleep disappear after neodecortication (see review by Kleitman, 1963) as well as some (see below) preparatory activities (i.e., searching for a comfortable place to sleep and grooming behavior).

It is clear, therefore, that after decortication an appreciable "dissolution" of sleep–wakefulness physiology occurs. Since the most sophisticated aspects of sleep appear to be those most affected by decortication, this leads to the belief that the neocortex is the "highest level" of integration for sleep physiology. It is not clear as yet if the "highest level" control is located in frontal cortical areas as postulated by Jackson for other CNS functions; however, some experimental findings suggest that this might be the case (Velasco and Lindsley, 1965; Villablanca and Schlag, 1968; Lynch, *et al.*, 1969; Lynch, 1970; Moorcroft, 1971).

When the neocortex and striatum are removed in the cat and the limbic system is extensively damaged, a serious quantitative unbalance in sleep–wakefulness occurs. Data have been presented (see Chapter 4 this volume) demonstrating that in this condition sleep is reduced such that the animals spend only 0.8% of the time in REMs and 6.3% of the time in NREMs (compared to 13.8% and 38.2% for REMs and NREMs respectively in control animals). This observation is important for the present hypothesis inasmuch as it reveals another typically Jacksonian trait in the organization of the physiological control of sleep–wakefulness, namely that a balanced control is exerted by "higher level" structures over "lower level" mechanisms with the occurrence of a functional "release" when one of the structures contributing to the balance is eliminated. In the discussion of those experiments, it was suggested that thiopental induced a "sleep-rebound" by cancelling the activity of the "released" structure (presumably the hypothalamus) thus demonstrating the functional nature of the "release."

Although more research is needed to clarify this point, it seems that not only is the neocortex involved in this balance but also the striatum and probably the limbic system as well. In experiments (Jouvet, 1962) in which structures above the diencephalon were not as extensively ablated (striatum and limbic system probably mostly intact) as in our experiments, NREMs was drastically reduced but REMs amount remained within normal range (15–20%). That pure neo-decortication affects sleep less than neodecortication plus striatal removal, is supported by the finding of a permanent behavioral activity in diencephalic cats (Wang and Akert, 1962) and rats (Sorenson & Ellinson, 1970) versus in-activity in striatal cats (Wang and Akert, 1962) and only moderate activity in striatal rats (Sorenson and Ellison, 1970). There are indications that the limbic system also contributes to the balance discussed above but the pertinent data are not yet conclusive. Thus, while Lena and Parmeggiani (1964) claim that lesions to the limbic system reduce the amount of REMs in the cat, Kim *et al.* (1971) found that hippocampectomy in rats significantly reduces NREMs but does not induce a significant reduction of REMs.

The threshold for arousal during NREMs is decreased in the diencephalic as compared to the intact cat (see Chapter 4), thus suggesting that the "tonicity" of the sleep state is likewise affected at this stage of CNS involvement.

When the lesion progresses to involve the thalamus, most of the remaining postural and behavioral concomitants of sleep are affected. Thus, in the "athalamic" (see Chapter 4) as well as in the mesencephalic cats, the crouching position becomes nonexistant or distorted and the typical curled up posture along with the post somnic signs (stretching, yawning) completely disappear.

A marked disruption in the coupling of behavior with the electrocortical activity is also seen in cats following total thalamic ablation. The EEG corre-lates of NREMs, which are at least fragmentarily present in the diencephalic cat (see Chapter 4) appear to be missing altogether in the mesencephalic animal (Jouvet, 1962b; Villablanca, 1966a) and it remains to be seen if in this experimental condition, NREMs retains any other electrophysiological cor-relate (e.g., changes in multi-unit activity).

In the high mesencephalic animal the only discrete behavioral manifestation of NREMs similar to that occurring in intact animals during this stage of sleep (Berlucchi *et al.*, 1964b) is the fluctuation in the pupillary diameter and posi-tioning of the eyeballs (Villablanca, 1966a). Otherwise, a slight increase in the arousal threshold (Villablanca, 1966a) and a decrease in muscle tonus devoid of any characteristic postural pattern, are the only other general manifestations of NREMs at this stage of sleep "dissolution." On the other hand, all REMs manifestations including oculo-pupillary behavior and the phasic EEG pontine, phenomena, distinctively persist in the high mesencephalic animal. In contrast to the dramatic REMs reduction in the "diencephalic" cat, the amount of REMs in the mesencephalic cat tends to be normal (Jouvet, 1962b; Villablanca, 1966a). I have interpreted this phenomenon to be the result of the free operation of caudal brain-stem mechanisms controlling REMs after elimination of *both* sleep-enhancing and sleep-suppressing rostral brain influences.

Finally, when the influence of the mesencephalon is eliminated (pontine animal), none of the manifestations of NREMs are evident except for a decrease in postural tonus. On the other hand, REMs occurs "automatically" (Jouvet, 1965b) and can even be reflexively evoked, as for instance, while tube-feeding the animals (Villablanca, 1966a). REMs is still accompanied by pontine EEG and postural events but not by any oculo-pupillary manifestations as seen in intact cats. Thus, the manifestations of sleep which are "represented" below the mesencephalic level are only fragmentary and elemental, which suggests that the caudal brain stem should be considered as a "lowest" Jacksonian level in sleep control.

In conclusion, in this brief review, I have attempted to demonstrate that sleep-controlling mechanisms are morphofunctionally organized in the context of the Jackson theory in such a way that they evolve caudorostrally from more organized (more fixed or rigid in Jackson's terminology) to less organized (more flexible and adaptive), from simple to complex, and from automatic to "voluntary." These organizational patterns are at the core of the Jacksonian theory (Walshe, 1961).

While this integrative hypothesis might be an oversimplification of the extremely complex processes underlying sleep physiology, I am hopeful, however, that it may have some practical value in promoting better understanding of the physiology and pathophysiology of sleep as well as in the evaluation of neurochemical approach and even in the study of the ontogeny of sleep mechanisms. Thus, it would not be surprising if different "levels" of organization operate on the basis of different neurochemical substrates and, in relation to development, it appears (see Moorcroft, 1971) that "lowest level" structures mature earlier than "highest level" areas.

DEVELOPMENTAL ASPECTS OF
SLEEP PATTERNS

CHAPTER SIXTEEN

Introductory Remarks on Sleep Ontogenesis

DOMINICK P. PURPURA

Purpura: There is much concern today about the understanding of the morphophysiological processes which underlie the ontogenesis of sleep–wakefulness activities in different species, including man. Much discussion has focused upon the characteristics of cortical and brain-stem activities in the immature animal and the factors responsible for their developmental features. Unfortunately we know very little as yet about the control mechanisms that influence the changing characteristics of sleep–wakefulness behavior in the mature animal. And even less is known concerning these mechanisms in the immature animal.

One approach to the problem of defining the nature of these mechanisms may be to consider morphophysiological factors which distinguish the maturational features of neuronal organizations at different neuraxial sites in the developing brain. For example, the question may be raised as to how elements of the cerebral cortex differ from elements of the brain-stem raphe nuclei or reticular regions at different postnatal stages. Some answers to this may be forthcoming from examination of the comparative structure–function relations of neurons in cerebral cortex and brain stem during the postnatal period.

It is now well established that the typical pyramidal neurons of neocortex have relatively well-developed apical dendrites but rather poorly developed basilar dendrites in the neonatal kitten. Axodendritic synapses are present on these neurons but they are confined to the superficial apical dendrites where they are seen on smooth trunks. During the first postnatal week there is a rapid growth of basilar dendrites along with the initial appearance of axosomatic synapses. Spine synapses on dendrites make their appearance during the second postnatal week. This indicates that the pattern of synaptogenesis in neocortex proceeds from axodendritic to axosomatic to axospinodendritic synaptic development, with considerable temporal overlap in the various stages of synapse formation.

Electron microscopy has confirmed Golgi work in showing a high packing density of apical dendrites in the superficial neocortex in the newborn kitten.

Dement: Can you say a little bit more about the fact that the electron microscopy shows such packed dendrites?

Purpura: Two points can be made. One, that glial elements are not interposed between dendrites in the early postnatal period. Second, that an important aspect of the maturation of cortex from the fine structural standpoint is the remarkable increase in fine processes of the neuropil which represent, in part, the postnatal elaboration of glial processes.

Dement: Is there anything that can be said about subcellular elements?

Purpura: Neurotubules are not well developed in dendrites in the early postnatal period in the kitten. There are relatively few mitochondria as well and the endoplasmic reticulum is poorly organized. Ribosomes are more scattered than attached to ER. The general impression one gets in looking at the cell body of a neuron in the neocortex of the newborn kitten is that the intracellular metabolic machinery is operating at a relatively low level. However, this is not the case for neurons of the hippocampus which appear to be more intensely active in the newborn kitten than the neurons of the neocortex. In the postnatal period there is a progressive increase in the number of synapses, the number of vesicles per synapse, the length and electron density of pre- and postsynaptic membranes and the number of mitochondria found in a synaptic complex. Some workers have suggested that there is also a distinct change in vesicle morphology in some synapses during development.

A question which immediately comes to mind is, are the synapses observed in the neonatal period functional and if so, how do they operate? To provide data relevant to these questions we have employed the intracellular recording technique in studies of the functional properties of neurons and synapses in immature neocortex and hippocampus. It is clear from these investigations that excitatory and inhibitory postsynaptic potentials (EPSPs and IPSPs) are detectable in the very early postnatal period following stimulation of appropriate afferent pathways to cortical neurons. What has been particularly interesting in these studies are observations indicating that inhibitory synaptic pathways are remarkably well developed in the immature cerebral cortex. This has led us to suspect that inhibitory neurons may be precociously developed in the immature brain, for reasons which remain obscure.

By way of comparison with the morphological studies of immature cerebral cortex it is possible to summarize our preliminary findings on the kitten brain stem by the following:

1. Neurons of the lower brain-stem raphe nuclei are extremely well developed at birth and exhibit large numbers of axodendritic and axosomatic synapses.
2. Neurons of the lower brain-stem reticular formation are not distinguishable from raphe neurons on the basis of the number and extent of synaptic relations.
3. Caudal raphe neurons are more mature in overt morphological appearance (as judged by dendritic growth, synaptic endings, etc.) than rostral raphe neurons. The same applies to caudal versus rostral reticular elements.
4. At mesencephalic levels reticular neurons are more mature in appearance than mesencephalic raphe neurons.

The ultimate significance of these light and electron microscopic observations is not known. What is required to complete this analysis is a detailed investigation of the physiological properties of different organization of brain-stem neurons at different postnatal developmental stages. Until these data are at hand, it will not be possible to define the relationships of the morphological data to physiological operations which are reflected in overt behaviors such as those observed during sleep–wakefulness activities. One point is quite certain, however. Compared to cortical neurons, many lower brain-stem neuronal organizations are quite mature in appearance and may well be as functionally mature as they will ever be. If such is the case, then it is necessary to look to the developmental properties of target elements in the forebrain which receive brain-stem projections in the search for factors which confer "immaturity" upon certain varieties of behaviors in the developing animal.

CHAPTER SEVENTEEN

Neuro-Ontogeny of Sleep in the Rat

ALBERT GRAMSBERGEN

Investigation of the functional development of the immature brain and its morphology and biochemistry may provide clues to understanding the relations between behavioral states and underlying brain mechanisms in the adult. This is the background for our interest in the ontogeny of the nervous system. The experimental animal selected for these studies was the rat (*Rattus norvegicus albinus*) which is in some respects an ideal animal for research in neuro-ontogeny. The rat is relatively immature at birth and its early development is analogous to the human fetus in the late prenatal period.

The morphological development of the rat brain, and particularly of the cortex, is well documented (Eayrs and Goodhead, 1959; Dvořák, 1968; Caley and Maxwell, 1968a,b, 1970; Johnson and Armstrong-James, 1970). A number of biochemical investigations on the development of the rat brain have been reported (Samson *et al.*, 1963; McIlwain, 1966; Samson and Quinn, 1967; Gregson and Williams, 1969). However, considerable differences in the regional maturation of the rat brain unfortunately were often neglected in these studies.

Differences in techniques employed in these studies, such as the use of different strains of rats, different breeding and housing conditions etc. make it impossible or hazardous at least to correlate most of the results. Multidisciplinary studies within one institute or in different institutes but with exactly the same experimental conditions are an essential prerequisite for studying the causal relations between morphology, biochemistry, and brain function during development. Our study on the development of behavioral states and on the development of EEG is only a first step in this direction.

I. Development of Behavioral States

Studies of the development of rat behavior are scarce. Tilney and Kubie (1931) and Bolles and Woods (1964) studied some qualitative aspects in the development of rat behavior. Gramsbergen *et al.* (1970) studied quantitatively the development of behavioral states in the rat. Recently, interest in the neurophysiology of sleep has led to a number of investigations into the ontogeny of EEG in relation to sleep–wakefulness cycles in different animals.

The development of different EEG patterns related to behavioral states in the rat has been extensively studied by Jouvet-Mounier (1968) and Jouvet-Mounier *et al.* (1970). In these studies, however, the main interest was directed toward the EEG and other physiological parameters, as indicators of the functional development of the brain.

The developmental course of behavioral states was studied between the 2nd and the 30th postnatal day. At a fixed time of each day (between 9.00 and 13.00) one young rat at a time was placed in the observation cage (38 × 25 × 16 cm) with sanitary absorbant material on the floor (lighting schedule in the rat room: lights on from 8.00 to 18.00). The rat was observed for 40 min each day from the 2nd to the 14th day, and for 120 min each day from the 15th to the 30th day. These observation periods were selected because they were long enough to observe at least one sleep–wakefulness cycle, but were presumably short enough not to be disturbed by hunger (Gramsbergen *et al.*, 1970). The rat was returned to his litter after the observation. The cage temperature was 33 °C during the first days of the observations, then gradually lowered to 26 °C during the last days. These ambient temperatures were thus maintained at 2 °C below the age-specific neutral temperature (Taylor, 1960).

From a pilot study on a group of eight rats, behavior was classified into behavioral states which were qualitatively different, that is, sets of well-defined behavioral conditions which could be recognized when they recurred. It is obvious however, that any classification of behavior into behavioral states is quite arbitrary because it is dependent upon the criteria chosen (Prechtl *et al.*, 1969). We designed the following scale of behavioral states, which appeared to be easily recognizable from the 2nd to the 30th day. This scale parallels to some extent the scale Prechtl designed for human babies (Prechtl, 1965; Prechtl *et al.*, 1969).

State 1, "quiet sleep." The animal is still, except for small, brief movements as well as startles (sudden phasic contractions of all body muscles). Eyelids are sealed until the 14th day; after this point the eyes must be closed. Respiration is regular. Neck muscle tone is actively maintained.

The head for instance may remain somewhat raised, which indicates tonic activity in the neck muscles.

State 2, "active sleep." A relaxation in the postural muscles occurs and the head rests on the floor. Twitches in limbs, tail, ears, and vibrissae occur. Eyelids are sealed until the 14th day; after this point the eyes must be closed. Eye movements can be observed after the 10th day. Respiration is irregular. Startles identical to the startles in state 1 occur.

State 3, "quiet wakefulness." The rat sits quietly with open eyes. This behavioral state is observed only after the 14th to 16th day. It occurs in general during the transition from awake to asleep.

State 4, "active wakefulness." Gross body activity occurs without movement away from a stationary position. The rat grooms, moves his head about, and sniffs. After the 14th day, the eyes must be open.

State 5, "locomotion." The rat walks or runs about. After the 14th day the eyes must be open.

In Fig. 17.1 a sequential record of behavioral states of one rat on the 4th, 8th,

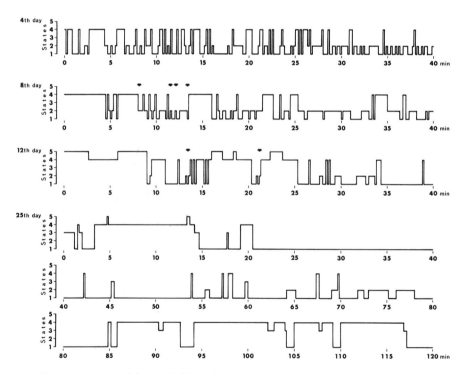

Fig. 17.1. Sequential record of behavioral states in one rat during 40 min of observation, on the 4th, 8th, and 12th day of life, and from another rat on the 25th day during 2 hr of observation. Behavioral states are indicated on the vertical scale. [From Fig. 2 (p. 272); Gramsbergen *et al.*, 1970, *Developmental Psychobiol.* **3** (267–280); by permission of John Wiley & Sons, Inc.]

and 12th day, and of another rat on the 25th day is shown. In the first 4 to 5 days only states 1, 2, and 4 can be observed. These states alternate rapidly and irregularly. After the first week of life, however, the number of oscillations decrease and sleep-wakefulness cycles can gradually be distinguished. At the 9th day the rat begins moving about on four legs (state 5) and at the 14th day the rat is able to open his eyes for brief periods in which the rat sits motionless with open eyes (state 3).

A. Quantitative Changes in the Distribution of States

Developmental trends in the quantitative distribution of the behavioral states and in the mean durations of single-state epochs were studied in two groups of 10 rats each (first group: postnatal ages 2–14 days, observation time 40 min daily; second group: postnatal ages 15–30 days; observation time 120 min daily). The behavioral state was recorded every 10 sec during these observation periods.

The quantitative distribution of the five behavioral states during the observation period changes markedly during development (Fig. 17.2).

During the first 4 to 5 days of life rats spend a high percentage of their time

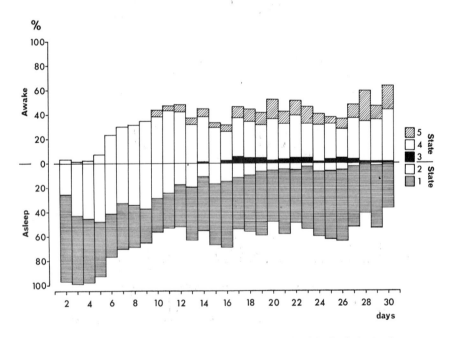

Fig. 17.2. Distribution of mean percentages spent in each of the five behavioral states as a function of age. Columns below the zero line indicate the two sleeping states, above the zero line the three awake states. [From Fig. 4 (p. 275); Gramsbergen *et al.*, 1970, *Developmental Psychobiol.* **3** (267–280); by permission of John Wiley & Sons, Inc.]

asleep. This percentage decreases gradually thereafter, until the 10th day, when rats spend about half of their time asleep and half of their time awake during the observation period. These proportions are then maintained until the 30th day. The increase in the percentage of wake time and a complementary decrease in the percentage of sleep time during the early postnatal period is a developmental phenomenon found in many mammals. Our findings in rats at 30 days of age are in accordance with the findings of Jouvet-Mounier (1968) and Jouvet-Mounier et al. (1970) in the 30-day-old, and in the adult rat. In disagreement with our findings, however, are Jouvet-Mounier's results about rat behavior in the early period of life (her rats were awake for about 25% of time in the first days). The surgical procedure (she made 24-hr polygraphic recordings of rats with implanted electrodes), the use of a different strain of rats, different criteria characterizing behavioral states, and perhaps other methodological differences might have effected this.

An interesting shift occurs in the distribution of total sleep time in the two sleep states. In the first days the percentage of time spent in state 1 decreases in favor of the percentage of time spent in state 2. From the 4th to the 11th day about half of sleeping time is spent in quiet sleep, whereas after the 11th day the percentage of time spent in quiet sleep increases again. A slight increase in the amount of active sleep in the first days of life, and a decline thereafter was described also in the rhesus monkey (Meier and Berger, 1965). Our finding that early in life a greater part of total sleep time is spent in active sleep than later on, seems to be a general phenomenon in mammals.

B. MEAN DURATION OF STATE EPOCHS

Remarkable developmental trends are also observed in the mean durations of single-state epochs (Fig. 17.3). The most dramatic change occurs in state 1 epochs. From less than 1 min they increase gradually up to an average duration of 6 to 8 min each. The relative amount of state 1 during the observation period remains about the same after the 10th postnatal day. This implies that state 1 epochs occur less and less frequently.

Only a slight increase is observed in the mean epoch length in state 2: (from 30 to 40 sec in the first days up to 60 to 80 sec later on). This means that the decrease in the total amount of state 2 is based on a decrease in the frequency of the occurence of state 2 epochs during development. The state 4 epoch length increases from a mean duration of less than 1 min in the first 4 days to about 2 min from the 10th day on. State 3 and state 5 epoch durations do not show a developmental trend. State 3 epochs occurring for the first time around the 14th to the 16th day have an average duration of 30 to 60 sec. State 5 occurring for the first time on the 10th day remains nearly constant around 90 sec. The steady increase in the mean epoch length of state 1, and the almost constant duration of state 2 epochs in the rat between the 2nd and the 30th day is a finding which has also been noted in the kitten and rabbit by Shimizu

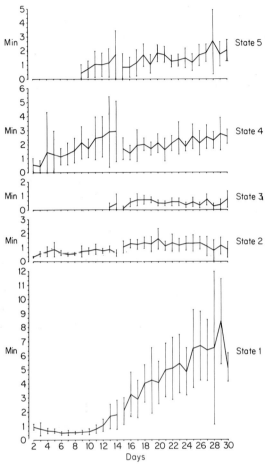

Fig. 17.3. Mean duration (ordinates) of single epochs for each state as a function of age; vertical bars indicate standard deviations. [From Fig. 5 (p. 176); Gramsbergen *et al.*, 1970, *Developmental Psychobiol.* **3** (167–280); by permission of John Wiley & Sons, Inc.]

and Himwich (1968). In the developing human infant, however, a decrease in the duration of the active sleep epochs occurs (Stern *et al.*, 1969; Dittrichová, 1969).

II. Development of the EEG

The development of EEG and of behavioral-state-specific EEG patterns in particular has been studied as a first step in the investigation of the relations between behavioral states and the underlying neurophysiological mechanisms.

Around the 4th to 6th day, an EEG signal is detectable for the first time (Crain, 1952; Schwartze, 1966; Deza and Eidelberg, 1967). We implanted 7-day-old rats under ether narcosis with two pairs of silver electrodes. One pair of electrodes was implanted over the area praecentralis agranularis (the sensorimotor cortex); another pair over the area striata (the visual cortex) (Krieg, 1946). Electrodes were connected to a miniature socket fixed to the skull with dental acrylic. After the surgical procedures the rats were replaced in their original nest. The first recording was made on the eighth day, one day after the implantation.

During the EEG recordings, the miniature socket on the rats head was connected with a supported lightweight cable to the polygraph (Offner Beckman dynograph type R). The rat was in a cage, which hung on a spiral string. Small movements of the rat induced cage movements, which were transduced into an actogram (Szabó et al., 1965). The behavioral state was recorded by an observer onto the polygram by means of a push-button system. The EEG recording, movements, and behavioral state were stored on magnetic tape (Ampex FR 1800), for off-line automatic analysis.

A. VISUAL ANALYSIS OF THE EEG

Visual analysis of the EEG from 8–10-day-old rats reveals predominantly frequencies up to 4 Hz. The EEG amplitudes remain low throughout the sleep–wakefulness cycle (Fig. 17.4).

Around the 10th day however, a remarkable development occurs. The EEG during state 1 shows bursts of high amplitude waves. In the course of a rapid development lasting 1 to 2 days these bursts grow longer and longer, until one burst runs into the next so that the high amplitude activity in state 1 becomes continuous. The EEG in state 2 and state 4, however, remains as low as before the 10th day (Fig. 17.4). From the 10th day onward, faster frequencies in the EEG develop as well. In contrast to the sudden development of amplitudes, the increase in the frequencies is gradual and continuous. The gradual increase in higher frequencies in the EEG is not specific for any one particular behavioral state or any one particular EEG pattern. It is rather a general phenomenon, which lasts until approximately the 20th day.

Jouvet-Mounier (1968) and Jouvet-Mounier et al. (1970) reported that the slow wave sleep pattern develops between the 12th and 14th day, 2 days later than in our rats. Genetic differences between her rats and our rats might be responsible for these differences.

After the 10th day specific EEG phenomena develop as well. After the high amplitude EEG pattern of state 1 has developed, brief episodes of attenuation of the EEG can be observed (Fig. 17.4, EEG on the 10th day, state 1). These flattenings, lasting only a few seconds, occur synchronously with short-lasting

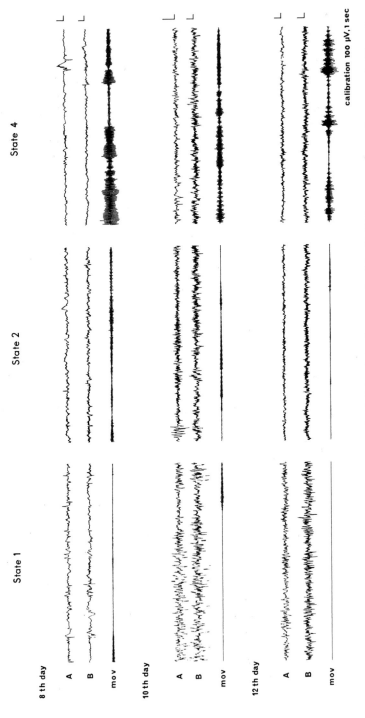

Fig. 17.4. EEG recorded from the motor cortex at the left side (A) and visual cortex at the right side (B) in state 1, state 2, and state 4, on the 8th, 10th, and 12th day. The lower trace in each record indicates movements. Calibration 100 μV, 1 sec. Time constant 0.3 sec.

346

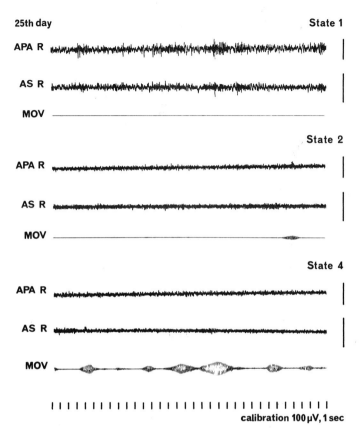

Fig. 17.5. EEG recorded on the 25th day from the motor cortex (APA) and visual cortex (AS), both on the right side in states 1, 2, and 4. The lower trace in each record indicates movements. Time constant 0.3 sec.

movements and startles. EEG spindles (14–18 Hz) occur in the state 1 EEG from the 16 to 18th day onward and a rhythm of 6–8 Hz is recorded from the occipital cortex during state 2 from about the same age (Fig. 17.5).

A rhythm of the same shape and of the same frequency can be recorded in state 2 from the dorsal hippocampus (Soulairac *et al.*, 1965; Timolaria *et al.*, 1970). This 6–8 Hz rhythm could be evoked by the dorsal hippocampus itself lying just beneath the occipital cortex in rats. Another possibility would be that the occipital cortex is driven via fiber connections from the dorsal hippocampus.

B. AUTOMATIC ANALYSIS OF THE EEG

Data which are quantitative and detailed to a high degree are essential for correlating the neurophysiological development with the morphological and

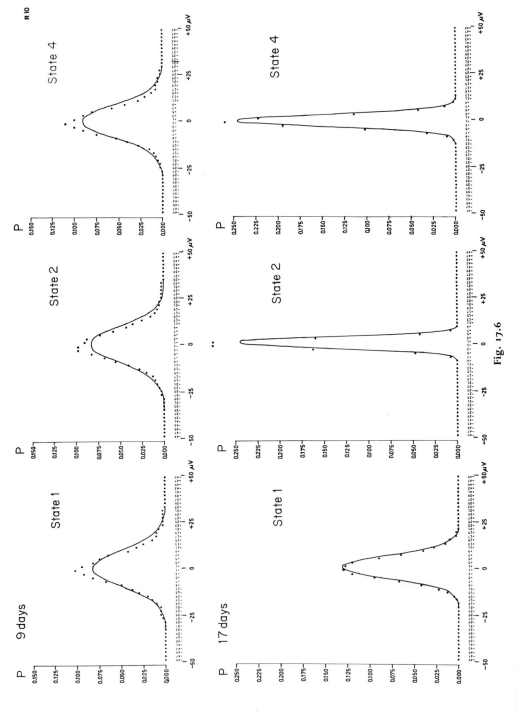

Fig. 17.6

biochemical development of the brain. Therefore automatic analysis of the EEG amplitudes and EEG frequencies was carried out. For automatic analysis $1\frac{1}{2}$-min artefact-free EEG samples recorded during states 1, 2, and 4 were chosen.

1. Amplitudes

The amplitudes were sampled at a rate of 250 Hz. An amplitude histogram of the converted values (amplitude to time converter TMC 606) was constructed (CAT 400B; TMC). The data of the histograms are punched onto paper tape, for further computation on a general purpose computer (Telefunken TR 4). The distributions were normalized, and the means and standard deviations were computed. Dividing the total power (the sum of the squared voltages) by the number of amplitude samples gave the mean power in microvolts squared. Finally, the probability density curve and the normal distribution belonging to the actual distribution were constructed. No differences are seen in the amplitude distributions of the EEGs recorded before the 10th day (Fig. 17.6). From that day on, however, the mean square voltages and the amplitude ranges of the EEG recorded in state 1 are higher when compared to these values in state 2 and state 4. The mean amplitude of the EEG fluctuates in one animal when in the same behavioral state but on different days. To be able to follow the developmental course of the mean-square voltages in the behavioral states in individual animals, we compared the mean-square voltage in state 1 with these values in the other behavioral states in the record of the same animal on the same day. The value of the mean-square voltage in state 1 was taken as 100% and the values of state 2 and state 4 compared with this value. Until the 10th day the values in state 2 and state 4 are scattered around the state 1 value (Fig. 17.7); after that day (in one case after the 11th day) the mean-square voltages in state 2 and state 4 are always lower than in state 1. After this relatively sudden change on the 10th and 11th day, no systematic development occurs in the mean-square voltage or the amplitude distributions.

2. Frequencies

Frequency analysis was carried out on a PDP-9 computer (Digital Equipment Corp.) by means of the direct Fourier analysis. The EEG signal was sampled at a frequency of 136.4 Hz and then filtered digitally at 40 Hz low

---

Fig. 17.6. Normalized nonsequential histograms of the amplitudes of the EEG recorded from the motorcortex in states 1, 2, and 4, on the 9th day (above) and on the 17th day (below). The empirical distribution (dotted line) is plotted on top of the theoretical normal distribution (solid line). P represents the probability density function; the horizontal scale indicates the amplitude in microvolts.

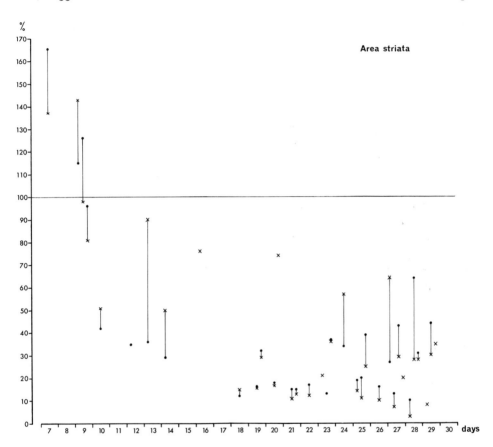

Fig. 17.7. Mean-square voltages computed from amplitude histograms of EEG recorded from the motor cortex. The mean-square voltages in state 2 (black dots) and in state 4 (asterisks) are expressed as percentages of the mean-square voltage in state 1 which was taken as the reference (100%). Values of state 2 and state 4, which are connected by a vertical line, are computed from the EEG recorded in the same session.

pass. The signal was transformed directly in pieces of 7.5 sec. The average power spectrum was plotted for each 1½-min sample in the range from 0 to 24 Hz with a graphical resolution of 0.4 Hz.

No substantial differences can be observed in the power spectra obtained from EEG recorded in states 1, 2, and 4 in the period between the 8th and 10th day (Figs. 17.8, 17.9, 17.10).

From the 11th day onward however, the frequency band broadens toward the higher frequencies. This development stops at about the 21st day. It should be noted that the development of higher frequencies in the EEG is a relatively

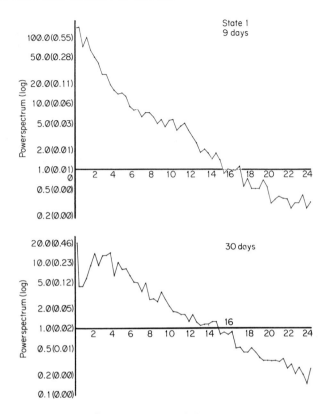

Fig. 17.8. Power spectra of state 1 EEG recorded in one rat on the 9th day (above) and in another rat on the 30th day (below). The horizontal scale gives the frequency in Hz; the vertical scale indicates the power (μV^2). Numbers in parentheses indicate values of the normalized power spectrum.

gradual process. It is apparently not linked to the rapid development of behavioral-state-specific EEG patterns, observed around the 10th day. In the EEG power spectra obtained in states 1, 2, and 4 of a 30-day-old rat (Figs. 17.8, 17.9, 17.10) it is obvious that lower frequencies (3–4 Hz) constitute a greater part in the state 1 power spectrum than in the power spectra of state 2 and state 4 in which relatively more power is concentrated at the higher frequencies.

Rapid developmental changes mark the period around the 10th postnatal day in the rat. Considerable shifts occur in the distribution of the behavioral states; behavioral state-specific EEG patterns develop suddenly after the 10th day; a broadening of the frequency band toward higher frequencies begins around this day. These developmental changes are accompanied by anatomical and biochemical changes as well. From the 10th day on, maturation of cortical neurons starts (Caley and Maxwell, 1968a), an enormous increase in the number of axons and dendrites can be observed (Eayrs and Goodhead, 1959) and adultlike synapses are seen in the rat cortex (Johnson and Armstrong-James, 1970). Myelination of cortical neurons (a relatively slow and gradual process) (Caley and Maxwell, 1968b) and vascularization (Craigie, 1925; Caley and Maxwell, 1970) begin to develop. In the same period enzyme systems develop: succinic dehydrogenase, playing a role in the aerobe glycolysis, increases considerably after the 10th day (Friede, 1959; Gregson and Williams, 1969) as well as cytochrome oxidase (Gregson and Williams, 1969) and ATPase (Samson and Quinn, 1967), enzymes which are crucial in the coupling of energy generation and consumption.

Each of these changes is related to functional development. It is extremely hazardous at this moment, however, to speculate about causal relationships

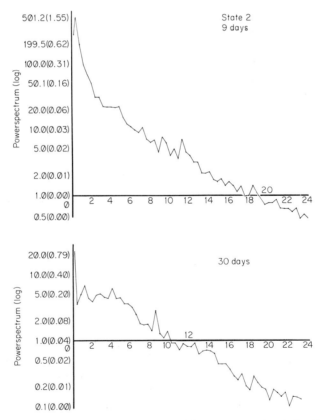

Fig. 17.9. Power spectra of state 2 EEG recorded in one rat on the 9th day (above) and in another animal on the 30th day (below). The horizontal scale gives the frequency in Hz; the vertical scale indicates the power (μV^2). Numbers in parentheses indicate values of the normalized power spectrum.

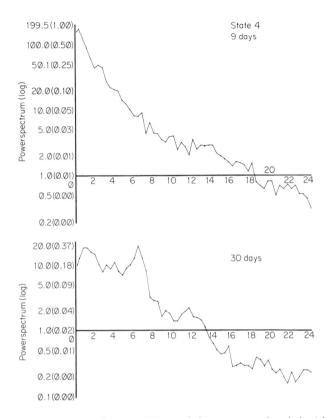

Fig. 17.10. Power spectra of state 4 EEG recorded in one rat on the 9th day (above) and in another animal on the 30th day (below). The horizontal scale gives the frequency in Hz; the vertical scale indicates the power (μV^2). Numbers in parentheses indicate values of the normalized power spectrum.

between functional, morphological, and biochemical neuro-ontogenesis. While taking into account the prerequisites about unity in methods, mentioned in the introduction, one should realize that relationships between these developmental changes may seem to be causally linked when they are actually merely coincidental because of the short developmental time scale in the rat. Investigations of disturbed developmental processes may be of further help in the future to untangle the causal relationships between function and structure during development.

ACKNOWLEDGMENTS

Part of this study was done in collaboration with Dr. P. Schwartze, Carl Ludwig Institut für Physiologie, Leipzig, G.D.R. The advice, criticism and comments of Professor H. F. R. Prechtl and Dr. Y. Akiyama as well as the assistance of Mrs. W. Gramsbergen, Mrs. H. Versteeg, Miss T. G. van der Sluis, and Miss T. Veenstra are gratefully acknowledged.

CHAPTER EIGHTEEN

Sleep in the Human Newborn[1]

OLGA PETRE-QUADENS

For a long time, sleep of the newborn attracted the attention of psychologists only (Wagner, 1939; Gesell and Amatruda, 1945; Wolff, 1959, 1965) who investigated it from a somatic and behavioral point of view. Studies on the electroencephalographic and polygraphic aspects of sleep are more recent (Parmelee *et al.*, 1961; Dreyfus-Brisac and Monod., 1965).

The individualization in the newborn, of a phase of eye movements (Delange *et al.*, 1962) was the first step of a series of investigations which eventually led to an objective classification of sleep patterns on the basis of behavioral criteria (Roffwarg *et al.*, 1964; Goldie and Velzer., 1965; Petre-Quadens, 1965). It is only recently that the significance of the behavioral state of the infant and its variations have been approached (Wolff, 1959, 1966; Escalona, 1962; Prechtl and Beintema, 1964; Eisenberg, 1965). In this regard, it is perhaps to Prechtl (1964, 1968) that we are indebted for the most systematic study of the different sleep parameters of the newborn. Our interest in the study of sleep of the newborn, and especially of the premature infant, has been motivated by considerations of the immaturity of his nervous system.

As for the ontogeny of sleep in man, the evolution of the complex constituted by the wakefulness and sleep states may be approached only by the study of the premature and newborn infant, the alternation of those two states

[1] Supported by grants from the FNRS (Fonds National de la Recherche Scientifique) and the FRE (Fondation Reine Elisabeth).

being a progressive acquisition. It is not only the duration of the sleep state which is destined to be modified during maturation but also that of the waking state. These durations regulated first only by subcortical mechanisms, later on depend on the circuits involving the cortex. We shall detail the particular characteristics of this evolution. The fast alternation of wakefulness and sleep will be seen to be progressively modified, finally to reach the usual nycthemeral rhythm in the adult.

How does the alternation of wakefulness and sleep appear in the early life of man? It is certain that in man, from the beginning of life, the wakefulness and sleep systems may function alone, even if they are submitted to cortical influences. They function probably by themselves in the newborn and certainly in the anencephalus. The features of the total sleep cycle in the newborn and the criteria allowing recognition, in this cycle, of the wakefulness and sleep phases have already been studied. Periodic awakening is very likely determined by the necessities of feeding. The total sleep cycle consists of the coalescence of numerous repose and activity periods varying from 50 to 60 min (Denisova and Figurin, 1926; Aserinsky and Kleitman, 1955). This fundamental organization never disappears, but the periods lengthen later on. The short periods of wakefulness in the newborn are probably under the influence of the mesencephalic reticular system. These primitive states of wakefulness and sleep are later modified in the 24 hr-nycthemeral rhythms, and with the occurrence of a critical reactivity of the newborn and the full diurnal consciousness of the adult, a series of intermediary states are observed. The maturation of the regime of wakefulness and sleep will be expressed not only by a progressive increase of wakefulness periods, but also by their consolidation into a "at one go" cycle, by greater critical consciousness and also by an adaptation of both states to the 24-hr-monophasic rhythm and to environmental and social conditions. We utilized both electroencephalographic and behavioral criteria to attempt to catch the "primitive aspect" of sleep. Among the behavioral criteria, the grouping of eye movements more particularly called our attention. Owing to the inconstancy of the relationships between the electroencephalographic and other physiological variables, we termed "paradoxical sleep" (PS) the sleep epochs presenting bursts of eye movements. It is with respect to the latter that we looked into the evolution of the other parameters, such as the electroencephalogram and the electromyogram.

Polygraphic records were made on 285 premature, mature, and postmature babies within a few hours of birth up to 7 days of age. The criteria utilized for the classification of sleep into various stages were both behavioral and electroencephalographic. Electroencephalographically, two variables were to be considered. One was the frequency: This is the pattern or stereotyped sequence of epochs of various critical frequencies. Among them are the spindles, the frequency of which is 13 or 14 Hz, and the stage *b* discharges at 5–6 Hz. The other variable was the amplitude. The latter led us to evaluate objectively electroencephalographic differences between the various stages of sleep by measuring the EEG amplitude.

From the behavioral point of view we considered the body movements, eye movements, smiling, and sucking movements.

I. Awakening

Distinctions were made by some investigators between several behavioral states, corresponding to the state of "awakening" (Prechtl *et al.*, 1968; Emde and Metcalf, 1968). In Fig. 18.1, the polygraphic characteristics are those of a quiet infant. First his eyes were open and he seemed to look around him (aw). Then, he was drowsy (St. *a*). All the time he had a pacifier in his mouth and

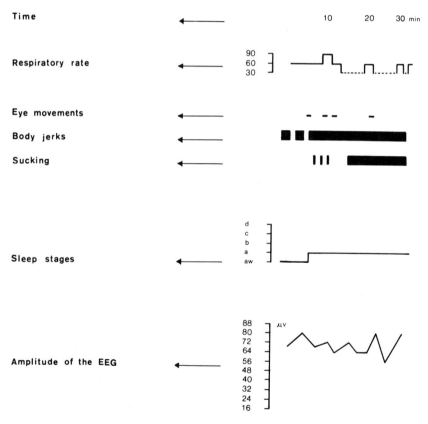

Fig. 18.1. Schematic representation of a polygraphic tracing of a 4-day-old baby; awakening, and stage *a*. From top to bottom: respiratory rate per minute (——regular; ..... irregular); presence of eye movements, body movements, and sucking movements; sleep stages; mean amplitude of the electroencephalogram.

sucked at intervals. The background rhythm was fast, of low voltage, with occasional slow waves. The mean amplitude of quiet awakening waves was similar to that of quiet sleep waves.

II. Sleep

Two types of sleep have been classified descriptively in the newborn: quiet sleep and active sleep (Delange *et al.*, 1962; Roffwarg *et al.*, 1964). We thought it appropriate to isolate an intermediary phase between awakening and active sleep: stage *a* or "undifferentiated sleep" which, from the behavioral as well as from the electroencephalographic point of view, presents its own features. It was, however, to be considered as a variety of active sleep. As for the term "awakening," the adequacy of the term "sleep" was questioned, because qualitative differences between neonatal "sleep" and "sleep" of older children and adults have been documented (Roffwarg *et al.*, 1966).

A. Quiet Sleep

Quiet sleep was subdivided into two stages, respectively called *b* and *c*, according to EEG criteria. Comparable from the somato-vegetative point of view, they were different from stages *a* and *d* on account of the regularity of the cardiac and respiratory rhythms, the absence of eye and facial movements and a body immobility interrupted by sudden startles.

Stage *b* was characterized in the EEG by the presence over the vertex of waves at 6 Hz standing out against a slow background tracing (Fig. 18.2).

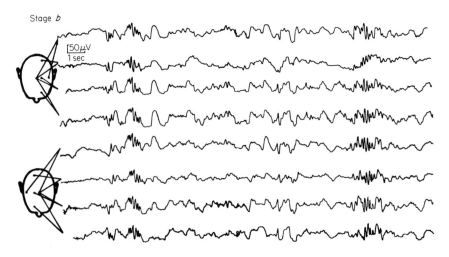

Fig. 18.2.   Van G. Mich.—age: 6 days—Stage *b*. [From Petre-Quadens, 1969]

Stage c differed from stage b by the presence of spindles of 12–14 Hz and slower and more ample waves (Fig. 18.3A,B). The mean amplitudes of the EEG were, however, similar in both stages b and c (Fig. 18.4).

The spindles appeared at certain moments of stage c and at the beginning of stage d. Their frequency was 12–14 Hz. They occurred over the vertex and in the temporo-parietal regions as shown in Fig. 18.3B. They were usually of low voltage and increased in amplitude during maturation. They were asynchronous in the newborn, whereas they appeared simultaneously in both hemispheres of the older infant.

Verley and Mourek (1962) emphasized the importance of the increase in amplitude of the electrocortical activity in the cat and the rabbit during ontogenesis, and particularly the importance of a "type of activity of sinusoidal aspect resembling that of the spindles (from 8 to 14 Hz) and of which various considerations allow us to think this type is similar to that of the spindles of the adult." In the newborn, the spindles had a frequency slightly lower (12–13 Hz) than those of the adult (14–15 Hz). Are we to link them up to those of the adult or are they due to two different mechanisms? We cannot do better than refer to the original description of Kellaway (1957): "poorly-defined sleep-spindles, maximal in the central regions are sometimes seen in the newborn. This is the first sleep pattern to appear and is the most stable and unchanging of all sleep characteristics throughout life. In succeeding months, the spindles gradually increase in amplitude and in duration." In the animal, a moderate but statistically significant increase of the frequency of the spindles during maturation has been described (Verley and Mourek, 1962). On the other hand, Valatx et al., (1964) distinguish in the kitten, a type of spindle at 11 Hz corresponding, in the adult animal, to quiet-awakening spindles. The other type, the sleep spindles, at frequencies of 15–18 Hz, would have a more tardy ontogenetic appearance.

It is probable that in the human newborn, the rarity of spindles, their frequency, and their lower amplitude compared to those of the adult, have led authors to neglect them and to place their appearance toward the age of 4 weeks (Metcalf, 1969) and even at the age of 3 months (Dreyfus-Brisac et al., 1958).

It is most likely that the spontaneous spindles and the recruiting phenomena in the sleeping animal are identical, and that the nonspecific nuclei of the thalamus are the substrate for it (Dempsey and Morison, 1942a; Jasper, 1949; Ralston and Ajmone-Marsan, 1956).

On the basis of these studies, Metcalf locates the origin of the spindles of the infant in the gray central nuclei. However, the studies in favor of the thalamic origin of the spindles do not exclude the participation of the cortex. Indeed, the ablation of the orbital cortex in the cat abolishes the spindles in the cortex and in the thalamus (Velasco and Lindsley., 1965), but only for a short period of time (see Chapter 4 by Villablanca).

Stage *c*

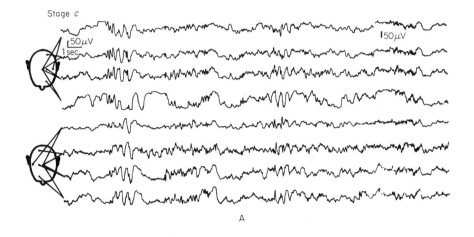

A

10 days

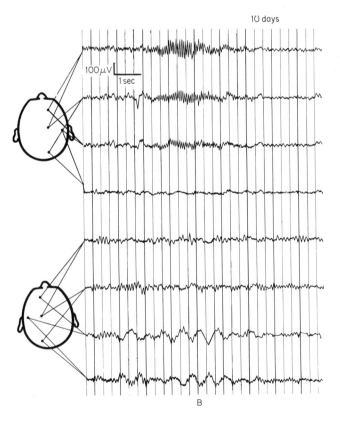

B

Fig. 18.3. A. Van D. Pat.—age: 3 days—Stage *c*. B. Spindles in a 10-day-old infant.

360

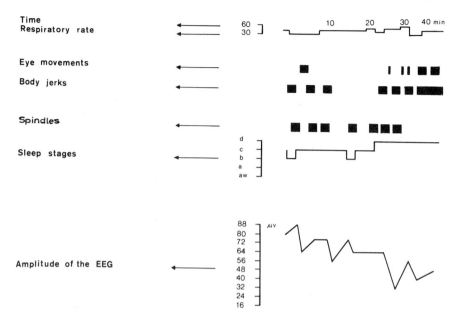

Fig. 18.4. Schematic representation of a polygraphic tracing of a 5-day-old baby. From the beginning of the recording, the infant was in a stage of quiet sleep (stages *b* and *c*). The appearance of PS (stage *d*) is marked by eye movements as well as by the increase of body movements and by a decrease of the EEG amplitude in spite of the persistence of spindles at the beginning of this stage. [From Petre-Quadens, 1969]

The discharges at 6 Hz characterizing stage *b* disappeared later on. They were also found in the sleep tracing of the pregnant woman where they immediately preceded paradoxical sleep. Slow rhythmic waves at 5 Hz in the newborn's EEG were observed earlier by Smith in 1938. He called them "periodic waves." Later on, they were designated by the name of "episodic sleep activity" (Harris and Tizard, 1960) and by "alternate tracing" (Dreyfus-Brisac and Monod 1956). Goldie and Velzer (1965) noticed the resemblance among this "episodic sleep activity," the activity in discharges of the isolated cortex (Bremer, 1938), and the complexes of the subacute sclerosing leukoencephalitis (Petre-Quadens *et al.*, 1968).

Stages *b* and *c* correspond from the behavioral point of view to "stage 1" of Prechtl and Beintema (1964), to "quiet sleep" of Parmelee *et al.* (1961), Dittrichová (1962), Monod and Pajot (1965), and to "phase 2" of Goldie and Velzer (1965).

However, the startles were numerous in quiet sleep. Wolff (1959) finds them more ample and more frequent than in active sleep and for that reason prefers to call this stage "regular sleep" rather than "quiet sleep." Because of its encephalographic aspects, this sleep is also called "synchronized sleep" or "slow sleep."

B. ACTIVE SLEEP

Active sleep was also subdivided into two stages, called a and d. This sub-division was based upon the various behavioral features, and essentially upon the differences between the patterns of eye movements. There were also electroencephalographic differences between the stages but they were not at once evident because of their variability.

Stage a was characterized electroencephalographically by a discrete slowing down of the awakening tracing. Its mean amplitude was similar to that of quiet awakening and of the quiet sleep tracing (Figs. 18.1 and 18.4). From the somato-vegetative and behavioral point of view, there were isolated eye movements, respiration was sometimes irregular but less so than in stage d, and sucking was present. (It will be recalled that the baby was recorded with a pacifier in his mouth.) The awakening threshold seemed low. Indeed, the least stimulation woke the infant up and he often began to cry.

Stage d, also called "paradoxical sleep," was characterized electroencephalographically by an activation of the electrocortical tracing. The mean amplitude was lower than during the other stages (Fig. 18.4). If it occurred after stage c, spindles appeared during the first minute. From the somato-vegetative and behavioral points of view, rapid eye movements appeared most often in discharges, with an irregular and superficial respiration, instability of the cardiac rhythm, little movements of the extremities, and a facial mimic rich in various expressions. The respiration accelerated considerably when eye movement discharges appeared. In this state, the presentation of a pacifier induced only a suspicion of sucking; the infant squeezed it between his lips a few seconds, then loosened it. This looseness may be due to the abolition of the muscle tone during paradoxical sleep. Even repeated auditive and tactile stimuli had no effect upon the course of stage d.

Stages a and d, which differed essentially by the absence or the presence of bursts of eye movements, correspond from the behavioral point of view to the "activated sleep" of Dittrichová (1962) and of Parmelee *et al.* (1962), to the "irregular sleep" of Wolff (1959), to "phase 2" of Goldie and Velzer (1965) and of Roffwarg *et al.* (1964). Electroencephalographically, they have been called "desynchronized sleep" and "fast sleep." We have separated them, whereas these authors have assimilated in one stage the sleep epochs where isolated eye movements appear and those where eye movements are grouped in bursts.

From the behavioral point of view, the absence of sucking during stage d was one criterion of differentiation with respect to stage a. This fact was confirmed by Prechtl's observation (1968) that sucking movements were absent during the phase characterized by eye movements. Stage *a* was distinct from stage *d* in the facility with which the infant woke up. The sucking movements are perhaps only a sign of a lowering of the awakening threshold. "Transitional sleep" which has been separated out by Parmelee and Wenner (1967) and by Emde and Metcalf (1968), seems to correspond to stage *a*. In the adult, the stage of polypnea occurs at the same time as the eye movement discharges (Aserinsky, 1965). But all the eye movement discharges are not necessarily accompanied by polypnea (Dement and Kleitman, 1957; Snyder *et al.*, 1964).

At present, the analysis of eye movements in man seems to indicate that bursts of eye movements and isolated eye movements are two distinct phenomena (Petre-Quadens and De Lee, 1970).

III. Smiling

The polygraphic criteria allowed us to limit to paradoxical sleep the stage of vigilance in which smiling appears for the first time (Petre-Quadens and Laroche, 1966). Its spontaneous appearance at birth has been described by Tcheng and Laroche (1965) and by Emde and Metcalf (1970). It is remarkable that smiling, long before it was induced at awakening by the image of the mother, appeared in "paradoxical sleep" in an organized form, and different from grins of a myoclonic type. The "smile to the angels" in sleep is a well-known phenomenon described in 1869 by Vogel (cited by Zipperling, 1913).

IV. Frequential Association of the Stages

The problem of the subdivision of active sleep into two distinct phases led us to search for other criteria of differentiation. With the aim of situating stage *d* in its relationship to other stages, we attempted to bring out a preferential order in the frequential association of the sleep stages.

We must bear in mind the symbols corresponding to the different stages of vigilance: A, awakening; *a*, active sleep; *b*, *c*, quiet sleep; *d*, paradoxical sleep, but we must attribute only a nominal value to these symbols.

In the analysis of these tracings, the frequential association of the stages has been taken into consideration without reference to their duration. Table 18.1 indicates the frequency with which a stage of vigilance is preceded or followed by another.

Considering, in its entirety, the succession of the stages between two awakenings, the standard form of a sleep cycle in the newborn has been disengaged. Its development is represented in Fig. 18.5.

As shown in this scheme, the sleep cycle of the newborn reveals a real organization.

TABLE 18.1

FREQUENTIAL ASSOCIATION OF THE VIGILANCE STATE COMBINED 2 BY 2[a]

A	*a*	*b*	*c*	*d*
aA : 10	Aa : 28	Ab : 0	Ac : 3	Ad : 4
bA : 3	ba : 0	ab : 5	ac : 14	ad : 10
cA : 5	ca : 5	cb : 0	bc : 0	bd : 4
dA : 17	da : 6	db : 2	dc : 11	cd : 18
Aa : 28	aA : 10	bA : 2	cA : 5	dA : 17
Ab : 0	ab : 5	ba : 0	ca : 5	da : 6
Ac : 3	ac : 14	bc : 0	cb : 0	db : 2
Ad : 4	ad : 10	bd : 4	cd : 18	dc : 11
$N = 35$	$N = 39$	$N = 7$	$N = 28$	$N = 36$

[a]From Petre-Quadens, 1969.

Paradoxical sleep, or stage *d*, appears during this cycle with a relative autonomy with regard to the other stages of vigilance (cf. Table 18.1). It may follow any stage and be followed by any stage. It may also interrupt awakening (sequence A*d*A is seen twice). It does, however, preferentially occur after quiet sleep: sequence *bd* is seen 4 times out of 7, and sequence *cd* 18 times out of 28, whereas sequence *ad* is only seen 10 times out of 29.

As regards stage *a*, sequence A*a*A (6 times) indicates that it may fill in the interval between two awakenings. This is not the case for stages *b* or *c*.

This investigation suggests some psychophysiological considerations.

A more subtle classification of sleep in the newborn than its subdivision into "quiet sleep" and "active sleep" seems to be needed. The amplitude of the electroencephalogram and the ocular aspects of stage *d* led us to distinguish it from stage *a*. Its particular situation in the sleep cycle confirms its individuality.

Paradoxical sleep (stage *d*) reveals a certain autonomy from the other sleep stages. Thus, we saw it appearing—although very seldom—between two awakenings (A*d*A). This interruption of the awakening by paradoxical sleep is characteristic in the newborn mammal and is even the only form of sequence remaining in the pontine cat (Jouvet, 1965b). In the human newborn, the preferential appearance of paradoxical sleep, after a quiet sleep stage (se-

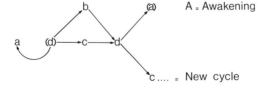

A = Awakening

Fig. 18.5. Sleep cycle in the newborn. [From Petre-Quadens, 1969]

c.... = New cycle

quences *bd* or *cd*) places his sleep in the maturation scale of the adult where this sequence is typical.

Let us recall that we have never seen the sequence A*b*, and the sequence A*c* was seen only 3 times out of 28. The appearance of quiet sleep, immediately after awakening, is improbable in the newborn.

V. Ontogeny of Paradoxical Sleep

The high percentage of paradoxical sleep in the newborn at the end of a normal gestation, and the much higher PS percentage of the newborn kitten are quite remarkable.

The simple observation of the premature shows us that his active sleep time is higher than that of the mature newborn. However, it is extremely difficult to discern whether a premature infant is awake or asleep (Gesell and Amatruda, 1945).

We tried to dissociate in the active sleep of the premature, as we did in the mature newborn, what belongs on one hand to paradoxical sleep, and on the other hand to this undefined stage which is stage *a* and which Parmelee and Wenner called "undifferentiated sleep" (1967). The distinction between the two aspects of active sleep, stage *a* on the one hand, and stage *d*, or paradoxical sleep, on the other hand, was given only by inspection of the oculogram. It was after 36 weeks of gestational age that paradoxical sleep, i.e., the phase where the eye movements are grouped, reached its highest proportion (Fig. 18.6).

Owing to the present state of controversy regarding the significance of both stages, *a* and *d*, we concentrated our attention on the eye movements only.

A. Eye Movements

During the past 3 years, a method of analysis of rapid eye movements in the infant has been developed which permits study of their density by measuring the time intervals separating them (De Lee and Petre-Quadens, 1968; Petre-Quadens *et al.*, 1969; Prechtl and Lenard, 1967).

Since it is not always clear—especially in premature infants—whether the baby is asleep or not, only the periods when the baby had his eye closed were taken into account. The periods with closed eyes in the premature and newborn babies were considered as "sleep."

The babies were grouped into three age groups according to the distribution of the data: 33–36, 37–39 and 40–41 weeks gestational age. There were 7 babies in the first, 12 in the second, and 14 in the third group.

Since the behavioral and EEG characterizations of states are continuously changing in premature and newborn babies, the extent of concordance between

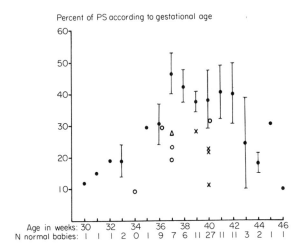

Percent of PS according to gestational age

Fig. 18.6. Percentage of paradoxical sleep with regard to gestational age. *Ordinate*: PS percentage per sleep cycle. *Abscissa*: (1) gestational age in weeks (2) number of normal cases corresponding to each term. The black circles correspond to the mean PS percentages in the prematures and normal neonates, and the vertical lines represent the standard deviations. The white circles correspond to dysmatures. The triangle corresponds to a case of microcephaly. The crosses represent the newborns with Down's syndrome. [From Petre-Quadens, 1969]

them was delineated by epochs of 40 sec. Therefore all the eye movements occurring during a complete sleep cycle of one interfeeding period were counted.

Rather than resort to an arbitrary method of determination of PS or REM sleep, we preferred to use the method of analysis of the time intervals, expressed in seconds, separating consecutive eye movements. With this method we obtained absolute frequencies, accounting for the occurrence of each interval during the consecutive PS epochs. These absolute frequencies have been converted into relative frequencies with respect to PS epochs of 40 sec for the above-mentioned reason and in order to control the time variable, i.e., the duration of each PS or REM epoch. We may thus consider the evolution of the intervals during sleep and also proceed with a graphic comparison of individual or group distributions.

Table 18.2 shows that the mean frequency per 40-sec epoch of the intervals (I) shorter than 1 sec, as well as those between 1 and 2 sec, and of those longer than 2 sec was similar in the 33–36 week prematures and in the full-term newborn. The density in I < 1 sec decreased in the 37–39 week gestational age group, and this decrease was also seen for the 1 sec ≤ I < 2 sec. This period coincides with the maturation of the cortical areas and their inhibitory functions. The delay between epochs in which a high eye movement density was detected was twice as long in the 33–36 and the 37–39 week age groups than

TABLE 18.2

FREQUENCY OF THE TIME INTERVALS BETWEEN THE EYE MOVEMENTS DURING PS[a,b]

Gest. age (weeks)	I < 1 sec		1 sec ≤ I < 2 sec		2 sec ≤ I	
	V	H	V	H	V	H
33–36	15.23	14.80	5.72	4.87	5.19	5.14
37–39	9.85	9.54	3.86	3.73	4.82	4.91
40–41	15.96	14.35	5.71	5.02	5.35	5.35

[a]From Petre-Quadens et al. 1971.

[b]Mean relative frequencies of I < 1 sec, 1 sec ≤ I < 2 sec, and I ≥ 2 sec for 40 sec paradoxical sleep, in premature and full-term babies. V = I between vertical eye movements. H = I between horizontal eye movements. The gestational age groups (in weeks) were determined according to the distribution of the data.

in the full-term neonates. Similarly, the delay between the onset of the recording and the first high density eye movement epoch diminished with increasing gestational age (cf. Table 18.3).

Different ways of approach were used in order to look into the organization of the eye movements within the different PS epochs during the sleep cycle. First, we observed a periodicity of the I < 1 sec between the consecutive PS epochs. In the premature babies, the variability in the frequency of these intervals between consecutive PS epochs was small. In the full-term neonates, there was a larger variability in those intervals from one PS epoch to the next one. These periodical changes stood out against a general tendency to a gradual increase of the I < 1 sec during the consecutive PS epochs of the same sleep cycle (Fig. 18.7). This observation might indicate that, towards birth, inhibitory functions are developing that exert their influence upon several parameters, of which the eye movements are one. The periodicity of the eye movement density reflects the periodicity of this function. Indeed, from full term on, the I < 1 sec showed periodical crests and troughs as if their

TABLE 18.3

LAPSE OF TIME BETWEEN THE PS PERIODS[a,b]

Gestational age (weeks)	Time interval before 1st REM (sec)	Time intervals between consecutive REMs (sec)
33–36	1364	668
37–39	1142	538
40–41	383	393

[a]From Petre-Quadens et al., 1971.

[b]Time lapse in seconds before the first PS stage (or REM), and between consecutive PS stages, where high-density eye-movement patterns have been found.

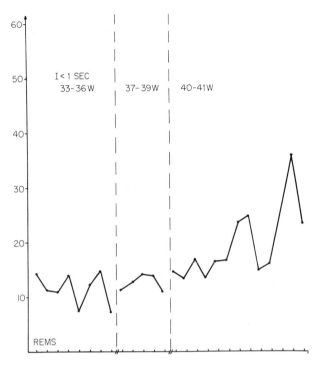

Fig. 18.7. Relative frequency of the I < 1 sec during consecutive PS stages (REMs) in premature babies of 33–36 weeks and 37–39 weeks gestational age; in full-term neonates (40–41 weeks). [From Petre-Quadens *et al.*, 1971]

appearance was inhibited alternatively. In premature infants, the small differences between the crests and troughs indicate a limited inhibitory power and a weak subsequent rebound.

Second, the correlation between the duration of the individual PS epochs of each age group and the various types of intervals showed that, for the I < 1 sec, the correlation became significant towards full term only. For the I ≥ 1 sec, this correlation was significant in each of the age groups. Among the variables that we investigated, in relation to maturation, the I < 1 sec were the only discriminative criterion (cf. Table 18.4).

What is then the meaning of PS? The question was raised whether PS in the newborn is just an artefact of the sleep-scoring method. Therefore, the intra-individual correlations between PS time and the intervals shorter than 1 sec were tested in each baby individually. In each of the three age groups, we took babies for which we had at least three PS epochs.

TABLE 18.4

CORRELATION BETWEEN FREQUENCY OF
THE I AND PS TIME[a,b]

Gest. age (weeks)	I < 1 sec	I ≥ 1 sec.
33–36	not signific.	$\alpha = 0.01$
37–39	$\alpha = 0.05$	$\alpha = 0.01$
40–41	$\alpha = 0.01$	$\alpha = 0.01$

[a]From Petre-Quadens *et al.*, 1971.
[b]Correlation coefficient between the relative frequency of I < 1 sec and I ≥ 1 sec and the duration of each PS stage in three age groups.

In the 33–36 week gestational age group, this correlation was significant at $\alpha = 0.05$ in only 1 baby out of 5. In the 37–39 week group, the correlation was significant at $\alpha = 0.05$ in 2 babies out of 6. But in the 40–41 week group, out of 13 babies, the correlation was significant at $\alpha = 0.01$ in 7 and at $\alpha = 0.05$ in 3 babies. It seems thus that PS reflects a process of physiological adaptation, reflecting the infant's ability to integrate the variations of the phasic phenomena—here the eye movements—which seem to be more sensitive to the process of maturation. The data thus indicate that there are two types of eye movement densities. It was also at full term that these high-density eye movement patterns had a periodicity within the consecutive PS epochs somewhat similar to the one in older age groups. We might conceive that the eye movements are originally a random phenomenon (Prechtl and Lenard, 1967). With the development of the cortical areas, nonspecific inhibitions occur, exerting their effects upon various physiological functions. It has been shown that the occurrence of eye movements in bursts, irregularities in respiration and heart rate, and the abolition of muscle tone, which characterize adult REM sleep, tend to coincide when the baby grows older (Petre-Quadens, 1969). There is is thus some evidence that with increasing maturation, the baby's brain becomes able to sustain larger periods of behavioral inhibition, responsible for the maintenance of both quiet and paradoxical sleep.

The mongoloid and microcephalic babies and three out of five dysmature newborns had a paradoxical sleep percentage inferior to that of the normal newborn of the same gestational age.

Mentally retarded subjects have fewer eye movements than normal subjects of the same age. The decrease of eye movement density in the mongoloid newborn, who later on become oligophrenic, poses the problem of ascertaining when, during intrauterine life, this abnormality appears and by which mechanism it occurs.

B. MUSCLE TONE

When eye movements occur during sleep in the adult, the muscle tone, at the level of the chin muscles, disappears. The abolition of the muscle tone is closely linked to paradoxical sleep in the adult (Jacobson *et al.*, 1964). The disappearance of electromyographic activity was seen in some mature neonates during the REM stage. It was less constant in the premature.

At 30 and 32 weeks gestational age, the electromyogram of the chin muscles showed a low-voltage background activity which did not vary during the recording. At 35 weeks' gestational age, this background activity was replaced by an electromyographic activity of the adult type. It was abolished in a low proportion during the REM stage. The proportion of abolition of muscle tone during this stage increased as the fetus appoached term. Thus we see appearing during ontogenesis, in active sleep, episodes corresponding to one only of the parameters of paradoxical sleep (Fig. 18.8). The electromyographic activity associated with smile and rapid eye movements was abolished in the instance of newborn *mature* infants whereas in *premature* infants EMG activity associated with smile and rapid eye movements might be conserved.

Figure 18.8 shows that in the premature, in the newborn and even in the

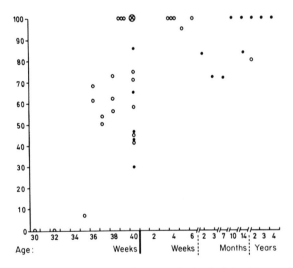

Fig. 18.8. *Ordinate*: abolition of the muscle tone at the level of the chin muscles, expressed in percentage according to the duration of the phase with rapid eye movements. *Abscissa*: on the left side of the black line, gestational age in weeks, calculated as from the probable date of conceiving. On the right side of the black line, actual age in weeks, months, and years. The black line on the x-axis indicates the moment of birth at term. The black circles refer to night recordings. The white circles refer to day recordings. ⊗ represents the results of the day sleep recordings in 15 full-term newborn infants. [From Petre-Quadens, 1969]

infant under 7 months (postnatal age), the abolition of the electromyogram at the level of the chin muscles was only linked up with eye movements in an irregular manner. Only at the age of 10 months, did the abolition of muscle tone coincide entirely with the occurrence of rapid eye movements. We do not know what goes on before the 10th week. In the postmature neonate, after the 42nd week of gestation, paradoxical sleep percentage decreased rapidly.

C. PARADOXICAL SLEEP AND THE CIRCADIAN CYCLE

In the newborn, most of the paradoxical sleep percentages were relative to day sleep recordings. The five tracings which have been made between 7:00 P.M. and 3:00 A.M. showed the lowest percentages of paradoxical sleep and the highest percentages of stage *a* (Fig. 18.9). Moreover, whereas during the day a recording of $2\frac{1}{2}$ to 3 hr was sufficient to obtain 60–90 min of behavioral sleep, 4–5 hr were necessary to obtain the same sleep time during the night. During the night, the neonates were much more excited, their sleep was frequently interrupted by awakening episodes, and stage *a* was quantitatively dominant.

At the age of 1 month, an infant had 21–22% paradoxical sleep per sleep cycle, and this proportion did not vary any further.

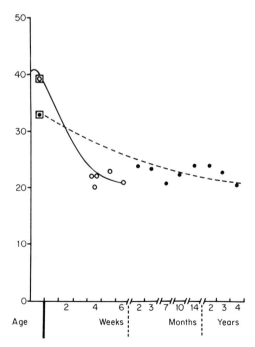

Fig. 18.9. Comparison between day and night sleep recordings. *Ordinate*: paradoxical sleep percentage. *Abscissa*: real age in weeks, in months and years. The white circles refer to day-recordings. The black circles refer to night recordings. The square with a white circle in it represents a PS percentage of day recordings in 21 full-term term neonates. The square with a black circle in it represents PS percentage of night recordings in 5 full-term neonates. [From Petre-Quadens, 1969]

It is important to emphasize here that these percentages of paradoxical sleep referred to a sleep cycle and not to a 24-hr cycle.

In the older child and in the adult, the proportions of paradoxical sleep per cycle and per 24 hr coincided.

From the age of 2 months, the day sleep periods were shorter and no longer comprised all the sleep stages. This is the reason why, from this age, our figures have been established on night recordings.

At the age of 10 months, night sleep resembled the adult's in its organization.

It appears from these data that the newborn infant sleeps more during the day than during the night. To this day sleep "facility" corresponded a higher proportion of REM stages. Our observations, although not numerous enough to affirm it, suggest that there exists during the first weeks of life an inversion of the circadian rhythm. Aserinsky and Kleitman (1955), basing their conclusions upon the protocols of Gesell, noted some differences between the day and night sleep cycles of the newborn. These differences were relative only to the length of the cycles "with eye movements." On the other hand, the mean length of the sleep stages "without eye movements" never varied. The length of the cycles with eye movements was 41.0 min during the night (from 3:00 to 6:00 A.M.), and 63.7 min during the day (from 3:00 to 6:00 P.M.)(Aserinsky and Kleitman, 1965).

VI. Conclusion

In what measure are the sleep stages of the adult derived from those of the newborn? It is not possible for us to answer this question. In one context, it does seem that stage *a* corresponds to an ontogenetically primitive state of sleep. It is characterized by a lack of behavioral inhibition and it disappears in the course of the first months of life. The presence in stage *a* of isolated ocular movements recalls those of stage 2 in the pregnant woman. Why is stage *a* present in greater proportion during the night? The study of fetal motility in the pregnant woman might clarify this problem somewhat. However, is it legitimate to suppose that a sleep stage would disappear and that new ones would establish themselves? As Dr. Prechtl pointed out, are the "stages" not merely entities arbitrarily delimited by our polygraphic criteria?

The study of sleep in the newborn and in the premature infant teaches us that the parameters are established independently of each other. In the course of maturation, the development of EEG activity, the abolition of the electromyogram and the appearance of rapid ocular movements tend progressively to become superposed and their coalescence results in the entity we call paradoxical sleep.

Hippocampal synchronization of paradoxical sleep—the most constant electrical sign in the adult cat—appears only at the 20th day after birth

(Cadilhac *et al.*, 1960). The stage of ocular movements in the newborn kitten, resembling so closely that of the adult cat, thus becomes defined and organized only tardily.

In drawing a distinction between paradoxical sleep and slow wave sleep, Jouvet (1963) attributed different origins to these two states, the reticular nucleus of the caudal pons being responsible for PS. Maturation of the fetal central nervous system occurring from below upwards, the more precocious development of midbrain and pons thus displayed (and displays) the fact that the very young premature infant manifests active sleep only (Roffwarg *et al.* 1964; Parmelee *et al.*, 1967).

However, active sleep in the very young premature infant is virtually entirely represented by stage *a* and embraces none of the EEG, EMG, or ocular characteristics of paradoxical sleep (REM sleep) properly speaking.

The ontogenetic significance of PS with rapid eye movements has been studied by Minkowski (1965). This author would interpret it as a fetal form reappearing in the adult. He postulates that eye movements exist in the fetus before the formation of the eyelids, either as accompanying movements of the head, or as a proprioceptive response of the eyeballs themselves. Minkowski emphasizes that the myelinization of the posterior longitudinal fasciculus is found quite early in the pons and tegmentum of the midbrain, that it appears at the fourth month of intrauterine life, and after a short time in a part of the reticular formation and adjoining oculomotor nuclei. The reappearance of a type of fetal motility would indicate that certain efferent pathways potentially survive in the deep levels of the nervous system, and remain liable, in some conditions, to appear again as functional pathways in the adult. That paradoxical sleep would represent the momentary reappearance of a vestige of a fetal sleep type is, however, questioned.

The notions of neuronal inhibition and excitation allow us to take account of the variations of the bursts of ocular movements observed during sleep in the course of maturation. Numerous neurophysiological studies plead in favor of the intervention of the frontal cortex in the genesis of PS. Hernández-Peón (1965) showed that PS can be induced by cholinergic stimulation both of the frontal lobes and of the pyriform cortex. Frontal lobe lesions in the preoptic area reduce the length both of quiet sleep and of active sleep. It is therefore logical to suppose that these two phases of sleep which have different awakening thresholds result from differences in the degree of inhibition produced upon neurons responsible for awakening, by the same hypnagogic system. But, over and above the inhibitory influences, there exist excitomotor phenomena in paradoxical sleep. Among them, and in first order, are the bursts of ocular movements with their train of associated signs: pupillary dilation at the moment of the ocular movements (Snyder, 1967), acceleration of respiratory rhythm, erection, and smiling. These excitomotor phenomena are precisely the ones which are reduced in neonates with mongolism and with microcephaly. The percentage of the stage of ocular movements is likewise diminished, although in less constant degree, both in dysmature and postmature infants in whom mental prognosis is at least in doubt (Grünewald, 1964) (Fig. 18.6). In the adult, the observation of ocular flickering movements during moments of intellectual concentration led Teitelbaum (1954) to come forward with the hypothesis that these ocular movements of the waking state are connected with those of sleep.

A great amount of experimental animal work and parallel investigations in the newborn and human infant have sought to define the precise relationship between the wakefulness–sleep cycle and learning capacities. Recent papers indicate that in such correlations we must take into consideration not only the state of maturation of the brain, but also general predisposing factors some of which are endocrine.

What is the meaning of the decrease in PS with respect to maturation? What are the nervous structures which are essential to the infant for the acquisition of longer periods of wakefulness and for reduction in sleep time? What are the structures responsible for the polyphasic aspect of neonatal sleep?

The biological rhythms to which we referred above perhaps play a role in the consolidation of the alternation of vigilance and sleep. We shall only invoke here the instance of temperature reflected at the level of the muscle tone. Also, the nycthemeral variations of the plasma corticosteroids and urinary ketosteroids suggest that the adrenocortical and hypophyseal activity may in turn influence not only the state of the muscle tone, but probably also the reactivity of the central nervous system. It becomes therefore difficult to consider the alternation of wakefulness and sleep as being the privilege solely of nervous mechanisms, and we must think also of the participation of endocrine mechanisms.

In place of the mesodiencephalic regulation that governs a polycyclic alternation of vigilance and sleep in the newborn will be substituted a stable alternation of these two states and a considerable prolongation of active vigilance due to a cortical regulation. Deficits in this regulation may also shed some light upon the significance of normal sleep ontogeny and, as Dr. Dement pointed out in this conference, emerge in a research area of considerable potential importance.

VII. Summary

The observations reported here indicate that both quiet and active sleep in the newborn infants are not homogeneous entities. Various data suggest that active sleep should be divided into two different stages on the basis of behavioral differences. One of them has been called stage *a* and represents a primitive sleep state. The other has been called stage d or paradoxical sleep (PS). Both stages differed by their EEG and EMG criteria and by the grouping of the eye movements.

During stage d or PS, eye movements appeared in bursts as in the adult. EEG amplitude was lowest. Muscle tone was often abolished in the mature newborn but this was not constant. Simultaneously with the rapid eye movements the chin EMG activity disappears progressively as the baby matures.

Stage a was a poorly defined sleep stage, interrupted by crying, with strong sucking movements, an active EMG at the level of the chin muscles and with isolated eye movements. This stage has also been called "undifferentiated sleep" (Parmelee and Wenner, 1967). It did not present any of the PS characteristics. The younger the premature, the more important was stage a quantitatively. For this reason, it is thought to represent a primitive state.

Quiet sleep has also been divided into two stages on the basis of their EEG characteristics. The spindle frequency was 6–7 Hz in stage b and 13–14 Hz in stage c. Both these EEG aspects were particular to quiet sleep. The babies had then only a few jerks and no eye movements. The muscle tone at the level of the chin was generally present. It was impossible to distinguish between those two EEG aspects of quiet sleep by means of any other parameter, either behavioral or linked to birth circumstances. Since the EEG and the behavioral aspects of the newborn infants changed continuously during the first 48 hr of life to become more steady later on, only sleep of 3–6-day-old babies has been analyzed.

In order to better situate stage d or PS with reference to the other sleep stages, the sequential association of the different sleep stages has been analyzed in mature neonates. Stage d was relatively independent from the other sleep stages. It might follow or be followed by any other stage. It might interrupt awakening. It preferentially followed quiet sleep. This characteristic situated stage d in the adult maturation scale where this is a frequent association.

PS or stage d, characterized by bursts of eye movements was rare in very young prematures. It increased progressively and reached its maximum proportion at about 36 weeks gestational age. The progressive organization of PS or REM sleep with maturation has been confirmed by measuring, in premature and newborn babies, the time intervals separating the consecutive eye movements. Results showed a decrease for the I $<$ 1 sec in the age group 37–39 weeks (gestational age). No change was seen for the intervals longer than 1 sec. This relative decrease in eye movement density coincides with the development of the cortical structures and their inhibitory function.

The time intervals between the eye movement periods decreased with maturation as did the time intervals between the beginning of the recording and the first sustained REM period.

In the full-term newborn babies, high-density eye movement patterns showed an organization within the consecutive REMs similar to those in older age groups.

The results indicate that the changes which occur do not concern the organization of the eye movements themselves. They seem to indicate that with increasing maturation, the baby is able to sustain longer periods of behavioral inhibition needed for both the development of quiet sleep and REMs.

Discussion

Purpura: It is certainly interesting to me that what we really have in the premature is a rather diffuse substrate for the production of the phenomenology of the eye movements. And even at this level, even though I show in the pictures in the newborn cat a fairly well-organized brain stem, it is obvious that there is so much more that is going on to resculpture the precision of the movements. The same thing is happening in the development of the cat, a change in density and distribution. Has anybody looked at that in the cat too? In other words, what Dr. Petre-Quadens is saying is that if you really put a fine microscope on the phenomena, you start to see additional aspects of the parameters which you could miss if you just looked at the global picture of eye movements. There is more to it in the microstructure of the eye movements, just as there is in every pattern.

Villablanca: I interpret Dr. Petre-Quadens' observations as a suggestion that the neocortex is introducing, as it matures, ordering and patterning in the function of the basic mechanisms of the caudal brain stem controlling rapid eye movements during REMs. This viewpoint appears to be supported by the finding in the cat that the pattern of rapid eye movements during REMs is markedly changed after neodecortication (Jeannerod *et al.*, 1965; Villablanca, see Chapter 4).

Purpura: I don't think you will confine it to the cortex. What I want to stress too is that within the brain stem, you are going to have a maturational sequence. Why just the cortex? Bear in mind that the medial longitudinal fasciculus is an early myelinated pathway in the newborn animal and human.

Petre-Quadens: My speculation of a cortical mechanism is based upon the fact that with increasing gestational age, the maturation of the central nervous system is extending from the brain stem upwards to the cortex (Larroche, 1962). But I do not know the nature of whatever may be responsible for the periodicity of the short eye movement interval frequencies. The point is that although there is no change in the total amount and in the relative density of the eye movement discharges in premature and full-term babies, they do occur in the prematures in an irregular manner. What seems to appear with increasing gestational age is a sort of frequency-limiting mechanism which groups the eye movement into bursts. The control which one sees with maturation in heart rate, respiration, etc. during slow wave sleep is not confined to slow wave sleep alone. There is a control in paradoxical sleep too. It may be that PS and eye movement density are two different entities. Paradoxical sleep, defined by the simultaneous occurrence of three parameters—abolition of the EMG, activation of the EEG, and occurrence of eye movements—may reflect a process of physiological adaptation. The variability observed in PS percentage in different babies may reflect their individual ability to integrate the variations of the phasic phenomena which seem to be more sensitive to various influences. Transition periods might occur this way.

Dement: There is perhaps one other important factor that appears to affect the physiological course of events during a transition period. We say that the major criteria of NREM sleep in the cat are the presence of EMG activity together with slow waves and spindles in the EEG; REM sleep is EEG activation together with EMG suppression. It would be nice if these, and other criteria, all changed simultaneously. However, they do not. If we must make a standard decision about the precise onset of the REM period, we tend to watch for EMG suppression and then score the REM onset at the point of EEG activation. If EEG activation occurs first, then we wait for EMG suppression. Dr. Ferguson in our laboratory analyzed these events as a function of the sleep schedule in which the cat was being maintained. He looked at successive 3-sec epochs before and after the onset of REM periods. More specifically, he identified the 3-sec epoch *in which* EEG activation occurred, and then asked where the EMG suppression took place in relation to it. If the cat was being forced to consolidate his sleep and wakefulness periods, so that, for example, he walked on a treadmill for 16 hr and then slept in a recording cage for 8 hr, *Ferguson found that EMG suppression took place in exactly the same 3-sec epoch as EEG activation in more than 50% of REM onset periods*! In animals who were allowed to sleep whenever they pleased and were simply recorded continuously 24 hr per day, less than 10% of REM onset period showed this simultaneity. In other words, the point of transition from NREM sleep to REM sleep was sharper and less ambiguous in animals who were consolidating their waking and sleeping periods. The point of all this is that newborn infants are sleeping *ad lib*. If they were forced to maintain clear-cut wakefulness for longer periods of time, would their sleep states be less ambiguous? In terms of all the things we have been discussing, it would be interesting to see if we could reduce the physiological disorganization in the infant by keeping him awake for somewhat longer periods. For example, an infant might be kept awake for 2 or 3 hr by gentle stimulation. I will hasten to add that this might be more difficult to accomplish than we expect. Dr. Howard Roffwarg has said that sleep deprivation in newborn infants is virtually impossible. The transition from one state to another is more clear-cut when you force the cat to consolidate.

Minard: Rapid eye movement deprivation has been done with newborns. There is at least some evidence it may occur with some infants for periods much longer than a few hours and it may even start earlier than birth, but there are problems in evaluating data. The future of sleep research may lie in moving beyond the globally defined sleep stages in various ways, particularly with the infant and with topics like REM deprivation. Cumulative records of rapid eye movements during sleep have provided one approach I believe is especially promising. The record is simply plotting the number of rapid eye movements, minute-by-minute, on the chart's ordinate, and the number of minutes on the abcissa. With other responses, the technique is common in animal and drug research. Order and change not readily seen by other methods become evident in such recordings. Individual differences also become evident. When we played tape-recorded normal nursery noise during the interfeeding sleep of seven 3-day- and 4-day-old infants, there was no consistent change in their cumulative REM records, nothing to make them consistently or significantly different from those obtained from the same infants under quiet conditions. One infant, however, a 3-day-old, who appeared to have less patterning than most in his initial cumulative record, showed a marked reduction in REM. When the infant was studied again at 8 days, the reduction was even more marked. Rapid eye movement was virtually abolished. It seems reasonable to infer that this infant was experiencing REM deprivation and general disruption of sleep and also to infer that deprivation might have been occurring in the nursery where our noise was recorded. Nevertheless, he did not appear to be sleeping badly according to either the reports of the nurses who saw him in the nursery or the research assistant who studied him. Three months later, he was diagnosed as "hyperactive." As with nearly all the infants we have studied, this infant showed day-to-day reduction in the amount of sleeping REM. The one exceptional infant we have recorded was the infant of a mother on phenothiazine-type medication during pregnancy. This infant showed three and fourfold *increase* in sleeping REM frequency from the first to the third day of life. The finding may have represented the "rebound" one regularly finds when REM deprivation is stopped. The rebound may have been from the REM-suppressing effects of the mother's medication reaching the relatively tiny nervous system of the infant. Support for this interpretation was provided by some studies of observed eye movements. Two studies by different observers watching 30 infants each have shown day-by-day increases in the time from the start of the first sustained lid closure to the first eye movement observed beneath the lid. (The observation suggests day-to-day decline in REM.) In the first study, average latency was 4.10 min; in the second it was 4.44 min. You can imagine our surprise when we observed an infant with a latency of 45 min when he was 12 hr old. The latency appeared to *decline* day-by-day. The mother of this infant was also on phenothiazine-type medication. A pediatric neurologist detected opisthotonus in the infant, a condition listed as a possible side effect of the medication which had been given the mother. Perhaps this infant allowed us to observe REM deprivation, due to medication effects remaining at 12 hr, as well as subsequent rebound.

Each of these observations is in need of further exploration. I believe this is the first such report of REM rebound in the infant. Perhaps most important in what I have reported is the suggestion that we must look beyond globally rated sleep stages. These stages showed none of the day-by-day reduction in the first week which was so evident in cumulative REM recording. Reduction in REM stage sleep has only been demonstrated later in development. The stages revealed little individual patterning, they showed none of the striking change produced by normal nursery noise in one of our infants, and they did not demonstrate the day-by-day increase in sleeping REM which provides evidence for REM rebound. For each of these observations, it was necessary to look at the eye movements themselves.

Dement: One problem is the relatively large duration of the scoring epoch induced. When we use scoring epochs of 60 sec, or 30 sec, or even 20 sec, it is absolutely clear that several state changes can occur within such a duration. Many investigators have encountered this problem when they have attempted to do all-night sleep recordings immediately following prolonged wakefulness. There is a commonly shared feeling that REM sleep is somehow unstable in this condition. Actually, we are often seeing a very rapid alternation between REM sleep and NREM sleep. For 5 sec the state is clearly REM with rapid eye movements, EEG activation, sawtooth waves, irregular respiration, and so on. However, in the next 5 sec, we see spindles, *slow* eye movements, and maybe even an upsurge of EMG activity. In the cat, we can see clear-cut behavioral correlates of very brief state changes. There is no question that such brief durations do not fundamentally alter the concept of state. Obviously, if one were trying to say that a state change occurred every 100 msec, it would be behaviorally ridiculous. However, the 30-sec epoch which is so popular is too long to be precise. This instability or rapid shift of states is more likely to occur at the end of REM periods. I am sure that a careful examination would reveal other correlates of this process, such as coherence change.

Metcalf: Dr. Petre-Quadens, did you count eye movements in small-for-date infants or postmature infants? Because of their particular features of maturation one might wonder about deviation from normality.

Petre-Quadens: We measured the intervals between the eye movements in three small-for-date infants. In two babies, the amount of intervals shorter than 1 sec was low, the periodicity between them was lacking, and the total amount of eye movement was decreased. Similar features were seen in mongoloid neonates. In the third baby, however, the results were quite normal.

Purpura: What happens to babies delivered naturally and by cesarian section? Do you see anything in the first couple of days?

Petre-Quadens: We did not measure the eye movement intervals when this study was made. Only the EEG was taken into account. When the cesarian section was made for mechanical reasons, about 50% of the babies had a normal EEG, and the other 50% had an EEG with predominant slow waves. Active sleep, however, was decreased in both groups and the babies were weaker. This might be an effect of the mother's medication. When the cesarian section was made because of fetal distress, the EEG was abnormal in all cases. Since the drugs given to the mother do get through the placenta, the interaction between their effect and the effect of anoxia due to fetal distress makes it difficult to clearly evaluate the influence of the method of delivery on the infant's brain (Petre-Quadens and Dubois-Dalcq, 1965).

Minard: I have a comment and two questions: my understanding from your data is that your time constant is long enough, so moderate reduction in corneoretinal potential will not have serious effects. My belief about this is partly based on recordings obtained from newborns and infants while simultaneously obtaining records with time constants like yours. There has been no evidence of serious problems so long as the experimental objective was the one you had. I have one trivial question and one I find more interesting, but so complex we may only be able to raise it rather than answer it here. First, in counting your vertical and horizontal eye movements, how do movements at an angle enter in? Could one movement contribute to both categories?

Second, I wonder about the possible theoretical significance of the oscillation you observe in certain REM interval frequencies. Could it mean some sort of feedback, integration, or "governor" is not quite working? Perhaps there is a "REM generator" and a "REM inhibitor" which are coordinated in the adult, but earlier in development there is delay in feedback relationships integrating them? The result of such a delay would be oscillation.

Petre-Quadens: In the case of oblique eye movements, the deflections on the horizontal and vertical leads would be simultaneous. This happens sometimes but it is rather rare. I do not have an explanation for the REM oscillation. Something is acting as a periodically recurrent eye movement-limiting mechanism which develops with maturation as shown in Fig. 18.7 of this paper. This frequency-limiting mechanism could account for the troughs of the REM rhythm. One might also think of a frequency-enhancing mechanism responsible for the crests of the curves. I am afraid that your question merely emphasizes our ignorance about the rhythmical nature of not only the eye movements but most of the biological events.

CHAPTER NINETEEN

Sleep Studies in Hormonal and Metabolic Diseases of Infancy and Childhood

HANS-GERD LENARD
FRANZ-JOSEF SCHULTE

In spite of the fact that infants and children sleep more the younger they are and though both pediatricians and parents assign great or even exaggerated importance to quantity and sometimes even quality of children's sleep, pediatricians were relatively late in entering the sleep business. There have been exceptions, to be sure: Czerny, as early as 1891, made an attempt to assess sleep depth in infants by means of electrical stimulation. Since, however, at that time he had no information on the importance of neutral temperature for a steady behavioral state and studied his subjects at a room temperature below 20° C, he encountered some difficulties in keeping them asleep and his results were rather inconsistent. By means of a plethysmograph attached to the fontanel he was still able to observe that during sleep there were periods of regular pulsations alternating with those of highly irregular patterns in the writeout. In 1913 the Austrian pediatrician Zipperling observed in his sleeping baby granddaughter spells of eye movements, body jerks, and irregular respiration. Concerned about her health, he decided to visit the Royal Saxonian Department of Obstetrics in Dresden, where he was able to find a similar phenomenon in about 50% of all healthy infants, and the experienced head midwife—whose name did not enter the literature—expressed the opinion that the percentage was in fact still higher. Zipperling's delicious and methodically perfect publication of these observations was, 40 years before Aserinski and Kleitman (1955), premature and not sufficiently appreciated.

So the physiologists, psychiatrists, and psychologists did the basic work on sleep physiology while eminent neuropediatricians like Peiper (1961) still considered sleep as an analogue to immaturity and the greater demand for sleep in infancy as the result of the immature brain's tendency to relapse into the state of nonfunctioning. Meanwhile the situation has changed. Pediatricians apply the information provided by modern sleep research for diagnostic purposes, and are sometimes able to themselves gather important data for the understanding of sleep mechanisms in man by studying physiology and pathology of the developing brain.

For the neuropediatrician polygraphic sleep recordings are an unique diagnostic tool. By taking into account sleep states and stages as defined by other recorded physiological parameters he can increase the reliability of his EEG evaluation in infants: a potential which is an epileptic spike during wakefulness or REM sleep may be a normal constituent of the trace alternant when it occurs during NREM sleep. Similarly, the correct interpretation of data on respiration or heart rate is impossible without the additional information on the baby's behavioral state as it is provided by the polygram. Moreover, it is possible by means of sleep recordings to study coordinative and homeostatic capacities of the brain developmental levels when these complex functions are not assessable by other diagnostic methods. Coordinative capacities are shown in the building up of a typical pattern of physiological variables which define a state, and homeostasis is expressed in the brain's ability to keep a certain state stable over time (Fig. 19.1).

Changes in these functions are a very sensitive indicator of brain disorders of developmental anomalies. When otherwise healthy prematures reach term, they show definite differences and even anomalies in their sleep pattern as compared to full-term newborns (Dreyfus-Brisac, 1970). Unfortunately, changes in the course of the sleep cycles and in the sleep states are not very specific in relation to clinical diagnosis. As shown by Prechtl (1968) and by Schulte et al. (1969, 1971), many different pathologic conditions result in an immature EEG pattern and in a disintegration of the sleep states. Usually NREM sleep, the state with the most complex and sensitive homeostasis, is affected first, which results in an increase of the ratio of REM to NREM sleep and in an increase of the amount of undefined or transitional sleep.

During the search for criteria in the polygraphic recordings which might be of more specific value for clinical diagnosis, it became obvious that alternations in the amount of sleep spindles are related to certain disease states. Schultz et al. (1968) found a decrease of spindle activity during NREM sleep in hypothyroid infants, and an increase in spindle activity was observed in

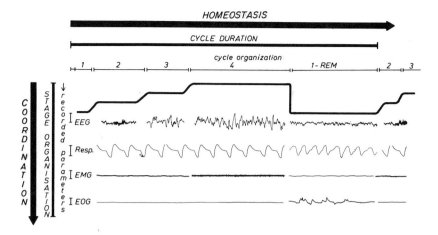

Fig. 19.1. Diagnostic possibilities of polygraphic sleep recordings in infants.

patients with phenylketonuria (Poley and Dumermuth, 1968; Gross and Schulte, 1969). In order to be able to assess changes in spindle activity quantitatively it appeared necessary to collect data on spindle activity and its developmental changes in normal infants and children.

In normal full-term babies the first traces of spindle activity appear at about 48–52 weeks (Metcalf, 1970). In prematures spindle development has already started at a conceptional age of 44–48 weeks; influences of extrauterine factors on spindle development can thus be assumed (Metcalf, 1969). When spindles first appear, they are of low amplitude, show the typical frequency for infants of 13–14 Hz but not yet the typical spindle shape, and are frequently interrupted by background activity. These are called grade 1 spindles by Metcalf; grade 2 spindles, the typical ones, appear at a conceptional age of 52 weeks. By measuring with a ruler the length of every spindle and the interval between successive spindles during the first two NREM epochs of normal night sleep we have analyzed the spindle development in a cross section of subjects between the ages of 3 months and 3 years (Lenard, 1970). The values obtained, accurate to about 1/15 sec, were plotted as histograms and median and interquartile ranges were computed for both spindle length and interval duration for each hemisphere of each subject. For the intervals we found minimal values at 4 months and an increase in the following months (Fig. 19.2). For spindle duration the situation is the reverse: The maximum length is found at 4 months, thereafter the length of the spindles decreases until the third year (Fig. 19.3). Interesting differences were found in the expression of spindle activity over the two hemispheres. In about 80% of the subjects more and longer spindles

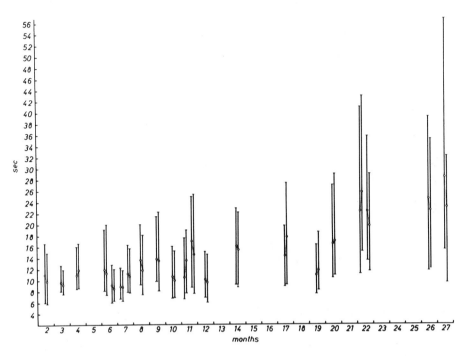

Fig. 19.2. Median and interquartile range of spindle intervals of 21 infants and children. The intervals are shortest at 3 months and increase in the following months.

are found over the right hemisphere. The hemispheric differences were very constant in infants studied longitudinally, e.g., in a hypothyroid group (Fig. 19.6). While in infancy spindles are present throughout the whole epoch of NREM sleep, in the following years they are found almost exclusively during stage 2 sleep at the beginning of an NREM epoch. There are some data pointing also to a slowing of the frequency within the spindles to 11–12 Hz in later stages of development.

These data on the development of spindles have been confirmed by spectral analysis of the EEG. With the generous help of the Health Sciences Computing facilities of UCLA we have analyzed, in a cross section of subjects, 3-min periods of REM sleep (active sleep = AS) and of NREM sleep (quiet sleep = QS). The designation QS II-IV corresponds to the sleep stages 2–4 in older infants and children; during the first 6 months of life and under pathological conditions, when Dement stages are not clearly distinguishable, the numbers II-IV refer to the first, middle, and last third of a NREM epoch. Figure 19.4 (pp. 386–388) shows the development of a power peak in the spindle frequency, beginning at 2 months, reaching maximum at 4 months, and decreasing thereafter. During the first year of life spindles are present in all three segments of NREM sleep; later they are restricted to QS II.

EEG changes in hypothyroid patients have been extensively investigated and are described as consisting of a slowing and flattening curve. It is generally held that restitution of the electroencephalographic activity to normality and normal intellectual and somatic development is obtained more easily the earlier therapy is initiated. No prognostic value has been assigned to alterations of the EEG (Raiti and News, 1971). From clinical observation it appeared that hypothyroid subjects sleep easier and more or are at least more frequently drowsy than normals. Objective sleep studies, performed by Kales *et al.* (1967a), could not confirm this observation. Hypothyroid patients do not sleep more, they only sleep differently. In adult patients Kales found quantitative changes in the sleep stages consisting in a reduced amount of stages 3 and 4 before treatment, and a tendency toward normalization under therapy. The authors discuss whether the reduction in stage 4 sleep, found similarly in depressed and in normal aged subjects, could be attributed to decreased levels of physical and mental activity.

Sleep recordings in hypothyroid patients under the age of 2 years showed

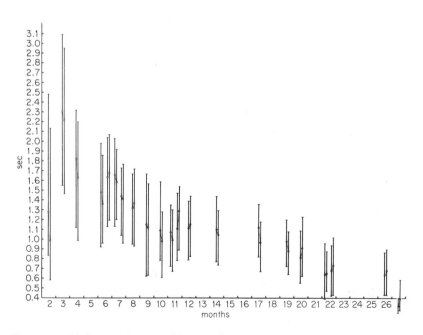

Fig. 19.3. Median and interquartile range of spindle duration of 21 infants and children. The spindles are longest at 3 months and decrease in the following months.

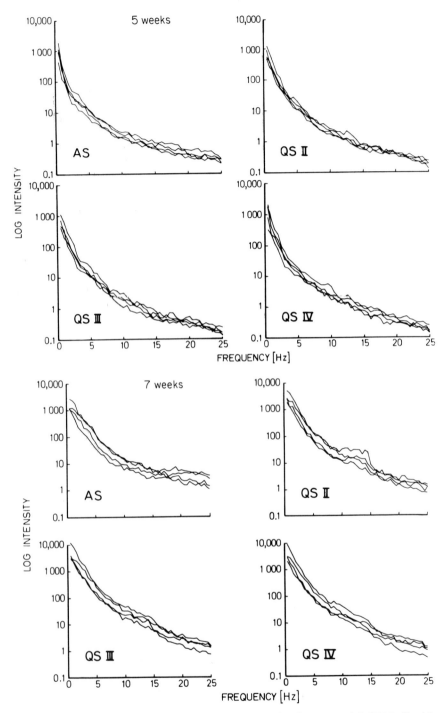

Fig. 19.4. Power spectra of right and left fronto-central and centro-occipital EEG of healthy infants and children during sleep. Time of analysis is 3 min. AS = REM sleep. QS II-IV first, second,

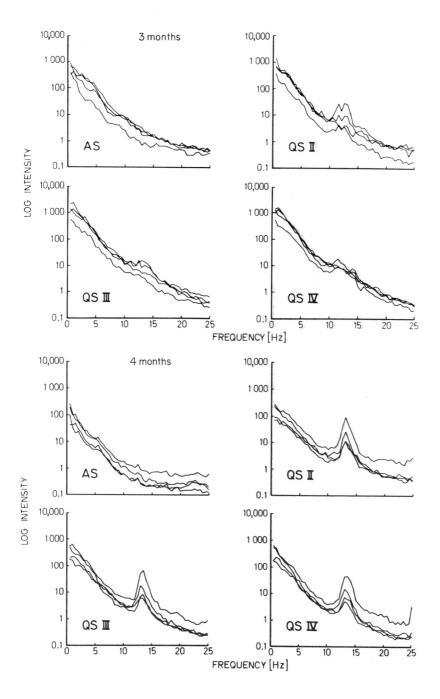

and third part of one NREM epoch. Spindles appear during the second month, are highest during the third and fourth months. At this age they are present throughout NREM sleep, later they are present throughout NREM sleep. Hypnagogic theta-activity appears during the second half of the first year and is highest around 2 years. (Continued on following page.)

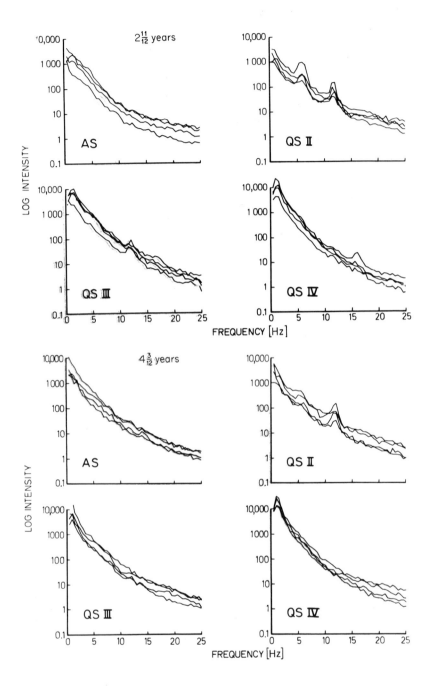

Fig. 19.4 (cont.)

388

a different situation from that reported by Kales in adults. Initially there was some increase in atypical or undefined sleep, usually with a flat EEG but with regular respiration and without REMs. However, the most striking changes in the sleep stage pattern were due to two facts: The almost complete lack of REMs which made it almost impossible to detect typical REM sleep before treatment, and the impressive lack of sleep spindles in spite of long periods of NREM sleep with high voltage EEG, regular respiration, and tonic EMG activity (Fig. 19.5).

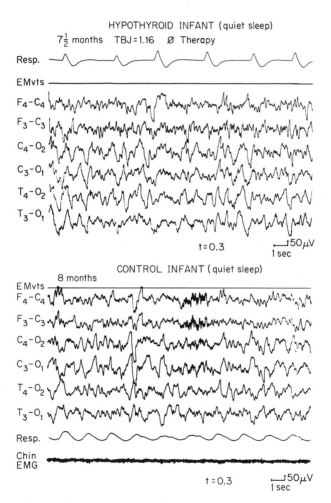

Fig. 19.5. The EEG during NREM sleep of hypothyroid infants is characterized by the lack of sleep spindles.

Schultz *et al.* (1968), using a semiquantitative method for analysis, found a delay of development or a decrease in the incidence of sleep spindles in all patients studied after the age of 3 months. All infants responded to thyroid therapy with different degrees of spindle development but not all of them reached the same amount of spindles as healthy controls. Developmental follow-up studies by means of the Gesell schedule appeared to be consistent with the hypothesis that a restitution or development of spindle rhythms occurs only in those children who develop relatively normally also on the intellectual level. The possibility of a correlation between spindle intensity and cerebral development, i.e., the possibility that exact quantitative data on spindle development might be used as a guideline for therapy and prognosis in addition to insufficient biochemical data and the slowly reacting bone maturation is exciting indeed. We have therefore started to carry out sleep studies in our hypothyroid patients using exact parameters for quantification. This program is still under way and far from its final aim—the guidance of therapy by means of electroencephalographic data. But it has already resulted in some interesting observations.

Handmade measurements of spindle length and spindle density in three patients before and under treatment showed striking increase in both parameters correlated with clinical and biochemical improvement (Fig. 19.6). This method of analysis appears to be very reliable but it is time-consuming and cumbersome. We have therefore carried out frequency spectral analysis of the EEGs of another nine patients which confirmed our earlier data. Figure 19.7 shows the results of this analysis in two patients before and under hormonal therapy. The most obvious change is a significant increase of the power in the frequency band of the spindles during NREM sleep. In some cases (Fig. 19.7B, p. 393) there was in addition a shift of the frequency of the spindles to the faster side. Follow-up studies are under way to establish the degree of correlation between the hormonal balance at a given moment, the developmental level, and the data of EEG analysis.

The neurophysiological basis for the increase of spindle activity under thyroid hormone is not known. There are, however, two hypothetical explanations suggesting either morphological or functional changes as the possible cause. Spindles are generated in the thalamus (Andersen and Andersson, 1968), but can be abolished by destruction of thalamic nuclei as well as by ablation of certain cortical areas (Velasco and Lindsley, 1965). It therefore appears that cortical spindles are the result of thalamocortical synchronizing mechanisms in a feedback system which requires extensive interneuronal connections. This assumption is supported by the observation that during ontogenesis the development of spindles coincides with the boom in the development of axons, dendrites, and synaptic connections in the brain. The development of dendritic arborization is delayed in hypothyroidism and

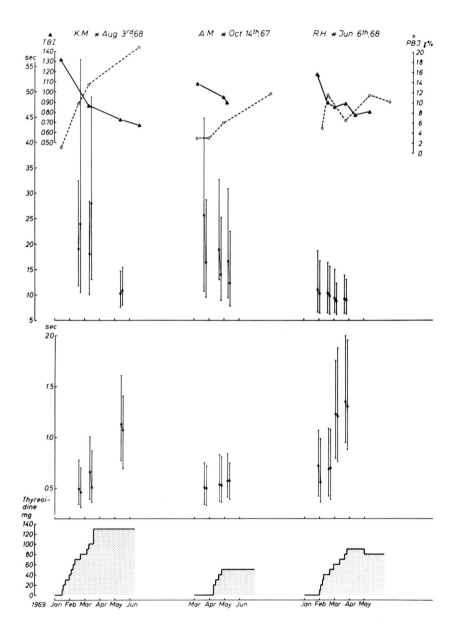

Fig. 19.6. Three hypothyroid patients before and under treatment. Upper line: Values for PBJ and thyroxine binding index. Second line: Median and interquartile range of spindle intervals. Third line: Median and interquartile range of spindle duration. Last line: Dose of hormonal substitution.

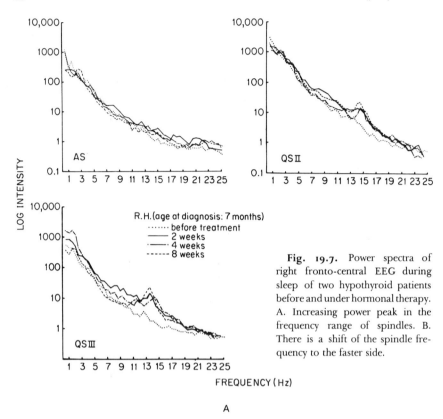

Fig. 19.7. Power spectra of right fronto-central EEG during sleep of two hypothyroid patients before and under hormonal therapy. A. Increasing power peak in the frequency range of spindles. B. There is a shift of the spindle frequency to the faster side.

induced by thyroxine (Eayrs, 1960, 1964; Legrand and Bout, 1970). Thus the lack of spindle activity in hypothyroid patients may be related to a lack of anatomical pathways and the appearance of spindles under hormonal substitution could be the result of a catching-up of morphological maturation of the development of intracortical, interhemispheric and thalamocortical synaptic interrelations. On the other hand, it is necessary to discuss possible functional influences of thyroid hormone on cortical and subcortical neurons. It is known that thyroxine increases cortical excitability by increasing the ratio of intracellular to extracellular sodium very rapidly over a period of 4–8 hr (Timiras and Woodbury, 1965) and that it increases, at least in early developmental stages, cerebral oxygen consumption (Fazekas *et al.*, 1951; Tirri *et al.*, 1968). These or similar factors may account for increased spindle activity immediately after the application of thyroxine as observed by Short *et al.* (1964) during their work on caudate spindles, and by Abbadessa and Montalbano (1968). We have seen an impressive increase in spindle amplitude only a few days after small doses of thyroid hormone in older children with hypopitui-

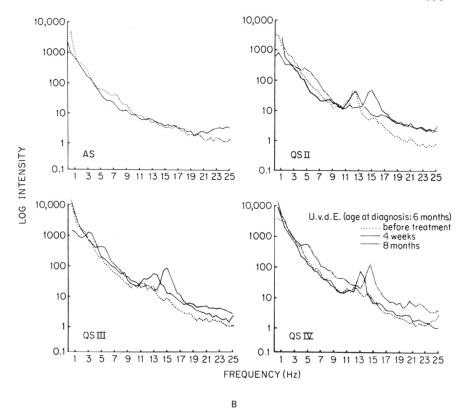

B

tarism, but with normal intellectual development and normal EEG. Vice versa, we have observed unusually high spindles in a hyperthyroid boy which decreased under thyrostatic treatment (Figs. 19.8 and 19.9). Since however, Kales *et al.* (1967a) were apparently unable to find a lack of sleep spindles in adult hypothyroid subjects, and because of the outstanding quantity of the increase in spindles not only in amplitude but also in number and duration occurring in treated hypothyroid infants, we think that structural immaturity rather than functional alteration is the main cause of spindle lack in infantile hypothyroidism. There are probably other conditions which can decrease spindle activity during quiet sleep; but none is known in which the decrease is equally obvious as in hypothyroidism and there is no other substance available which is so powerful in enhancing spindle development during early life as thyroid hormone.

Hypothyroid infants are usually quiet, friendly, and sociable. Only rarely do they develop convulsive disorders. Exactly the opposite is the case in infants and children with phenylketonuria (PKU) which are hyperactive, difficult to

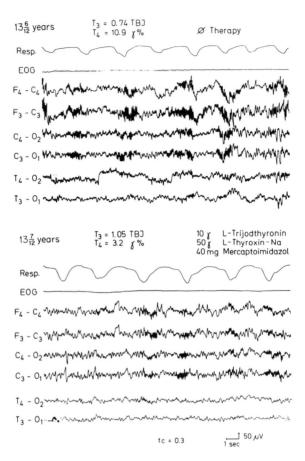

Fig. 19.8. Pronounced spindle activity in the EEG during stage 2 sleep in a hyperthyroid patient. Decrease of spindle activity under treatment.

handle, and frequently get seizures. Whereas hypothyroid patients lack spindles, PKU patients have exceeding amounts of electroencephalographic activity in the frequency range of spindles. Gross and Schulte (1969) analyzed polygraphic sleep recordings from PKU patients and compared them with those of normal controls matched for age. The records of PKU patients showed more pages containing spindles; the average length of spindles was longer and the number of spindles during NREM epochs was higher in the patient group than in the control group. During the past 2 years we have obtained EEG frequency spectra from sleep records of a larger group of PKU patients both before and during dietary treatment. Figure 19.10 gives examples from this study: It shows the appearance of spindles at NREM sleep onset already at the age of

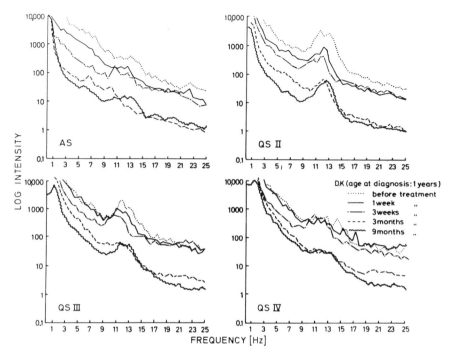

Fig. 19.9. Power spectra of right fronto-central EEG during sleep in a hyperthyroid patient before and under therapy. The spindle peak decreases to hypothyroid values simultaneously with the appearance of biochemical signs of iatrogenic hypothyroidism.

5 weeks, spindles throughout the whole NREM epoch at the age of 8 weeks, and a maximal spindle peak at 3 months. Sometimes an energy peak in the frequency range of spindles was found during sleep states which, by all other criteria such as presence of rapid eye movements, irregular respiration, and absence of muscle tone, had to be classified as REM sleep. During the third year of life, when spindle activity is normally diminished and restricted to stage 2, PKU patients show peaks in the spindle range throughout the whole NREM sleep. It is also apparent that the spindle peaks in PKU patients are more irregular and extend sometimes over a broader frequency range than the normal 13–14 Hz.

During observation periods of up to 3 months, dietary treatment which normalized phenylanlaine and 5-HT (serotonin) levels in the blood neither changed the pathological EEG pattern nor the abnormal frequency spectrum. As yet we have no idea whether the early institution of long-term dietary treatment over years can finally normalize EEG spindle activity. As an explanation of the increased spindle activity in PKU, morphological changes in the brain are not as readily available as in hypothyroidism. The myelination defects,

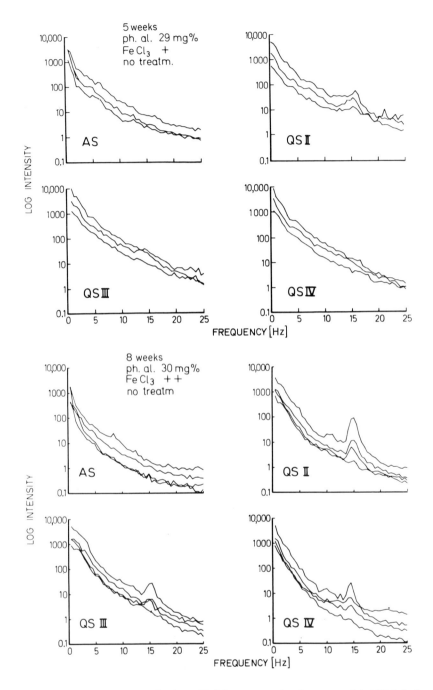

Fig. 19.10. Power spectra of right and left fronto-central and centro-occipital EEG during sleep in patients with phenylketonuria. The spindle peak appears abnormally early, is very high,

396

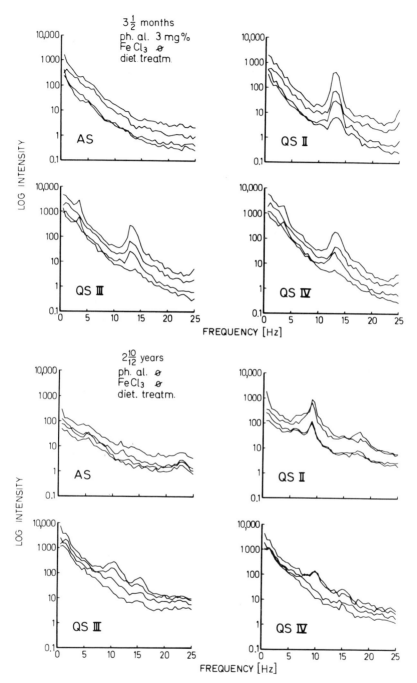

and sometimes abnormally broad-based. Biochemical normalization under dietary treatment does not change the abnormal EEG spectrum within the observation period of up to 3 months.

shown by Scholz (1957), Poser, and van Bogaert (1959) and Crome *et al.* (1962) are probably not yet developed at the very early stages of the disease; they would not help to explain the excessive spindle activity anyway. It has been suggested by Neame (1961) and by Linneweh *et al.* (1963) that competitive inhibition by other amino acids, by high levels of phenylalanine, or an impairment of their transport through cell membranes can occur, causing deficient composition of nerve cells. But why should this increase spindle activity? It it necessary to look for possible functional disorders in the brain caused by the metabolic defect.

High levels of phenylalanine interfere with several enzyme systems, one of which is glutaminic acid-decarboxylase, an enzyme essential for the formation of gamma-aminobutyric acid (GABA). Since GABA has a strong influence on inhibitory neurons (Elliot and Jaspers, 1959; Roberts and Eidelberg, 1960), a lack of this substance could increase cerebral excitability and the brain's tendency for rhythmic discharges. On the other hand, high phenylalanine levels lead to disturbances in tryptophan metabolism. Either the hydroxylation of tryptophan, or the active transport of 5-hydroxytryptophan into the brain, or—less likely (Hsia *et al.*, 1963)—the 5-hydroxytryptophan decarboxylase activity is inhibited by the elevated blood levels of phenylalanine and its metabolites (Pare *et al.*, 1958; Davison and Sandler, 1958). By one or more of these mechanisms the amount of 5-HT in blood and brain is diminished in PKU (Hsia *et al.*, 1963). Serotonin, a substance of high synaptic activity, is supposed to increase cortical synchronization (Koella and Czicman, 1966). In our patients the blood levels of 5-HT were decreased to half the normal values or less. Thus a decrease of cortical synchronization should be expected and it is surprising to find instead an increase in spindle activity and no change in the amount of spindle activity under a treatment which quickly normalizes the 5-HT level. It is also uncertain whether a great variability in the electrical power over different cortical areas found in our PKU patients can be explained by the lack of 5-HT.

Infants and children with PKU appeared to be a unique natural model to test the theory of a humoral sleep regulation via serotonergic and monoaminergic neurons in the brain stem (Jouvet, 1966, 1970; Koella, 1970). Because of decreased 5-HT levels, the ratio of NREM sleep to REM sleep was expected to be low in untreated patients and to return to normal after initiation of dietary treatment and normalization of blood 5-HT levels.

In order to test this hypothesis we recorded polygraphically the first two cycles of normal night sleep in 22 infants and children (aged 16 days to $3\frac{9}{12}$ years) with untreated PKU and in 22 age-matched controls. Moreover, 13 patients with treated PKU (aged 45 days to $3\frac{10}{12}$ years, treated for periods between 10 days to 18 months, all with blood phenylalanine levels below 8 mg/100 ml) were compared with untreated patients matched for age. Sleep state scoring was carried out by three different methods: (1) by subjective visual analysis of the record, using mainly EEG pattern and oculogram as indicators of sleep state (paradoxical sleep versus slow wave sleep); (2) by determining the presence or absence of rapid eye movements in 20-sec period (REM versus NREM sleep); (3) by computer analysis of punch cards containing data on respiration, limb and body movements, EEG pattern and eye movements (codes according to Parmelee *et al.*, 1968). At least three out of four criteria describing active sleep or quiet sleep had to be present to classify a 20-sec period as either state; those periods with less than three fitting criteria were scored undifferentiated sleep. The results obtained by the three methods of analysis (Figs. 19.10 and 19.11) showed no significant differences in the amount of the two sleep states between patients and controls, and between untreated and treated patients (a full report of these results by Schulte *et al.* is in press). To meet the argument that changes in the ratio of sleep states in PKU patients may become obvious only in all-night recordings, we carried out such recordings in another three untreated patients and three controls matched for age. Again, no significant differences could be detected.

Our results are at variance with earlier reports on sleep state changes in PKU patients by Petre-Quadens and Jouvet (1966) and by Feinberg *et al.* (1969). This discrepancy may be due to the fact that the above-mentioned authors investigated adult subjects in whom long-lasting mental retardation with convulsions and myelination defects rather than an impaired serotonin/norepinephrine balance could account for the reported decrease in REM sleep. Moreover, our results do not confirm the hypothesis that 5-HT influences the destribution of NREM versus REM sleep. Even the rapid rise of 5-HT after the

	PKU untreated N = 22	control infants N = 22	PKU untreated N = 13	PKU treated N = 13
NREM SLEEP	65.5 ± 21.0 n = 29	65.4 ± 18.2 n = 29	70.1 ± 22.7 n = 17	69.7 ± 18.0 n = 17
QUIET SLEEP	61.2 ± 20.0 n = 29	60.7 ± 21.5 n = 29	68.0 ± 17.8 n = 17	65.4 ± 16.7 n = 17
SLOW WAVE SLEEP	59.6 ± 19.8 n = 29	57.4 ± 18.5 n = 29	63.5 ± 16.7 n = 17	62.0 ± 17.7 n = 17

Fig. 19.11. Ratio of the two sleep states in phenylketonuric patients versus healthy controls and in treated versus untreated phenylketonuric patients. No significant difference in this ratio could be demonstrated by three different methods of analysis (see text) in spite of very low blood 5-HT values in untreated patients. N, number of infants; n, number of cycles analyzed.

institution of low phenylalanine diet, almost simulating an acute experiment for the evaluation of 5-HT as a sleep hormone, did not alter the ratio of the two sleep states. It is conceivable that alterations of the plasma levels of norepinephrine and epinephrine which occur in PKU (Nadler and Hsia, 1961) have contaminated our results, thus weakening their relevance for the biochemical theories of sleep. However, animal studies with intravascular, intracerebral, or intraventricular administration of 5-HT, PCPA, or MAO inhibitors do not provide a more convincing experimental approach since most of the applied drugs also act upon both serotonin and catecholamines (Jouvet, 1970). Long-term follow-up studies in PKU will be necessary to answer the questions whether data on sleep behavior and the EEG during sleep can be used to evaluate the effect of dietary treatment.

Sleep studies have provided new aspects for diagnosis and control of the effect of therapy. Concerning the mechanisms of sleep in man, the study of these pathological conditions has resulted in some new questions which are still unanswered.

Discussion

Petre-Quadens: How long after onset of the treatment did you record from the hypothyroid children? And how long does the increase in spindle intensity last?

Lenard: Initially, we made control recordings 1 week after onset of therapy. The EEG, however, showed only little change after this interval, and we decided to control the EEG—as a routine—in monthly intervals. There are fluctuations in spindle intensity. A slight decrease may occur after the initial increase if the biochemical situation changes again toward the hypothyroid side.

Petre-Quadens: We did some studies on the effects of 5-HTP on sleep in mongoloid children. Recordings were taken before onset of therapy, during the first week and 2 months later. We noticed an increase in the frequency of the eye movement intervals shorter than 1 sec, which reached a peak a few days after onset or after increase of 5-HTP (Petre-Quadens et al., 1971). The amount of spindles increased at the same time. Two months after onset of therapy, no changes could be detected any more either in the eye-movement frequency or in the spindles. When we stopped the therapy, both the amount of eye movements and the spindles decreased dramatically.

The same sequence was seen during pregnancy. There was a simultaneous increase in the spindles and in the density of the eye movements (Petre-Quadens,

1969). It might be related to the gradual increase of blood progesterone levels during pregnancy (Zander, 1955; Short and Eton, 1959). One should remember the experiments of Kawakami and Sawyer (1964). They showed that in rabbits, hormones produce an EEG afterreaction including a sequence of spindle sleep and paradoxical sleep. It has been speculated that hormone levels may act on the brain via some highly localized brain amines (Meyerson, 1964).

Villablanca: I would like to ask Dr. Perte-Quadens a question related to her interesting observation concerning changes in REMs in mongoloid children after treatment with 5-HTP. Do you have any information regarding the thyroid gland activity in your children before and after the administration of 5-HTP? In other words, could the influence of 5-HTP upon REMs be due to an action of the drug upon the thyroid?

Petre-Quadens: We do not have any information about it but maybe Dr. Lenard could answer this question.

Lenard: There is probably no influence of thyroxine on 5-HTP, 5-HTP decarboxylase, and 5-HT in the brain (Skillen *et al.*, 1961), and little, if any, on cerebral MAO (Zile, 1960; Ho Van Hap *et al.*, 1967; Lisch and Aigner, 1968). If thyroxine and 5-HTP act independently, I do not quite see why their effect on the electrical brain activity should be so similar.

Question: Is the decrease in eye-movement frequency, Dr. Petre-Quadens, after the end of the treatment significantly lower than the initial level?

Petre-Quadens: It is lower but not significantly.

Question: Would you say that after increase of serotonin there is an increase in cortical synchronization?

Metcalf: It is said to increase synchronization.

Question: What happens to patients with alkaptonuria? There, the metabolic defect does not result in severe morphological damage.

Metcalf: The EEG changes in alkaptonuria are said to be very variable. Disagreement about the existence of these changes suggests that they may, in fact, not exist.

Question: We sometimes see that spindles alternate from one side to the other. Do you consider this as pathological? Spindles are also more stable on one side than on the other.

Lenard: This is correct. Spindles are usually less frequent over the left hemisphere.

Metcalf: Dr. Lenard has microscopically examined spindle development in the period of time we are talking about; he told us that spindles characteristically alternate from side to side in the same child. I think that he and I find that alternating spindles, voltage asymmetry, and phase asynchrony are normal at least up through adolescence. So that we would not treat an alternating spindle, whether it is in amplitude or in phase or in frequency as an abnormality. Now we would get concerned clinically if there is a persistence of voltage asymmetry or frequency disturbance or a particular phasing of spindles always within one hemisphere. If you see peculiar persistent asymmetries in infants, a second EEG must be done with absolutely perfect technique because it is the technical problem which most often leads us to diagnose an EEG as being abnormal. I think that the real job of the pediatric encephalographer is to recognize artefacts.

Question: What is the data epoch you use for your spectral analysis, Dr. Lenard?

Lenard: Three minutes.

Question: Why did you take 3-min epochs for spindle analysis? Why not 10 or 20 sec?

Metcalf: I agree. I think you do yourself a disservice, Dr. Lenard, by using such long data epochs to show your spindle frequency. When there are few spindles you may "wash out" data by this averaging. If you took smaller data epochs, selected by visual inspection of the record, you may be able to demonstrate with greater precision differences between amounts of spindles as well as their frequency range in normal versus abnormal cases. I believe that the autocorrelogram is one of the best mathematical transforms for evaluating synchronization and rhythmicity. With the spectral display you really do not know about the organization of the rhythms. Whereas if you use autocorrelation, specifically designed to evaluate some aspects of organization of the rhythms, you will obtain quantitative data about periodicity. I realize that autocorrelograms are difficult to evaluate. They are confusing and difficult to compare, but they do depict how much rhythmicity is present and what the primary rhythm is. This is just the place for it. I am impressed that there is a loss of rhythmicity in children with PKU and that rhythmicity is improved when treatment succeeds. Our two major EEG findings in PKU are alterations in rhythmicity and just what you are seeing, which is the amount and quality of spindling. I agree completely with what you describe. This makes me feel that we would also see the same things if we look at organization per se. You have such excellent computer display techniques; the rest of us have not yet caught up with you. We must have better ways of getting at the statistics of EEG organization; the autocorrelogram should not be neglected because it is so easy to do with modern instrumentation. It can be accomplished in a number of different ways. There are orthodox ways of treating the data which would make it impossible to see small amounts of spindling. With time averaging versus smoothing, you get different displays: Each is of particular value, but we have demonstrated that spindle frequencies (with rudimentary spindles) are poorly detected with spectral time averaging as compared to smoothing.

All of us who are doing this work are beginning to learn that we must vary our ways of using the computer, to show the data to its best advantage. Often one must know in advance what he is trying to show. This is really what we are arguing about. Many programs are designed to show long-term trends in the EEG. These methods are not suitable for analysis of short-term events. Then, other, more relevant and specific techniques must be used.

CHAPTER TWENTY

General Discussion: Significance of the Sleep Parameters in Early Behavioral Development

Metcalf: We are interested in clarifying the relationships between the sleep EEG as an epiphenomenon of brain maturation in relation to behavioral development. We assume that in early infancy, particularly prior to 6–9 months of life, behavioral development has strong organismic roots which gradually evolve and emerge in terms of interactions with developing cyclic functions. I will try to relate some things we have found and some speculations which might generate discussion.

We are interested in looking at EEG development in terms of Spitz's organizing principals of infant development. He has indicated that there are nodal points in infant development that are important for emerging cyclic functions. He conceptualizes three such major points in the first year. We have elected to axiomize these from the viewpoint of EEG development. One is the beginning of social smiling at about 3 months; the other is the onset of a special kind of of anxiety. All infants show this anxiety behavior between 6 and 9 months. The development of smiling and the onset, development, and fate of infantile anxiety have been heavily researched by many people; these facts of behavioral development are well known and well accepted. It has been posited that the development of social smiling has important organismic roots resting upon foundations of brain maturation. We therefore search for points in brain maturation (using the EEG) that might lock into this. We find that at about the time infants begin to smile socially (maturing past the period of endogenous, automatic smiling to any stimulus, or preponderance of smiling during REM sleep with little smiling awake) a number of CNS physiological developments occur: (1) A changeover from the infantile type of sleep onset via a REM state to sleep onset into a non-REM state. (2) Very strong voltage modulation of the EEG: this is not present before about age 3 months. (3) The beginning of hypersynchronous drowsy patterns in the EEG. These are merely time-dependent correlations. We are not in a position to talk about causal relationships between brain and sleep maturation as seen in the EEG and the beginning of smiling. Second, with regard to the development of anxiety in infants we have carried out two projects:

1. We have attempted to relate EEG development to fussiness in the first 3 months of life. Infants at about the age of 4 or 5 weeks tend to go through a phase of fussiness lasting about a week or two. On the average, this fussy period is believed to wane by 3 months. It has been postulated that this fussy period is related to processes of brain maturation. It has been suggested that until the age of 5 weeks, sensory input is processed in a way that is different from the way it is processed later on. Specifically, there is the suggestion that there is a kind of barrier to the input of sensory stimulation in infants up to the age of about 5 weeks. For a short period of time between 4 to 6 weeks of age CNS maturation permits increased sensory input. The organism can be flooded by stimuli, but the infants do not yet have the capacity to handle, shut out, modulate, or process sensory input. During this time there is an increase of fussiness. After about age 6 weeks there is a gradual development of information-processing, inhibitory capacity on the part of the infant. Sensory input begins to be "filtered." We have attempted to investigate this by means of sensory testing of infants, neurological examinations, careful interviews of mothers, EEG sleep studies, etc. Our hypothesis was that the onset of sleep spindles was a landmark in brain maturation which would relate to the upsurge of fussiness. We failed to demonstrate this. We were not able to demonstrate a relationship between any landmark of EEG development and this so-called organismically based fussy period during infancy. However, what we did find was that there is a variable period in all infants (sometimes during the fussy period), when the EEG for about a week becomes quite disorganized. This has led us to look for other periods of disorganization during the course of normal EEG development. It appears to be something that all of us have neglected out of ignorance and out of an assumption that EEG development should be smoothly straightforward in its adult-bound trajectory. We expected EEG development to work this way; it does not. There are periods when there must be step-function changes among various aspects of brain maturation, wherein processes become temporarily out of synchrony. It is very important for people studying sleep

and sleep physiology developmentally to look for periods of desynchrony or asynchrony among processes that are ordinarily well entrained and well patterned. Our previous work on the entrainment of sleep patterns of early infancy into later infancy represents a case in point. We now know that the sleep EEG of the infant shows many episodes of lack of synchrony, a lack of expected patterning among the various parameters that we choose to examine. Eye movements, respiration, EEG, EMG, etc., are poorly patterned and entrained early and better patterned in older infants. How are these various processes driven, synchronized, and entrained?

At $2\frac{1}{2}$ or 3 months there is a brief period when the EEG and behavioral parameters become desynchronized for a time. There is another such period just before spontaneous K-complexes emerge. They develop at about 4 to 6 months. There is another such period at about 9 months. All of these are best seen in the slow sleep EEG. We have speculated on the basis of Piaget's findings about memory development and what has been said about the infant's ability to differentiate its mother from strangers and mothers from all other people (plus our old notion that spontaneous K-complexes represent an information-processing signal in terms of self-generating central nervous system processes), that the capacity, or organismic substrate for dreaming becomes organized at about 6 months. In terms of memory and infant behavior we would guess that dreaming as such may begin to take place at about 9 months. This speculation may not be researchable. In our present work we are attempting to examine infant behavior and EEG development to see if we can make rational and intelligent interpretations about possible dreams from infant behavior. The earliest verbal report from an infant about a dream is at age 19 months. There are also reports of infant's self-reported dreams at age 22 months. These reports, although rare up to the age of $2\frac{1}{2}$ years, indicate that young children can dream and report dreams between age 19 months and $2\frac{1}{2}$ years. Sleep "terror" arousals begin at about 9 to 12 months. There are sleep laughing reports from age 9 months. I think that sleep terrors at about 9 months should be given serious scientific attention. They cannot easily be "explained away" as being due to somatic causes. Terror awakenings are even more common after age 18 months (dream reports begin at 19 months).

Minard: I tend to disagree with Dave in a friendly way. Like "sleep" and "dreaming," "social" is a word in popular use and having connotations difficult to work with experimentally. Much harm has been done by not substituting functional definitions for popular definitions in experimental work, where we must deal with the functional relationships of observables and cannot fully explore popular belief. In terms of observable functional relationships, "social" has been redefined as meaning *behavior reinforcing another person's behavior*, as in the case of a "thank you" or an effective smile. "Social" could also refer to the fact that a response is elicited by "social" stimulation. If we accept the first of these definitions, neonate smiling is clearly social because, if you show appropriate audiences the smiles of neonates, audience members can be reinforced in quite evident ways. Young nurses will express pleasure and want to see films of neonate smiling over again. Now some experimenters point out differences between muscles involved in neonate and adult smiling or differences in time of occurrence, but, still, a response capable of reinforcing another's behavior, and therefore capable of exerting control over another's behavior, is "social" in an important sense.

With regard to the second definition, we should consider the probability that most previous researchers have used inappropriate "social" stimuli, establishing only that a stimulus which is "social" for one audience may not be "social" for another. They have used nodding smiling faces when they should have used a woman's voice. Studies by our group have indicated a tape-recorded female voice significantly increased the frequency of smiling during a newborn's active sleep, while noises continuously present in the nursery were not associated with increased smile frequency.

Sander: Sleep must be thought of also in terms of its adaptive function. The rhythmicity of sleep would have an adaptive significance in terms of the relation between timing of environmental cycles and of the infant's intrinsic sleep–waking cycle. Using day-by-day observations "around the clock" of distributions of neonatal states of sleeping and waking under three different infant caretaking situations, we have measured a number of variables relevant to infant and to caretaker, some by observation of time of onset of major sleep and wake epochs, some by time-sampled event recording, and some by a continuous 24-hr automatic monitoring bassinet which registers in real time changes in infant motility and crying, along with the caretaker's approach, removal from and return of the infant to the bassinet.

The determinants of the time course of the various transitional and awake states during a single awake epoch also have been of interest. The matter of how the caretaker interprets the neonate's smile in sleep-onset REM makes a noteworthy difference in the time course of an awake epoch. The smile occurs actually as the baby is falling asleep, but when the mother sees it, she may read it as an opportunity for social interaction, stimulate the baby, and arouse it at the very moment it is heading for sleep. We have seen a number of caretakers disrupt the natural time course of awake cycles by trying to play with the baby at the wrong time.

The periods of disorganization, of which you spoke, have also been of interest to us as we tried to determine the beginning of stability in the actual clock time of onset of naps and of longest sleep epoch per 24 hr. The first step in the process of temporal stabilization appears to be the settling of the longest sleep epoch per 24 hr in the night hours. Then, in the natural mother caretaking situation, three daytime naps may settle for a few days into a clock time occurrence which shows *relative* stability for a number of days only. This relative stability then disappears for 48 hr or so with the infant now reemerging with *two* naps per day, which again will show a relative stability in clock time of onset for a number of days, to be followed later by a next epoch of relative disorganization and so on.

In one of our paradigms, infants who have had one individual as sole foster mother in the first 10 days of life will be given a second individual as a new sole foster mother on the 11th day of life. Immediately with this change and in spite of the experience of the second foster mother, these infants will show a significant increase in crying, especially in the daytime 12 hr, and an increase in frequency of feeding distress events.

We are working with the hypothesis that within the first days of life key connections are established via the infant–caretaker interaction between regulation of infant state and specific maternal cues, among which may be time characteristics of caretaking exchanges.

The evidence in the three groups of neonates is that the duration per 24 hr of awake states during the first 3 days is greater than at any time until the end of the first month of life. We have interpreted this as an indication possibly of these first hours as a time of key adaptation between caretaker and infant. We are most keen to understand better the critical interactional parameters of this first adaptation.

Question: Is it your impression, Dr. Metcalf, that the 8-month anxiety is related to dreaming?

Metcalf: No, the 8-month anxiety really starts at 6 months. There are actually two kinds of infantile anxiety." One starts at about 6 months and one starts at about 9 to 12 months. The 9 to 12 month anxiety, separation anxiety, may involve dreaming. We have not looked at our children from that particular point of view; it should be done.

Question: When is the onset of K-complexes? of drowsiness? the onset of sleep stages?

Metcalf: Spontaneous sleep K-complexes are occasionally seen at 4 months. Never earlier. For most infants, K-complex inception is around 6 months. One of the reasons we do not see spontaneous K-complexes under 6 months is because K-complexes cover the same frequency spectrum as the NREM sleep EEG. The K-complexes are buried in the "noise" of the ongoing EEG when they first develop. We can actually differentiate EEG sleep and stage 2A, 2B, 2C. Stage 2A would be a relative low amplitude EEG with spindles and K standing out. You just don't see that kind of sleep until the infant is about 7–8–9 months old: It is a pattern-recognition, pattern-differentiation problem. My speculation is that when K-complexes as spontaneous events develop, there is some internal information processing taking place in the central nervous system and that the K-complex as an internally evoked event is an information-processing signal. We should see some other changes perhaps in eye movements, or EMG activity, or some EEG spectral changes coincident with the development of spontaneous K-complexes. We keep looking because we think these changes should be there.

There are two ways of looking at drowsiness. One is drowsy behavior and the other is what is seen in the EEG that correlates with drowsiness, i.e. the hypersynchrony. Drowsy behavior, depending upon the criteria, can be seen from earliest infancy. I am unaware of EEG drowsy hypersynchrony being present much before 3 months. It starts between 3–4 to 6 months but you really do not see it very clearly until 9 to 12 months; it lasts until about 7 years. Now, if it does not start before 6 months it is probably because of the immaturity of the central nervous system. But why does it stop at 7 years and why is it individual? Why do some children have more EEG activity? In children, there is a special pattern of EEG arousal (or prearousal) which you cannot easily differentiate from stage 4 EEG. And therefore I have always somewhat disagreed with the Kales-Jacobson work on stage 4 sleep-walking. Therefore, I think this is another stage of consciousness in addition to transcendental meditation as a possible additional state. As far as the four sleep stages are concerned, it is my experience that you cannot identify all of them before 6 months. After 6 months you are able to identify stage 1, stage 2, and something that is a mixture of stages 3 and 4.

Question: Do you see a modification or a change in the slow waves of the K-complexes with age?

Metcalf: In the typical K-complex at 6–8 years, the first component, which is at about 250 msec, is of very high amplitude and very sharp. The slower component often is not seen because the typical K-complex in that age group consists of a series of K-complexes in close proximity. They push in upon, and include the following slow wave. Usually, you do not see the following slow waves before age 3 years or after age 7 or 8 years in the row EEG.

Dement: What about spontaneous K-complexes? Can you evoke a K-complex?

Metcalf: Yes, you can, especially as computer-derived sensory-evoked responses. You do not see spontaneous K-complexes in a soundproof room before 5 to 6 months.

Dement: What does it mean when an organism has a great predominance of NREM sleep as opposed to REM sleep, or vice versa? Sometimes we like to think of NREM sleep as the ultimate central behavioral inhibition. In cats that we treated chronically with *p*-chlorophenylalanine, we saw an upsurge of many specific behaviors in association with the reduction of NREM sleep. Just as a speculation, suppose serotonergic neurons were only concerned with the inhibitory regulation of specific behavioral tendencies such as sexual behavior, aggressive behavior, eating behavior, etc. The absence of this behavior, i.e., intense serotonergic activity, would be NREM sleep. REM sleep is a special case in this regard because it is, in a sense, behavioral facilitation in association with specific peripheral motor inhibition. It should be included with the behavioral facilitation of wakefulness, and both are opposed to the behavioral inhibition of NREM sleep.

From this point of view, what does it mean that a 5-year-old child or a 10-year-old child has such an incredible predominance of NREM sleep, particularly stage 4? REM sleep is definitely decreased, at least from the standpoint of percentage. Why does this change after puberty?

Some people contend that the REM-NREM ratio in the elderly predicts something about wakefulness. In other words, if the REM percent is high, the elderly person is likely to be energetic, sexually active, etc. If REM sleep is low, he may be lethargic, distinterested, near the end. Again, we must ask, how do these developmental shifts in the organization of sleep relate to other aspects of the life situation?

Metcalf: It is an interesting idea. It makes me think that there are energy levels in people. I never thought of it as a division between serotoninergic and catecholamine processes. One wonders where constitution enters, and we might think that some people may be genetically endowed to be serotonergic individuals, as it were. Our longitudinal EEG studies have some children who for years have usually large amounts of slow wave sleep; this is compatible with what you suggest.

Dement: I wonder if we could make some comments on the functional or adaptive significance of sleep stage organization in the very young animal? Why do newborn kittens have virtually 100% active sleep? Does quiet sleep fulfill a function in the human infant that is not relevant in the newborn kitten?

Metcalf: Active sleep and quiet sleep are both present in full-term neonates. In quiet sleep, the human infant looks as if it is "really out" except for the facial muscles which are tonic. If you observe an infant in quiet sleep, the body and face are immobile. In active sleep the eyes, limbs, face, and body are all working.

Lenard: I want to come back to the correlation between behavioral and electroencephalographic parameters. It would be extremely important for pediatricians to know whether the development of premature babies is influenced by external stimulation and is different from that of full-term newborns spending the same developmental phase *in utero*. It has not been easy to demonstrate such differences. On the behavioral side, it has been shown that social smiling develops earlier in prematures than in full terms (Joppich and Michaelis, 1967). Dr. Metcalf could show that spindles develop earlier in prematures (at about 44 weeks conceptional age) than in full terms (where they appear around the 48th week). This may be a symptom of advanced or changed cerebral maturation.

Purpura: Is this the same morphology of the spindles that appears later on in the adult or is it an entirely different kind of spindle that we see in non-REM sleep stage 2?

Metcalf: The same topographic, morphological, and frequency characteristics and the same relationship to sleep stage.

Dement: I would like to emphasize one point. We are often very imprecise when we talk about spindles. We oversimplify. For example, people are always talking about 12 *to* 14 Hz spindle activity as if this were one process. It has been clearly demonstrated that there are at least three kinds of sleep spindles in the adult human EEG. One kind is a 14 Hz spindle, one is a 12 Hz spindle, and one is a 10 Hz spindle. There is not one spindle which smears out in frequency from 9 to 15 Hz! There are three different frequencies which separate very nicely. Furthermore, they have functional significance. First, they have different topographic distribution over the scalp. Second, as Gibbs and Gibbs demonstarted very well in their *Atlas* (1950), they tend to be associated with different background EEG patterns. Finally, it has been demonstrated that they are differentially effected by prefrontal lobotomy (Lennox and Coolidge, 1949). In the old days when we scored all the miles and miles of sleep recordings by eye and hand, it was just too difficult to make these differentiations. Now, with the use of the high speed computer for processing EEG data, it is no longer appropriate to disregard the complexity of the spindle process. I wonder if the human infant also has three different kinds of spindles. There do seem to be differences between infants and adults. Often, the infant spindles appear to be monophasic, whereas in the adult they are clearly sinusoidal. I do not know what this means.

There is also another functional relationship in the cat that is worth mentioning. It is analogous to the so-called spindle-tripping phenomenon reported years ago by Dempsey and Morison (1942a). They found that a spindle shock to the thalamus in the barbiturate animal could trip a full-blown barbiturate spindle (6–8 Hz). There is often a transitory period during sleep in the cat where, quite clearly, a spindle PGO spike in NREM sleep is tripping the occurrence of a sleep spindle in the sensorimotor cortex. At other times there are either no discernible PGO spikes, or there are no clear temporal relationships between PGO spikes and sleep spindles. Nonetheless, it is possible that phasic activity is involved in producing what we usually think of as a sign of NREM sleep. I would like to raise two questions for consideration. First, in the human infant, is there any evidence that phasic activity is related to the occurrence of sleep spindles? In the adult, we think of the K-complex as a kind of NREM phasic event. The K-complex is related to the phasic EMG suppression described by Pivik and Dement (1970). Is there any sign that phasic activity, EMG suppression if not K-complexes, occurs at all in NREM stage 2 containing no discernible spindles as it does for epochs containing several spindles?

Metcalf: The first spindle bursts we see are around 14 Hz; they then settle down and lock in at 12 Hz. The faster 16–18-Hz rhythm is something we have recently discovered. It is difficult to state whether or not they represent the same process that is generating spindle bursts, other than the fact that they relate to sleep in the same way, in the same scalp region. They do not have the same burst characteristics; they are continuous fast activity which we feel merge, developmentally, into subsequent "true" spindle bursts.

Villablanca: I wonder whether there will be any correlation between hemispheral lateralization of sleep spindles and the future handedness in the babies. In relation to this it would be interesting to know if there is a "dominant" side concerning spindle lateralization and what is the percentage of children in this category. It would be thrilling indeed to be able to predict to mothers the future handedness of their offspring.

Lenard: In about 80% of our children we have seen more and longer spindles over the right hemisphere. In the other 20% there were more spindles over the left side.

Purpura: I suspect that the immaturity of the corpus callosum among other things is allowing the differences on different sides. I am not saying that the callosum is responsible for allowing one hemisphere or another to lead. We do not know really in man when the callosum matures. But one of the things I would suspect happens with callosum maturation is the development of inhibition. One function the callosum seems to have is not so much to excite but to inhibit neurons in projection cortex.

Metcalf: I would agree with the inhibitory hypothesis but I would place it in higher systems in relation to the mechanisms underlying alternation of spindling between the hemispheres.

Bremer: There is a possibility that the maturation of the callosum would have an importance for the organization of the bilateral symmetry of the cortical electrogenesis in the infant. In cats the callosum is just one factor in this symmetry which is shown only in the acute experiment. When you cut it, this disorganizes the symmetry momentarily. But studies by Adey and Creutzfeldt have shown that in chronic cats and monkeys bilateral symmetry, after the callosum section, reappears entirely.

Villablanca: Would you say that REM sleep episodes may be reflexly produced? Dr. Metcalf, is it just the nipple or do you need the feeding? Observations of REM episodes occurring after feeding in babies reminds me of a similar finding in animal experiments. Before REMs was fully recognized, Bard and Macht (1958) described in chronic pontine and mesencephalic cats "a sudden postural collapse which in many respects resembled the clinical syndrome of 'cataplexy'" could often be induced by feeding. Later we demonstrated that in chronic mesencephalic cats such episodes have all the behavioral and polygraphic features of REMs (Villablanca, 1966). Recently Sorenson and Ellison (1970) found that tube feeding chronic thalamic rats induced sleep in these otherwise insomniac animals. These observations suggest that this is a brain-stem reflex phenomenon which, upon maturation, is brought under control by rostral brain mechanisms.

Metcalf: Our data are confusing. We thought at one time that we could drive the infant into a REM state with feeding. At this point I would conceptualize the REM state in the human as being a less deep level of consciousness, i.e., lighter sleep. Putting something in the baby's mouth will not, in itself, drive the infant into any specific state.

This goes back to what Dr. Dement was saying about forcing cats' sleep cycles. Even nurseries where babies are fed on "self-demand" do not really do it that way. Babies are not fed on their own schedule, they are fed on the nurse's schedule. Furthermore, when we get a baby into our lab, we may have difficulty putting electrodes on. The babies are excessively handled, become disturbed, and respond by being driven into NREM sleep by these manipulations. Thus, the need for long-term recording (at least feeding-to-feeding) with infants.

CHAPTER TWENTY-ONE

Final Remarks

GIUSEPPE MORUZZI

To realize how great the progress of our knowledge on sleep has been during the past 40 years it is enough to review mentally what we have learnt during this week and the main steps of the literature pertaining to the different approaches. It is fitting to recall that a major line of endeavor started here in Belgium, with Bremer's classical works on the *encéphale isolé* and the *cerveau isolé*.

Instead of making an attempt to give a summation—an almost impossible task also in view of the time available—it is perhaps advisable to insist on what we do not know or we are little informed about.[1] Maybe some answer to questions which are now coming to our minds will be given by the experimental work of the next few years.

First of all, we know very little about the *physiological significance* of sleep, although we conceal our ignorance with terms such as sleep recovery or sleep debt. We might perhaps say tentatively that sleep is concerned with cerebral homeostasis. However, there are several neurons and synapses which do not

[1] The literature on the data recalled in these final remarks may be found in two recent reviews by Moruzzi (1969, 1972).

need the slow recovery processes occurring during sleep; and there is as yet little evidence that the structures in which there is such a need are able to control, through appropriate feedback mechanisms, the centers concerned with the sleep–waking cycle. We are probably dealing with mechanisms basically different from those which control Claude Bernard's *milieu intérieur* (Cannon's homeostasis).

A second difficulty is represented by the fact that we are unable to measure the slow *processes of recovery* which go on during sleep. The time which is spent in sleep, as determined by behavioral or EEG criteria, is not an index of the real amount of these recovery processes. It is probably incorrect to state that some mammals, such as the cow or the antelope, never sleep. However, one must concede that in these herbivores the periods of sleep are so infrequent and short-lasting that they are likely to escape the attention of the observer. With respect to brain recovery, the needs are of course likely to be different in different mammals; this fact, however, is unlikely to explain by itself the striking differences in sleep behavior one observes between herbivores and carnivores. It is almost certain, moreover, that some animals, like the domestic cat, oversleep with respect to their needs. The lack of correlation between sleep duration and the amount of recovery is also shown by studies on sleep deprivation in man. The duration of synchronized sleep providing an almost complete recovery is, in fact, out of proportion to the duration of a preceding sleep deprivation.

Third, and finally, we have the tendency to forget that sleep recovery may be obtained only at the heavy price of a temporary *loss of consciousness*: a state that implies serious problems for the survival of the species. All known examples of instinctive behavior, in both mammals and birds, are in fact disrupted during sleep. Therefore the animals must adapt their requirements in terms of defense, food, and water supply to the sleep–waking cycle. An appropriate control of sleep behavior must have great survival value for the species, as it becomes apparent when one considers the implications of a temporary loss of consciousness in the herbivores living in the wild state. Perhaps the control of sleep is taken over by another instinctive behavior, one antagonistically oriented with respect to those occurring during the waking state.

References

Abbadessa, S., and Montalbano, M. E. (1968). Strutture ipotalamiche sensibili alla tiroxina. *Boll. Soc. Ital. Biol. Sper.* **44**, 1906–1908.

Adey, W., Kado, R., and Rhodes, J. (1962). Sleep: cortical and subcortical recordings in the chimpanzee. *Science* **414**, 932–933.

Adrian, E. D. (1941). Afferent discharges to the cerebral cortex on peripheral sense organs. *J. Physiol.* **100**, 159–191.

Adrian, E. D., and Moruzzi, G. (1939). Impulses in the pyramidal tract. *J. Physiol.* **97**, 153–199.

Akert, K., Koella, W., and Hess, R. (1952). Sleep produced by electrical stimulation of the thalamus. *Amer. J. Phsyiol.* **168**, 260–267.

Akimoto, H., and Saito, Y. (1966). Synchronizing and desynchronizing influences and their interactions on cortical and thalamic neurons. *In Progr. brain Res.* **21A**, 323–351.

Akimoto, H., Yamaguchi, N., Okabe, K., Nakagawa, T., Nakamura, I., Abe, K., Torii, H., and Masahashi, K. (1956). On the sleep induced through electrical stimulation of the dog thalamus. *Folia Psychiat. Neurol. Japan.* **10**, 117–146.

Akindele, M. O., Evans, J. I., and Oswald, I. (1969). Monoamine oxidase inhibitors, sleep and mood. *Electroenceph. Clin. Neurophysiol.* **29**, 47–56.

Albe-Fessard, D., and Liebeskind, J. (1966). Origine des messages somato-sensitifs activant les cellules du cortex moteur chez le singe. *Exp. Brain Res.* **1**, 127–146.

Allison, T., and Goff, G. D. (1968a). Potentials evoked in somatosensory cortex to thalamo-cortical radiation stimulation during waking, sleep and arousal from sleep. *Arch. Ital. Biol.* **106**, 41–60.

Allison, T., and Goff, W. R. (1968b). Sleep in a primitive mammal, the spiny anteater, *Psychophysiology* **5**, 200–201.

Allison, T., and Van Twyver, H. (1970). The evolution of sleep. *Nat. Hist.* **79**, 56–65.

Amassian, V. E., and Weiner, H. (1966). Monosynaptic and polysynaptic activation of pyramidal tract neurons by thalamic stimulation. *In* "The Thalamus" (D. P. Purpura and M. D. Yahr, eds.), pp. 255–282. Columbia Univ. Press, New York.

Anders, T., Emde, R., and Parmelee, A. (eds.) (1971). *A Manual of Standardized Terminology, Techniques, and Criteria for Scoring of States of Sleep and Wakefulness in Newborn Infants.* UCLA Brain Inform. Service, BRI Publ. Office, Los Angeles, California, NINDS, Neurolog. Inform. Network.

Andersen, P., and Andersson, S. A. (1968). "Physiological Basis of the Alpha Rhythm." p. 235. Appleton, New York.

Andersen, P., and Eccles, J. C. (1962). Inhibitory phasing of neuronal discharge. *Nature (London)* **196**, 645–647.

Andersson, S. A., and Manson, J. R. (1971). Rhythmic activity in the thalamus of the unanaesthetized decorticate cat. *Electroenceph. Clin. Neurophysiol.* **31**, 21–34.

Andersen, P., Brooks, C.McC, Eccles, J. C., and Sears, T. A. (1964a). The ventro-basal nucleus of the thalamus: potential fields, synaptic transmission and excitability of both presynaptic components. *J. Physiol.* **174**, 348–369.

Andersen, P., Eccles, J. C., and Sears, T. A. (1964b). The ventrobasal complex of the thalamus: Types of cells, their responses and their functional organization. *J. Physiol.* **174**, 370–399.

Andersen, P., Andersson, S. A., and Lomo, T. (1967a). Some factors involved in the thalamic control of spontaneous barbiturate spindles. *J. Physiol.* **192**, 257–281.

Andersen, P., Andersson, S. A., and Lomo, T. (1967b). Nature of thalamo-cortical relations during spontaneous barbiturate spindle activity. *J. Physiol.* **192**, 283–307.

Andersson, S. A., Holmgren, I., and Manson, J. R. (1971) Synchronization and desynchronization in the thalamus of unanaesthetized decorticate cat. *Electroenceph. Clin. Neurophysiol.* **31**, 335–345.

Angeleri, F., Marchesi, G. F., and Quattrini, A. (1969). Effects of chronic thalamic lesions on the electrical activity of the neocortex and on sleep. *Arch. Ital. Biol.* **107**, 633–667.

Arduini, A., Berlucchi, G., and Strata, P. (1963). Pyramidal activity during sleep and wakefulness. *Arch. Ital. Biol.* **101**, 530–544.

Armstrong, D. M. (1965). Synaptic excitation and inhibition of Betz cells by antidromic pyramidal volleys. *J. Physiol.* **178**, 37P–38P.

Asanuma, H., and Brooks, V. B. (1965). Recurrent cortical effects following stimulation of internal capsule. *Arch. Ital. Biol.* **103**, 220–246.

Asanuma, H., and Okamoto, K. (1959). Unitary study on evoked activity of callosal neurons and its effect on pyramidal tract cell activity on cats. *Jap. J. Physiol.* **9**, 473–483.

Asanuma, H., and Okuda, O. (1962). Effects of transcallosal volleys on pyramidal tract cell activity of cat. *J. Neurophysiol.* **25**, 198–208.

Aschoff, J. (1969). Desynchronization and resynchronization of human circadian rhythms. *Aerosp. Med.* **40**, 844–849.

Aserinsky, E. (1965). Periodic respiratory pattern occurring in conjunction with eye-movements during sleep. *Science* **150**, 763–766.

Aserinsky, E., and Kleitman, N. (1953). Regularly occurring periods of eye motility, and concomitant phenomena, during sleep. *Science* **118**, 273–274.

Aserinsky, E., and Kleitman, N. (1955). A motility cycle in sleeping infants as manifested by ocular and gross bodily activity. *J. Appl. Physiol.* **8**, 11–18.

Astic, L., and Jouvet-Mounier, D. (1969). Mise en évidence du sommeil paradoxal in utero chez le cobaye. *C. R. Acad. Sci. Paris* **264**, 2578–2581.

Bach-y-Rita, G., and Baurand, C. (1966). Comparaison entre les effets de destruction localisée du sous-thalamus et de la formation réticulée mésencéphalique. *Rev. Neurol.* **115**, 591.

Bach-y-Rita, G., Trevasten, C., and Poncet, M. (1966). Effets des lesions thalamiques unilatérales associés á une section interhémisphérique sur le comportement et l'activité EEG au cours de la veille et du sommeil et après injection de pentetrazol chez le chat. *J. Physiol.* **58**, 452–453. 453.

Baker, M. A. (1971). Spontaneous and evoked activity of neurones in the somatosensory thalamus of the waking cat. *J. Physiol.* **217**, 359–379.

Baldissera, F., Broggi, G., and Mancia, M. (1964). Spinal reflexes in normal unrestrained cats during sleep and wakefulness. *Experientia* **20**, 577.

Baldissera, F., Broggi, G., and Mancia, M. (1966a). Monosynaptic and polysynaptic spinal reflexes during physiological sleep and wakefulness. *Arch. Ital. Biol.* **104**, 112–133.

Baldissera, F., Cesa-Bianchi, M. G., and Mancia, M. (1966b). Responses of visual cortex to transcallosal and geniculate stimulations during sleep and wakefulness. *Arch. Ital. Biol.* **104**, 231–246.

Baldridge, B., Whitman, R., and Kramer, M. (1965). The concurrence of fine muscle activity and rapid eye movements during sleep. *Psychosom. Med.* **27**, 19–26.

Bard, Ph., and Macht, M. B. (1958). The behaviour of chronically decerebrate cats. *In* "Neurological Basis of Behavior" (G. E. W. Wolstenholme and C. M. O'Connor, eds.), pp. 55–75. Churchill, London.

Bard, Ph., and Rioch, McK. D. (1937). A study of four cats deprived of neocortex and additional portion of the forebrain. *Bull. John Hopkins Hosp.* **60**, 73–147.

Batini, C., Moruzzi, G., Palestini, M., Rossi, G. F., and Zanchetti, A. (1958). Persistent patterns of wakefulness in the pretrigeminal midpontine preparation. *Science* **128**, 30–32.

Batini, C., Moruzzi, G., Palestini, M., Rossi, G. F., Zanchetti, A. (1959). Effects of complete pontine transection on the sleep–wakefulness rhythm: The midpontine pretrigeminal preparation. *Arch. Ital. Biol.* **97**, 1–12.

Batsel, H. L. (1960). Electroencephalographic synchronization and desynchronization in the chronic "cerveau isolé" of the dog. *Electroenceph. Clin. Neurophysiol.* **12**, 421–430.

Baum, J. (1900). Beiträge zur Kenntnis der Muskelspindeln. *Anat. Hefte I Abt.* **13**, 249–305.

Baust, W., and Bohnert, B. (1969). The regulation of heart rate during sleep. *Exp. Brain Res.* **7**, 169–180.

Baust, W., Niemczyk, H., and Vieth, J. (1963). The action of blood pressure on the ascending reticular activating system with special reference to adrenaline induced EEG arousal. *Electroenceph. Clin. Neurophysiol.* **15**, 63–72.

Baust, W., Berlucchi, G., and Moruzzi, G. (1964). Changes in the auditory input during arousal in cats with tenotomized middle ear muscles. *Arch. Ital. Biol.* **102**, 675–685.

Bazett, H. C., and Penfield, W. G. (1922). A study of the Sherrington decerebrate animal in the chronic as well as the acute condition. *Brain* **45**, 185–265.

Beaudreau, D. E., Daugherty, W. F., Jr., and Masland, W. S. (1969). Two types of motor pause in masticatory muscles. *Amer. J. Physiol.* **216**, 16–21.

Benoit, O. (1970). Spontaneous repetitive discharge of thalamic units during sleep in cats. *Psychophysiology* **7**, 310–311.

Berger, H. (1930). Ueber das Elektroen Kephalogram des Menschen. *J. Psychol. Neurol.* **40**, 160–179.

Berger, R. J. (1961). Tonus of extrinsic laryngeal muscles during sleep and dreaming. *Science* **134**, 840.

Bergonzi, P., Cianchetti, C., Ferroni, A., and Marchesi, G. (1970). (Deprivation of REM sleep in epileptic patients—modification of discharges and of organization of nocturnal sleep Privazione della v fase di sonno in soggetti epilettici—modificazione delle scariche e dell organizzazione del sonno notturno. *Riv. Neurol* **40**, 344–348. (It.)

Bergonzi, P., Cianchetti, C., Merchesi, G., and Ferroni, A. (1971). "Dream deprivation" in epileptics: changes in seizures and night sleep organization *Electroenceph. Clin. Neurophysiol.* **31**, 182. (Abstract)

Berlucchi, G. (1965). Callosal activity in unrestrained unanesthetized cats. *Archi. Ital. Biol.* **103**, 623–634.

Berlucchi, G., Maffei, L., Moruzzi, G., and Strata, P. (1964a). EEG and behavioral effects elicited by cooling of medulla and pons. *Arch. Ital. Biol.* **102**, 372–392.

Berlucchi, G., Moruzzi, G., Salvi, G., and Strata, P. (1964b). Pupil behavior and ocular movements during synchronized and desynchronized sleep. *Arch. Ital. Biol.* **102**, 230–244.

Björklund, A., and Stenevi, U. (1971). Growth of central catecholamine neurons into smooth muscle grafts in the rat mesencephalon. *Brain Res.* **31**, 1–20.

Blake, H. (1937). Brain potentials and depth of sleep. *Amer. J. Physiol.* **119**, 273–274.

Blake, H., and Gerard, R. (1937). Brain potentials during sleep. *Amer. J. Physiol.* **119**, 692–703.

Blake, H., Gerard, R., and Kleitman, N. (1939). Factors influencing brain potentials during sleep. *J. Neurophysiol* **2**, 48–60.

Blondaux, C., Juge, A., Sordet, F., Chouvet, G., Jouvet, M., and Pujol, J. F. (1973). Modification du métabolisme de la sérotonine cérébrale induite chez le rat par administration de 6-Hydroxy-dopamine. *Brain Res.* **50**, 101–114.

Bolles, R. C., and Woods, P. J. (1964). The ontogeny of behaviour in the albino rat *Anim. Behav.* **12**, 427–441.

Bonvallet, M. (1966). "Système nerveux et vigilance," p. 130. Presses Univ. de France, Paris.

Bonvallet, M., and Allen, M. B. Jr. (1962). Localisation de formations bulbaires intervenant dans le controle de différentes manifestations de l'activation réticulaire. *C. R. Soc. Biol.* **156**, 597–601.

Bonvallet, M., and Allen, M. B. (1963). Prolonged spontaneous and evoked reticular activation following discrete bulbar lesions. *Electroenceph. Clin. Neurophysiol.* **15**, 969–988.

Bonvallet, M., and Bloch, V. (1961). Bulbar control of cortical arousal. *Science* **133**, 1133–1134.

Bonvallet, M., Dell, P., and Hiebel, G. (1954). Tonus sympathique et activité électrique corticale. *Electroencephal. Clin. Neurophysiol.* **6**, 119–144.

Bovet, D., Bovet-Nitti, F., and Oliverio, A. (1969). Genetic aspects of learning and memory in mice. *Science* **163**, 139–149.

Bowe-Anders, C., Adrien, J., and Roffwarg, H. (1972). The ontogenesis of PGO waves in the kitten. Presented at the Association for the Psycho-physiological Study of Sleep, New York, May 1972.

Bowsher, D. (1967). Etude comparée des projections thalamiques de deux zones localisées des formations réticulées bulbaires et mésencéphaliques. *C. R. Acad. Sci. (Paris)* **265**, 340–342.

Bradley, P. B. (1958). The effects of 5-hydroxytryptamine on the electrical activity of the brain and on behaviour in the conscious cat. *In* "5-Hydroxytryptamine," (G. P. Lewis, ed.), pp. 214–220. Pergamon, Oxford.

Bremer, F. (1935). Cerveau "isolé" et physiologie du sommeil. *C. R. Soc. Biol. (Paris)* **118**, 1235–1241.

Bremer, F. (1936). Nouvelles recherches sur le mécanisme du sommeil. *C. R. Soc. Biol. (Paris)* **122**, 460–463.

Bremer, F. (1937). L'activité cérébrale au cours du sommeil et de la narcose. Contribution à l'étude du mécanisme du sommeil. *Bull. Acad. Roy. Méd. Belg.* **4**, 68–86.

Bremer, F. (1938a). L'activité électrique de l'écorce cérébrale. *Actual. Sci. Ind.* **658**, 46.

Bremer, F. (1938b). Effets de la déafférentation complète d'une région de l'écorce cérébrale sur son activité électrique spontanée *C. R. Soc. Biol. (Paris)* **127**, 355–359.

Bremer, F. (1938c). L'activité électrique de l'ecorce cérébrale et le problème physiologique du sommeil. *Boll. delle Soc. Ital. di Biol. Sper.* **13**, 271–290.

Bremer, F. (1958). Cerebral and cerebellar potentials. *Physiolog. Rev.* **38**, 357–388.

Bremer, F. (1960). Les régulations nerveuses de l'activité corticale. *P. Schweig. Arch. Neurol. Neurochir. Psychiat.* **86**, 34–48.

Bremer, F. (1961). Neurophysiological mechanisms in cerebral arousal. *In* "The Nature of Sleep" (G. E. W. Wolstenholme and M. O'Connor, eds.), Ciba Symposium, pp. 30–50. Churchill, London.

Bremer, F. (1970a) Preoptic hypnogenic focus and mesencephalic reticular formation. *Brain Res.* **21**, 132–134.

Bremer, F. (1970b). Inhibitions intrathalamiques récurrentielles et physiologie du sommeil. *Electroencephal. Clin. Neurophysiol.* **28**, 1–16.

Bremer, F., and Stoupel, N. (1959). Facilitation et inhibition des potentiels évoqués corticaux dans l'éveil cérébral. *Arch. Int. Physiol. Biochim.* **67**, 240–275.

Bricolo, A. (1967). Insomnia after bilateral stereotactic thalamotomy in man. *J. Neurol. Neurosurg. Psychiat.* **30**, 154–158.

Bronzino, J. D. (1968). Verification of a neural feedback pathway in the brain stem of the cat between the midbrain reticular formation and the nucleus of the tractus solitarius. Diss., Worcester Polytechnic Inst.

Bronzino, J. D. (1971). Effect of serotonin and xylocaine upon evoked responses established in neural feedback circuits associated with sleep-waking process. *Biol. Psychiat.* **3**, 217–226.

Brooks, D. (1967). Localization of the lateral geniculate nucleus monophasic waves associated with paradoxical sleep in the cat. *Electroenceph. Clin. Neurophysiol.* **23**, 123–135.

Brooks, D., and Bizzi, E. (1963). Brain stem electrical activity during deep sleep. *Arch. Ital. Biol.* **101**, 648–665.

Brooks, V. B., and Asanuma, H. (1965). Recurrent cortical effects following stimulation of medullary pyramid. *Arch. Ital. Biol.* **103**, 247–278.

Brooks, V. B., Rudomin, P., and Slayman, C. C. (1961). Peripheral receptive fields of neurons in the cat's cerebral cortex. *J. Neurophysiol.* **24**, 302–325.

Broughton, R. (1968). Sleep disorders: Disorders of arousal? *Science* **159**, 1072–1078.

Brunelli, M., Magni, F., Moruzzi, G., and Musumeci, D. (1971a). The sleep-waking cycle in the acute thalamic pigeon. *Proc. Int. Physiolog. Congr. 25th, München* **9**, 247.

Brunelli, M., Magni, F., Moruzzi, G., and Musumeci, D. (1971b). Effetti di stimolazioni elettriche localizzate del ponte sulla attivita istintiva del piccione talamico e del piccione integro. *Atti Acc. Naz Lincei, Cl. Sci. Fis. Mat. Nat., sez. VIII* **50**, 603–606.

Brunelli, M., Magni, F., Moruzzi, G., and Musumeci, D. (1972). Brain-stem influences on waking and sleep behaviors in the pigeon. *Arch. Ital. Biol.* **110**, 285–321.

Buchwald, J. S., and Eldred, E. (1961). Relations between gamma efferent discharge and cortical activity. *Electroenceph. Clin. Neurophysiol.* **13**, 243–247.

Buguet, A., Petitjean, F., and Jouvet, M. (1970). Suppression des pointes PGO du sommeil par lésion ou injection in situ de 6-Hydroxydopamine au niveau du tegmentum pontique. *C. R. Soc. Biol. (Paris)* **164**, 2293–2298.

Burns, B. D. (1950). Some properties of cat's isolated cerebral cortex. *J. Physiol.* **111**, 50–68.

Burns, B. D. (1951). Some properties of isolated cerebral cortex in the unanaesthetized cat. *J. Physiol.* **112**, 156–175.

Buser, P., and Imbert, M. (1961). Sensory projections to the motor cortex in cats: a microelectrode study. *In* "Sensory Communication" (W. A. Rosenblith, ed.), pp. 607–626. M.I.T. Press, Boston, Massachusetts and Wiley, New York.

Cadilhac, J., Passouant-Fontaine, Th., and Mihailovic, Lj. (1960). Modifications selon l'âge de o a 45 jours des postdécharges corticales hippocampiques, thalamiques et réticulaires ainsi que des crises cardiazoliques chez le chaton. *C. R. Soc. Biol.* **154**, 169–172.

Cajal, S. R. (1911). "Histologie du système nerveux de l'homme et des vertébrés." Maloine, Paris.

Caley, D. W., Maxwell, D. S. (1968a). An electron microscopic study of neurons during postnatal development of the rat cerebral cortex. *J. Comp. Neurol.* **133**, 17–43.

Caley, D. W., and Maxwell, D. S. (1968b). An electron microscopic study of the neuroglia development of the rat cerebrum. *J. Comp. Neurol.* **133**, 45–70.

Caley, D. W., and Maxwell, D. S. (1970). Development of the bloodvessels and extracellular spaces during postnatal maturation of rat cerebral cortex. *J. Comp. Neurol.* **138**, 31–48.

Calvet, J., Calvet, M. C., and Scherrer, J. (1964). Etude stratigraphique corticale de l'activité EEG spontanée, *Electroenceph. Clin. Neurophysiol.* **17**, 109–125.

Cannon, W. B., and Rosenblueth A. (1949). "The supersensitivity of denervated structures. A law of denervation" pp. 1–245. New York, MacMillan Company.

Capon, A. (1959). Nouvelles recherches sur l'effet d'éveil de l'adrénaline, *J. Physiolog.* **51**, 424–425.

Carreras, M., Lechi, A., and Passera, S. (1966). L'organization anatomo-fonctionelle des noyaux thalamiques chez l'animal décortiqué. *Rev. Neurol.* **115**, 67–78.

Castellucci, V. F., and Goldring, S. (1970). Contribution to steady potential shifts of slow depolarization in cells presumed to be glia. *Electroenceph. Clin. Neurophysiol.* **28**, 109–118.

Chase, M. H. (1970). The digastric reflex in the kitten and adult cat: paradoxical amplitude fluctuations during sleep and wakefulness. *Arch. Ital. Biol.* **108**, 403–422.

Chase, M. H. (1971a). Cerebral cortical control of jaw reflexes in the squirrel monkey (Saimiri sciureus). *Neurosci. Bull.* 160.

Chase, M. H. (1971b). Brain stem somatic reflex activity in neonatal kittens during sleep and wakefulness. *Physiol. Behavior* **7**, 165–172.

Chase, M. H. (1972). Patterns of reflex excitability during the ontogenesis of sleep and wakefulness. *In* "Sleep and the maturing nervous system" (C. D. Clemente, D. P. Purpura and F. E. Meyer, eds), pp. 253–285. Academic Press, New York.

Chase, M. H., and McGinty, D. J. (1970a). Modulation of spontaneous and reflex activity of the jaw musculature by orbital cortical stimulation in the freely-moving cat. *Brain Res.* **19**, 117–126.

Chase, M. H., and McGinty, D. J. (1970b). Somatomotor inhibition and excitation by forebrain stimulation during sleep and wakefulness: Orbital cortex. *Brain Res.* **19**, 127–136.

Chase, M. H., and Nakamura, Y. (1968). Inhibition of the masseteric reflex by vagal afferents. *Experientia* **24**, 918–919.

Chase, M. H., McGinty, D. J., and Sterman, M. B. (1968). Cyclic variation in the amplitude of a brain stem reflex during sleep and wakefulness. *Experientia* **24**, 47–48.

Chase, M. H., Nakamura, Y., and Torii, S. (1970a). Afferent vagal modulation of brain stem somatic reflex activity. *Exp. Neurol.* **27**, 534–544.

Chase, M. H., Torii, S., and Nakamura, Y. (1970b). The influence of afferent vagal fiber activity on masticatory reflexes. *Exp. Neurol.* **27**, 545–553.

Chow, K. A., Dement, W. C., and Mitchell, S. N. (1959). Effects of lesions of the rostral thalamus on brain waves and behavior in cats. *EEG Clin. Neurophysiol.* **11**, 107–120.

Claes, E. (1939). Contribution à l'étude physiologique de la fonction visuelle. I. Analyse oscillographique de l'activité spontanée et sensorielle de l'aire visuelle corticale chez le chat non anesthésié. *Arch. Int. Physiolog.* **48**, 181–237.

Clemente, C. D., and Sterman, M. B. (1963). Cortical synchronization and sleep patterns in acute restrained and chronic behaving cats induced by basal forebrain stimulation. *Electroenceph. Clin. Neurophysiol.* **24**, 172–187.

Clemente, C. D., and Sterman, M. B. (1967). Basal forebrain mechanisms for internal inhibition and sleep. *In* "Sleep and Altered States of Consciousness" (S. S. Kety, E. V. Evarts and H. L. Williams, eds.), Publ. Ass. Res. Nerv. Ment. Dis., Vol. XLV, pp. 127–147. Baltimore, Maryland. Williams and Wilkins.

Clemente, C. D., Sterman, M. B., Wyrwicka, W. (1963). Forebrain inhibitory mechanism: Conditioning of basal forebrain induced EEG synchronization and sleep. *Exp. Neurol.* **7**, 404–417.

Clemente, C. D., Chase, M. H., Knauss, T. A., Sauerland, E. K., and Sterman, M. B. (1966). Inhibition of a monosynaptic reflex by electrical stimulation of the basal forebrain or the orbital gyrus in the cat. *Experientia (Basel)* **22**, 844–848.

Cohen, B., Housepian, E. M., and Purpura, D. P. (1962). Intrathalamic regulation of activity in a cerebellocortical projection system. *Exp. Neurol.* **6**, 492–506.

Coleman, P. D., Gray, F. E., and Watanabe, K. (1959). EEG amplitude and reaction time during sleep. *J. Appl. Physiol.* **14**, 397–400.

Collins, E. H. (1954). Localization of an experimental hypothalamic and midbrain syndrome simulating sleep. *J. Comp. Neurol.* **100**, 661–697.

Coombs, J. S., Eccles, J. C., and Fatt, P. (1955). The electrical properties of the motoneurone membrane. *J. Physiol. (London)* **130**, 291–325.

Couch, J. R. (1970). Responses of neurons in the raphé nuclei to serotonin, norepinephrine and acetylcholine and their correlation with an excitatory synaptic output. *Brain Res.* **19**, 137–150.

Courville, J., Walsh, J., and Cordeau, J. P. (1962). Functional organization of the brain stem reticular formation and sensory input. *Science* **138**, 973–975.

Cowan, W. M., Guillary, B. W., and Powell, T. P. S. (1964). The origin of the mamillary peduncle and other hypothalamic connexions from the mid-brain. *J. Anat.* **98**, 345–363.

Craigie, E. H. (1925). Postnatal changes in vascularity in the cerebral cortex of the male albino rat. *J. Comp. Neurol.* **39**, 301–324.

Crain, S. M. (1952). Development of electrical activity in the cerebral cortex of the albino rat. *Proc. Soc. Exp. Biol. Med.* **81**, 49–51.

Creutzfeldt, O., and Grüsser, O. J. (1959). Beeinflussung der Flimmerreaktion einzelner corticaler Neurone durch elektrische Reize unspezifischer Thalamuskerne. *Proc. Int. Congr. Sci.*, *1st* **1/3**, 349–355.

Creutzfeldt, O. D., Watanabe, S., and Lux., H. D. (1966). Relations between EEG phenomena and potentials of single cortical stimulation. *Electroenceph. Clin. Neurophysiol.* **20**, 1–18.

Crome, L., Tymms, V., and Woolf, L. I. (1962). A chemical investigation of the defects of myelination in phenylketonuria. *J. Neurol. Neurosurg. Psychiat.* **25**, 143–148.

Crosby, E. C., Humphrey, T., and Lauer, E. W. (1962). "Correlative Anatomy of the Nervous System." p. 731. Macmillan, New York.

Czerny, A. (1891). Physiologische Untersuchungen ueber den Schlaf. *Jb. Kinderheilk.* **33**, 1–29.

Dahl, D. R. (1968). Short-chain fatty acid inhibition of rat brain NA–K adenosine triphosphatase. *J. Neurochem*, **15**, 815–820.

Dahlstrom, A., and Fuxe, K. (1964). Evidence for the existence of monoamines containing neurons in the central nervous system. *Acta Physiolog. Scand. Suppl. 232*, **62**.

Davis, H., Davis, P., Loomis, A., Harvey, N., and Hobart, G. (1938). Human brain potentials during the onset of sleep. *J. Neurophysiol.* **1**, 24–38.

Davis, H., Davis, P., Loomis, A., Harvey, N., and Hobart, G. (1939). Electrical reactions of human brain to auditory stimulation during sleep. *J. Neurophysiol.* **2**, 500–514.

Davison, A. N., and Sandler, M. (1958). Inhibition of 5-hydroxytryptophan decarboxylase by phenylalanine metabolites. *Nature (London)* **181**, 186–187.

DeArmond, S., and Fusco, M. M. (1971). The effect of preoptic warming on the arousal system of the mesencephalic reticular formation. *Exp. Neurol.* **33**, 653–670.

Delange, M., Castan, Ph., Cadilhac, J., Passouant, P. (1962). Les divers stades du sommeil chez le nouveau-né et le nourrisson. *Rev. Neurol.* **107**, 271–276.

De Lee, C., and Petre-Quadens, O. (1968). Les mouvements oculaires du sommeil. *Acta Neurol. Belg.* **68**, 327–331.

Delius, J. D. (1970). Irrelevant behaviour, information processing and arousal homeostasis. *Psycholog. Forsch.* **33**, 165–188.

Dell, P. (1971). Lower brain stem mechanisms and sleep induction. *Proc. Int. Congr. Physiolog. Sci. Munich* **8**, 29–30.

Dell, P., and Padel, Y. (1964). Endormissement rapide provoqué par la stimulation sélective d'afférences vigiles chez le chat. *Rev. Neurolog.* **111**, 381.

Delorme, F., Jeannerod, M., and Jouvet, M. (1965). Effets remarquables de la réserpine sur l'activité EEG phasique pontogeniculo occipitale. *C.R. Soc. Biol. (Paris)* **159**, 900–903.

Delorme, J. F., Riotte, M., and Jouvet, M. (1966a). Conditions de déclenchement du sommeil paradoxal par les acides gras à chaine courte chez le chat pontique chronique, *C. R. Soc. Biol. (Paris)* **160**, 1457–1460.

Delorme, F., Froment, J. L., and Jouvet, M. (1966b). Suppression du sommeil par la p-chloromethamphetamine et p-chlorophenylalanine. *C.R. Soc. Biol. (Paris)* **160**, 2347–2351.

Dement, W. (1958). The occurrence of low voltage fast electroencephalogram patterns during behavioral sleep in the cat. *Electroenceph. Clin. Neurophysiol.* **10**, 291–296.

Dement, W. (1960). The effect of dream deprivation. *Science* **131**, 1705–1707.

Dement, W. (1964). Eye movements during sleep. *In* "The Oculomotor System" (M. Bender, ed.), pp. 366–416. Harper (Hoeber), New York.

Dement, W. (1965). Studies on the function of rapid eye movement (paradoxical) sleep in human subjects. *In* "Aspects Anatomofonctionnels de la Physiologie du Sommeil" (M. Jouvet, ed.). CNRS, Paris.

Dement, W. (1969). The biological role of REM sleep. *In* "Sleep, Physiology and Pathology" (A. Kales, ed.), pp. 245–265. Lippincott, Philadelphia, Pennsylvania.

Dement, W. (1972). Sleep deprivation and the organization of the behavioral states. *In* "Sleep and the Maturing Nervous System" (C. Clemente, D. Purpura, and F. Mayer, eds.), pp. 319–361. Academic Press, New York.

Dement, W. (1973). The biological role of REM sleep. *In* "Sleep as an Active Process" (W. Webb, ed.) 33–58. Scott Foresman, Chicago, Illinois.

Dement, W., and Kleitman, N. (1957). Cyclic variations in EEG during sleep and their relation to eye movements, body motility and dreaming. *Electroenceph. Clin. Neurophysiol.* **9**, 673–690.

Dement, W., and Rechtschaffen, A. (1968). Narcolepsy: Polygraphic aspects, experimental and theoretical considerations. *In* "The Abnormalities of Sleep in Man" (H. Gastaut, E. Lugaresi, G. Berti Ceroni, and G. Coccagna, eds), pp. 147–164. Aulo Gaggi Editore, Bologna.

Dement, W., and Wolpert, E. A. (1958). The relation of eye-movements, body motility, and external stimuli to dream content. *J. Exp. Psychol.* **55**, 543–553.

Dement, W., Rechtschaffen, A., Gulevich, G. (1966). The nature of the narcoleptic sleep attack. *Neurology* **16**, 18–33.

Dement, W., Henry, P., Cohen, H., and Ferguson, J. (1967). Studies on the effect of REM deprivation in humans and animals. *In* "Sleep and Altered States of Consciousness" (S. S. Kety, E. V. Evarts, and H. L. Williams, eds.), pp. 456–468. Williams and Wilkins, Baltimore, Maryland.

Dement, W., Kelley, J., Laughlin, E., Carpenter, S., Simmons, J., Sidoric, K., and Lentz, R. (1972a). Life on "The Basic Rest-Activity Cycle". *Psychophysiology* **9**, 132.

Dement, W., Mitler, M., and Henriksen, S. (1972b). Sleep changes during chronic administration of parachlorophenylalanine. *Rev. Can. Biol., Suppl.* **31**, 239–246.

Dement, W., Zarcone, V., Hoddes, E., Smythe, H., and Carskadon, M. (1973). Sleep laboratory and clinical studies with flurazepam (Dalmane). *In*: Proc. Int. Symp. Benzodiazepines (S. Garattini and L. Randall, eds.). pp. 599–611. Raven Press, New York.

Demetrescu, M., and Demetrescu, M. (1962). Ascending inhibition and activation from the lower brain stem. The influence of pontine reticular stimulation on thalamo-cortical evoked potentials in cat. *Electroenceph. Clin. Neurophysiol.* **14**, 602–620.

Demetrescu, M., Demetrescu, M., and Iosif, G. (1966). Diffuse regulation of visual thalamo-cortical responsiveness during sleep and wakefulness. *Electroenceph. Clin. Neurophysiol.* **20**, 450–469.

Dempsey, E. W., and Morison, R. S. (1942a). The production of rhythmically recurrent cortical potentials after localized thalamic stimulation. *Amer. J. Physiol.* **135**, 293–300.

Dempsey, E. W., and Morison, R. S. (1942b). The interaction of certain spontaneous and induced cortical potentials. *Amer. J. Physiol.* **135**, 301–308.

Denisova, M. P., and Figurin, N. L. (1926). Periodic phenomena in the sleep of children. *Nov. Refl. Fiziol. Nerv. Syst.* **2**, 338–345.

Derbyshire, A. J., Rempel, B., Forbes, A., and Lambert, E. F. (1936). The effects of anaesthetics on action potentials in the cerebral cortex of the cat. *Amer. J. Physiol.* **116**, 577–596.

Desiraju, T., and Purpura, D. P. (1970). Organization of specific-nonspecific thalamic internuclear synaptic pathways. *Brain Res.* **21**, 169–182.

Dewan, E. E. (1969). The programming (P) hypothesis for REMS. *Phys. Sci. Res. Papers* N° 388. Air Force Cambridge Res. Lab.

Dewson, J., Dement, W., and Simmons, F. (1965). Middle ear muscle activity in cats during sleep. *Exp. Neurol.* **12**, 1–8.

Deza, L., and Eidelberg, E. (1967). Development of cortical electrical activity in the rat. *Exp. Neurol.* **17**, 425–438.

Dittrichová, J. (1962). Nature of sleep in young infants. *J. Appl. Physiol.* **17**, 543–546.

Dittrichová, J. (1969). Development of sleep in infancy. *In* "Brain and Early Behaviour" (R. J. Robinson, ed.), pp. 193–204. Academic Press, New York.

Dormont, J. (1972). Patterns of spontaneous unit activity in the ventrolateral thalamic nucleus cats. *Brain Res.* **37**, 223–239.

Doty, R. W. (1969). Electrical stimulation of the brain in behavioral context. *Ann. Rev. Psychol.* **20**, 289–320.

Dreyfus-Brisac, C. (1970). Ontogenesis of sleep in human prematures after 32 weeks of conceptional age. *Develop. Psychobiol.* **3**, 91–97.

Dreyfus-Brisac, C., and Monod, N. (1956). Veille, sommeil et réactivité chez le nouveau-né à terme. *Electroenceph. Clin. Neurophysiol. Suppl.* **6**, 425–431.

Dreyfus-Brisac, C., Samson-Dollfuss, D., Blanc, C., and Monod, N. (1958). L'électroencéphalogramme de l'enfant normal de moins de 3 ans. Aspect fonctionnel bioélectrique de la maturation nerveuse. *Biol. Néonat. (Basel)* **7**, 143–175.

Dumont, S. (1964). Contribution à l'étude du contrôle réticulaire des intégrations sensorimotrices au cours de la vigilance. Faculté des Sci. de l'Univ. de Paris.

Dumont, S., and Dell, P. (1960). Facilitation réticulaire des mécanismes visuels corticaux. *Electroenceph. Clin. Neurophysiol.* **12**, 769–796.

Dunleavy. D. L. F., Brezinova, V., Oswald, I., MacLean, A. W., and Tinker, M. (1972). Changes during weeks in effects of tricyclic drugs on the human sleeping brain. *Brit. J. Psychiat.* **120**, 663–672.

Dvořák, K. (1968). Die postnatale Differenzierung des Golgi Apparates in den Neuronen der Grosshirnrinde bei der Ratte. *Z. Zellforsch.* **85**, 225–236.

Eayrs, J. T. (1960). The influence of the thyroid on the central nervous system. *Brit. Med. Bull.* **16**, 122–127.

Eayrs, J. T. (1964). Endocrine influence on cerebral development. *Arch. Biol. (Liege)* **75**, 529–565.

Eayrs, J. T., and Goodhead, B. (1959). Postnatal development of the cerebral cortex of the rat. *J. Anat.* **93**, 385–402.

Eccles, J. C. (1969). The inhibitory pathways of the central nervous system. The Sherringtonian Lectures IX, p. 135. Thomas, Springfield, Illinois.

Eckhard, H., Hess, E. H., and Polt, J. M. (1964). Pupil size in relation to mental activity during simple problem solving. *Science* **143**, 1190–1192.

Eisenberg, R. (1965). Auditory behavior in the human neonate. Methodologic problems and the logical design of research procedures. *J. Audit. Res.* **5**, 159–177.

Elliot, K. A. L., and Jaspers, H. H. (1959). Gamma-aminobutyric acid. *Physiol. Rev.* **39**, 383–386.

Emde, R. N., and Metcalf, D. R. (1968). Behavioral and EEG correlates of undifferentiated eye movement states in infancy. *Psychophysiology* **5**, 227.

Emde, R. N., and Metcalf, D. R. (1970). An electroencephalographic study of behavioral rapid eye movement states in the human newborn. *J. Nerv. Ment. Dis.* **150**, 370–376.

Emmers, R., Chung, R. M. W., and Wang, G. H. (1965). Behavior and reflexes of chronic thalamic cats. *Arch. Ital. Biol.* **103**, 178–193.

Escalona, S. K. (1962). The study of individual differences and the problem of state. *J. Amer. Acad. Child Psychiat.* **1**, 11–37.

Euler, C. V., and Söderberg, U. (1956). The relation between gamma motor activity and the electroencephalogram. *Experientia* **12**, 278–279.

Evans, J. I., and Lewis, S. A. (1969). Dose effects of chlorpromazine on human sleep. *Psychopharmacologia (Berlin)* **14**, 342–348.

Evans, J. I., and Oswald, I. (1966). Some experiments in the chemistry of narcoleptic sleep. *Brit. J. Psychiat.* **112**, 401–404.

Evarts, E. V. (1960). Effect of sleep and waking on spontaneous and evoked discharge of single units in visual cortex. *Fed. Proc. Suppl.* **4**, **19**, 828–837.

Evarts, E. V. (1963). Photically evoked responses in visual cortex units during sleep and waking. *J. Neurophysiol.* **26**, 229–248.

Evarts, E. V. (1964). Temporal patterns of discharge of pyramidal tract neurons during sleep and waking in the monkey. *J. Neurophysiol.* **27**, 152–171.

Evarts, E. V. (1965). Relation of cell size to effects of sleep in pyramidal tract neurons. *In* "Sleep Mechanisms" (K. Akert, C. Bally, and J. P. Schadé, eds.), pp. 81–89. Elsevier, Amsterdam.

Evarts, E. V., Fleming, T. C., and Huttenlocher, P. R. (1960). Recovery cycle of visual cortex of the awake and sleeping cat. *Amer. J. Physiol.* **199**, 373–376.

Faber, M. (1955). "Pathogenisis of Poliomyelitis." Oxford, London.

Falk, B., Hillarp, M., Thieme, G., and Torp, A. (1962). Fluorescence of catecholamines and related compounds condensed with formaldehyde. *J. Histochem. Cytochem.* **10**, 348–364.

Famaglietti, E. V., Jr. (1970). Dendro-dentritic synapses in the lateral geniculate nucleus of the cat. *Brain Res.* **20**, 181–191.

Favale, E., Loeb, C., and Manfredi, M. (1964). Modifications of calloso-cortical response by sleep. *Arch. Int. Physiolog. Biochim.* **72**, 863–870.

Favale, E., Seitum, A., Tartaglione, A., and Tondi, M. (1971). Presynaptic and postsynaptic changes in the ventrolateral thalamic nucleus during natural sleep and wakefulness. *Brain Res.* **29**, 351–353.

Fazekas, J. R., Graves, F. B., and Alman, R. W. (1951). The influence of the thyroid on cerebral metabolism. *Endocrinology* **48**, 169–174.

Feinberg, I., Braun, M., and Shulman, E. (1969). EEG sleep patterns in mental retardation. *Electroenceph. Clin. Neurophysiol.* **27**, 128–141.

Feldberg, W., and Myers, R. D. (1964). Temperature changes produced by amines injected into the cerebral ventricles during anaesthesia. *J. Physiol.* **175**, 464–470.

Feldberg, W., and Myers, R. D. (1966). Appearance of 5-hydroxytryptamine and an unidentified pharmacologically active lipid acid in effluent from perfused cerebral ventricles. *J. Physiol.* **184**, 837–845.

Feldberg, W., and Sherwood, S. L. (1954). Injections of drugs into the lateral ventricle of the cat. *J. Physiol.* **123**, 148–156.

Feldman, M. H., and Purpura, D. P. (1970). Prolonged conductance increase in thalamic neurons during synchronizing inhibition. *Brain Res.* **24**, 329–332.

Feldman, S. M., and Waller, H. J. (1962). Dissociation of electrocortical activation and behavioural arousal. *Nature (London)* **196**, (4861), 1320–1322.

Ferguson, J., and Dement, W. (1968). Changes in the intensity of REM sleep with deprivation. *Psychophysiology* **4**, 380–381.

Ferguson, J., and Dement, W. (1969). The behavioral effects of amphetamine on REM deprived rats. *J. Psychiat. Res.* **7**, 111–118.

Ferguson, J., Cohen, H., Barchas, J., and Dement, W. (1969a). Sleep and wakefulness: a closer look. Presented at a meeting of the Federation of Amer. Soc. for Exp. Biol., Symp. on "Neurohumoral aspects of sleep and wakefulness". Atlantic City, New Jersey.

Ferguson, J., Cohen, H., Henriksen, S., McGarr, K., Mitchell, G., Hoyt, G., Barchas, J., and Dement, W. (1969b). The effect of chronic administration of PCPA on sleep in the cat. *Psychophysiology* **6**, 220–221.

Ferrier, D. (1876). "The Functions of the Brain," XV + 323 pp. Smith Elder, London.

Filion, M., Lamarre, Y., and Cordeau, J. P. (1971). Neuronal discharges of the ventrolateral nucleus of the thalamus during sleep and wakefulness in the cat. II. evoked activity. *Exp. Brain Res.* **12**, 499–508.

Fisher, C., Gross, J., and Zuch, J. (1965). Cycle of penile erection synchronous with dreaming (REM) sleep. *Arch. Gen. Psychiat.* **12**, 29–45.

Foulkes, D. (1962). Dream reports from different stages of sleep. *J. Abnorm. Soc. Psychol.* **65**, 14–25.

Friede, R. L. (1959). Histochemical investigations on succinic dehydrogenase in the central nervous system. The postnatal development of rat brain. *J. Neurochem.* **4**, 101–110.

Friedman, S., and Fisher, C. (1967). On the presence of a rhythmic, diurnal, oral and instinctual drive cycle in man. *J. Amer. Psychoanal. Ass.* **15**, 317–343.

Frigyesi, T. L., and Purpura, D. P. (1964). Functional properties of synaptic pathways influencing transmission in the specific cerebellothalamocortical projection system. *Exp. Neurol.* **10**, 305–324.

Fulton, J., and Bailey, P. (1929). Contribution to the study of tumors in the region of the third ventricle: their diagnosis and relation to pathological sleep. *J. Nerv. Mental Dis.* **69**, 145–164.

Fuster, J. M. (1958). Effects of stimulation of brain stem on tachistoscopic perception. *Science* **127**, 150.

Fuster, J. M., and Uyeda, A. A. (1962). Facilitation of tachistoscopic performance by stimulation of midbrain tegmental points in the monkeys. *Exp. Neurol.* **6**, 389–406.

Galambos, R., Sheatz, G., and Vermier, V. G. (1956). Electrophysiological correlates of a conditioned response in cats. *Science* **123**, 376–377.

Gamper, E. (1926). Bau und Leistungen eines menschlichen Mittelhirnwesens (Arhinencephalie mit Encephalocele) zugleich ein Beitrag zur Teratologie und Fasersystematik. *Z. Ges. Neurolog. Psychiat.* **104**, 67–120.

Gassel, M. M., and Pompeiano, O. (1965). Fusimotor function during sleep in unrestrained cats. An account of the modulation of the mechanically and electrically evoked monosynaptic reflexes. *Arch. Ital. Biol.* **103**, 347–368.

Gassel, M. M., Marchiafava, P. L., and Pompeiano, O. (1964a). Phasic changes in muscular activity during desynchronized sleep in unrestrained cats. An analysis of the pattern and organization of myoclonic twitches. *Arch. Ital. Biol.* **102**, 449–470.

Gassel, M. M., Marchiafava, P. L., and Pompeiano, O. (1964b). Tonic and phasic inhibition of spinal reflexes during deep, desynchronized sleep in unrestrained cats. *Arch. Ital. Biol.* **102**, 471–499.

Gassel, M. M., Ghelarducci, B., Marchiafava, P. L. Pompeiano, O. (1964c). Phasic changes in blood pressure and heart rate during the rapid eye movement episodes of desynchronized sleep in unrestrained cats. *Arch. Ital. Biol.* **102**, 530–544.

Gassel, M. M., Marchiafava, P. L., and Pompeiano, O. (1965). An analysis of the supraspinal influences acting on the motoneurons during sleep in the unrestrained cat. Modification of the recurrent discharge of the alpha motoneurons during sleep. *Arch. Ital. Biol.* **103**, 25–44.

Gayet, M. (1875). Affection encéphalique (encéphalite diffuse probable) localisée aux étages supérieurs des pédoncules cérébraux et aux couches optiques, ainsi qu'au plancher du quatrième ventricule et aux parois latérales du troisième. Observation recueillie. *Arch. Physiol. Brown Séquard*, **7**, 341–351.

Genovesi, U., Moruzzi, G., Palestini, M., Rossi, G. F., and Zanchetti, A. (1956). EEG and behavioral patterns following lesions of the mesencephalic reticular formation in chronic cats with implanted electrodes. *Abstr. Comm. XX Int. Physiolog. Congr. Bruxelles*, 335–336.

George, R., Haslett, W., and Jenden, D. (1964). A cholinergic mechanism in the brain stem reticular formation: induction of paradoxical sleep. *Int. J. Neuropharm.* **3**, 541–552.

Gerebtzoff, M. A. (1948). Recherches sur l'inhibition généralisée de Richet. *Arch. Int. Physiol.* **LVI**, 286–310.

Gesell, A., and Amatruda, C. J. (1945). "The Embryology of Behavior", p. 289. Hobber, New York.

Giaquinto, S., Pompeiano, O., and Somogyi, I. (1963). Reflex activity of extensor and flexor muscles following muscular afferent excitation during sleep and wakefulness. *Experientia* **19**, 481–482.

Giaquinto, S., Pompeiano, O., and Somogyi, I. (1964). Descending inhibitory influences on spinal reflexes during natural sleep. *Arch. Ital. Biol.* **102**, 282–307.

Giarman, N. J., and Schmidt, K. F. (1963). Some neurochemical aspect of the depressant action of 4-butyrolectone on the central nervous system. *Brit. J. Pharmacol. Chemother.* **20**, 563–568.

Gibbs, F., and Gibbs, E. (1950). "Atlas of Electroencephalography," 2nd ed., Vol. I, Methodology and Normal Controls. Addison-Wesley, Cambridge, Massachusetts.

Glaesser, A., and Mantegazzini, P. (1960). Action of 5-hydroxytryptamine and of 5-hydroxytryptophan on the cortical electrical activity of the midpontine pretrigeminal preparation of the cat with and without mesencephalic hemisection. *Arch. Ital. Biol.* **98**, 351–366.

Globus, G. G. (1970). Quantification of the REM sleep cycle as a rhythm. *Psychophysiology* **7**, 248–253.

Goldie, L., and Velzer, C. (1965). Innate sleep rhythms. *Brain* **88**, 1043–1056.

Goldstein, L., and Beck, R. A. (1965). Amplitude analysis of the electroencephalogram. *Int. Rev. Neurobiol.* **8**, 265–312.

Goltz, F. (1892). Der Hund ohne Grosshirn. *Pfluegers Arch.* **51**, 570–614.

Gramsbergen, A., Schwartze, P., Prechtl, H. F. R. (1970). The postnatal development of behavioural states in the rat. *Develop. Psychobiol.* **3**, 267–280.

Granit, R. (1955). "Receptors and Sensory Perception." Yale Univ. Press, New Haven, Connecticut.

Granit, R., and Kaada, B. R. (1952). Influence of stimulation of central nervous structures on muscle spindles in cat. *Acta Physiol. Scand.* **27**, 130–160.

Greenberg, R. (1970). Dreaming and memory. *Int. Psychiat. Clin.* **7**, 258–267.

Gregson, N. A., and Williams, P. L. (1969). A comparative study of brain and liver mitochondria from new-born and adult rats. *J. Neurochem.* **16**, 617–626.

Gross, H. P., and Schulte, F. J. (1969). Über die vermehrte Spindelaktivität im Schlaf-EEG bei Kindern mit Phenylketonurie. *Z. Kinderheilk.* **105**, 324–333.

Grünwald, P. (1964). Infants of low birth weight among 500 deliveries. *Pediatrics* **34**, 157–163.

Guglielmino, S., and Strata, P. (1971). Cerebellum and atonia of the desynchronized phase of sleep. *Arch. Ital. Biol.* **109**, 210–217.

Guilleminault, C., Eldridge, F., and Dement, W. (1972). Narcolepsy, insomnia and sleep apneas. *Bull. Physio-pathol. Respirat.* **8**, 1127–1138.

Hackett, J. T., and Marczynski, T. J. (1969). Postreinforcement electrocortical synchronization and enhancement of cortical photic evoked potentials during instrumentally conditioned appetitive behavior in the cat. *Brain Res.* **15**, 447–464.

Haider, I., and Oswald, I. (1970). Late brain recovery processes after drug overdose. *Brit. Med. J.* **2**, 318–322.

Halberg, F. (1953). Some physiological and clinical aspects of 24-hour periodicity. *Lancet* **73**, 20.

Halberg, F., Anderson, J. A., Ertel, R., and Berendes, H. (1967). Circadian rhythm in serum 5-hydroxytryptamine of healthy man and male patients with mental retardation. *Int. J. Neuropsychiat.* **3**, 379–390.

Harper, R. M., and McGinty, D. J. (1973). A technique for recording single neurons from unrestrained animals. *In* "Brain Unit Activity During Behavior" (M. I. Phillips, ed.), pp. 82–104. Thomas, Springfield, Illinois.

Hartmann, E. (1966). Reserpine: its effects on the sleepdream cycle in man. *Psychopharmacologia (Berlin)* **9**, 242–247.

Hartmann, E. (1967). "The Biology of Dreaming," p. 53. Thomas, Springfield, Illinois.

Hassler, R. (1959). Anatomy of the thalamus. *In* "Introduction to Stereotaxis with an Atlas of Human Brain" (G. Schaltenbrand and P. Bailey, eds.), Vol. 1, pp. 230–290. Grune and Stratton, New York.

Head, H. (1923). The conception of nervous and mental energy (II) ("Vigilance": a physiological state of nervous system). *Brit. J. Psychol.* **14**, 126–147.

Henriksen, S., Jacobs, B., and Dement, W. (1972). Dependence of REM sleep PGO waves on cholinergic mechanisms. *Brain Res* **48**, 412–416.

Hernández-Peón, R. (1962). Sleep induced by localized electrical or chemical stimulation of the forebrain. *Electroenceph. Clin. Neurophysiol.* **14**, 423–424.

Hernández-Peón, R. (1965). Central neuro-humoral transmission in sleep and wakefulness. *In* "Sleep Mechanisms." (K. Akert, C. Bally, and J. P. Schadé, eds.), pp. 96–117. Elsevier, Amsterdam.

Hernández-Peón, R., and Chavez-Ibarra, G. (1963). Sleep induced by electrical or chemical stimulation of the forebrain. *Electroenceph. Clin. Neurophysiol. Suppl.* **24**, 188–198.

Hess, W. R. (1927). Stammganglien Reizversuche. Tagg. Dtsch. Ges. in Frankfurt a. M., 27 bis 30 sept. 1927. *Ber. Ges. Physiolog.* **42**, 554–555.

Hess, W. R. (1943). Symptomatik des durch elektrischen Reiz ausgelosten Schlafes und die topographie des Schlafzentrums. *Helv. Physiol.* **1**, C 61.

Hess, W. R. (1944). Das Schlafsyndrom als Folge diencephaler Reizung. *Helv. Physiolog. Pharmacolog. Acta.* **2**, 305–344.

Hess, W. R. (1954). "Diencephalon Autonomic Extrapyramidal Function." Grune and Stratton, New York.

Hess, W. R. (1968). "Hypothalamus und Thalamus." 2. Aufl. Thieme, Stuttgart.

Hess, R., Jr., Koella, W. P., and Akert, K. (1953). Cortical and subcortical recordings in natural and artificially induced sleep in cats. *EEG Clin. Neurophysiol.* **5**, 75–90.

Hinde, R. A. (1966). "Animal Behavior." p. 534. McGraw-Hill, New York.

Hobson, J. A. (1965). The effects of chronic brain-stem lesions on cortical and muscular activity during sleep and waking in the cat. *Electroenceph. Clin. Neurophysiol.* **19**, 41–62.

Hobson, J. A. (1967). Electrographic correlates of behavior in the frog with special reference to sleep. *Electroenceph. clin. Neurophysiol.* **22**, 113–121.

Hobson, J. A. (1972). Cellular neurophysiology and sleep research. *In* "The Sleeping Brain" (M. H. Chase, ed.), p. 59–83. Vol. 1, Perspectives in the Brain Sciences, BIS/BRI, Los Angeles.

Hobson, J. A., Goin, O. B., Goin, C. J. (1968). Electroencephalographic correlates of behaviour in tree frogs. *Nature (London)* **220**, 386–387.

Hoddes, E., Zarcone, V., Dement, W. (1972). The cross-validation of the Stanford Sleepiness, Scale, *Sleep Res*, **1**, 91.

Hodes, R., and Dement, W. (1964). Depression of electrically induced reflexes ("H-reflexes") in man during low voltage EEG "sleep". *Electroenceph. Clin. Neurophysiol.* **17**, 617–629.

Hodges, J. R. (1970). The hypothalamus and pituitary ACTH release. *Prog. Brain Res.* **32**, 12–18.

Hodgkin, A. L., and Huxley, A. F. (1952). The dual effect of membrane potential on sodium conductance in the giant axon of Loligo. *J. Physiol.* (London) **116**, 497–506.

Hoffman, P., and Tonnies, J. F. (1948). Nachweis des vollig konstanten vorkommens des Zungenkieferreflexes beim Menschen. *Pflügers Arch. Ges. Physiol.* **250**, 103–108.

Hongo, T. M., Kubota, K., and Shimazu, H. (1963). Electroencephalographic spindle and depression of gamma motor activity. *J. Neurophysiol.* **26**, 568–580.

Hösli, L., and Monnier, M. (1962). Schlaf-und Weckwirkungen des intralaminaren Thalamus. "Reizparameter und Koagulationsbefunde beim Kaninchen. *Pflügers Arch. Ges. Physiol.* **275**, 439–451.

Hosokawa, H. Proprioceptive innervation of striated muscles in the territory of cranial nerves. *Texas Rep. Biol. Med.* **19**, 405–464.

Ho van Hap, A., Babineau, L. M., and Berlinguet, L. (1967). Hormonal action on monoamine oxidase in rats. *Can. J. Biochem.* **45**, 355–358.

Hsia, D. Y., Nishimura, K., and Brenchley, Y. (1963). Mechanisms for the decrease of brain serotonin. *Nature (London)* **200**, 578.

Hubel, D. H. (1960). Single unit activity in lateral geniculate body and optic tract of unrestrained cat. *J. Physiol.* **150**, 91–104.

Hubel, D. H., and Nauta, W. Y. H. (1960). Electrocortigram of cats with chronic lesions of the rostral mesencephalic tegmentum. *Fed. Proc.* **19**, 287.

Hubel, D. H., and Wiesel, T. N. (1963). Receptive fields of cells in striate cortex of very young, visually inexperienced kittens. *J. Neurophysiol.* **26**, 994–1002.

Hugelin, A. (1961). Intégrations motrices et vigilance chez l'encéphale isolé. II. Contrôle réticulaire des voies finales communes d'ouverture et de fermeture de la gueule. *Arch. Ital Biol.* **99**, 244–269.

Hugelin, A., and Bonvallet, M. (1957). Etude oscillographique d'un réflexe monosynaptique cranien (réflexe massétérin). *J. Physiol. (Paris)* **49**, 210–211.

Hughes, J. R. (1964). Responses from the visual cortex of unanesthetized monkeys. *Int. Rev. Neurobiol.* **7**, 99–152.

Humphrey, D. P. (1968a). Re-analysis of the antidromic cortical response. I. Potentials evoked by stimulation of the isolated pyramidal tract. *Electroenceph. Clin. Neurophysiol.* **24**, 116–129.

Humphrey, D. P. (1968b). Re-analysis of the antidromic cortical response. II. On the contribution of cell discharge and PSPs to the evoked potentials. *Electroenceph. Clin. Neurophysiol.* **25**, 421–442.

Hunter, J., and Jasper, H. H. (1949). Effects of thalamic stimulation in unanesthetized animals. *Electroenceph. Clin. Neurophysiol.* **1**, 305–324.

Ingram, W. R., Knott, J. R., Wheatley, M. D., and Summers, T. D. (1951). Physiological relationships between the hypothalamus and the cerebral cortex. *Electroenceph. Clin. Neurophysiol.* **3**, 37–58.

Ingvar, D. H. (1955). Electrical activity of isolated cortex in the unanaesthetized cat with intact brain stem. *Acta Physiolog. Scand.* **33**, 151–168.

Itil, T. (1969) Automatic classification of sleep stages and the discrimination of vigilance changes using digital computer methods. *Agressologie* **10**, 603–610.

Itil, T. (1970). Digital computer analysis of the electroencephalogram during rapid eye movement sleep state in man. *J. Nerv. Ment. Dis.* **150**, 201–208.

Jackson, J. H. (1931–32). "Selected writings of John Hughlings Jackson." (J. Taylor, ed.), 2 vols. Hodder and Stroughton, London.

Jacobs, B., Henriksen, S., and Dement, W. (1972). Neurochemical bases of the PGO wave. *Brain Res.* **48**, 406–411.

Jacobson, A., and Kales, A. (1967). Somnambulism: All-Night EEG and related studies. *In* "Sleep and Altered States of Consciousness" (S. S. Kety, E. V. Evarts, and H. L. Williams, eds.), pp. 424–455. Williams and Wilkins, Baltimore, Maryland.

Jacobson, A., Kales, A., Lehmann, D., and Hoedemaker, F. S. (1964). Muscle tonus in human subjects during sleep and dreaming. *Exp. Neurol.* **10**, 418–424.

Jansen, J., and Jansen, J. K. S. (1955). On the efferent fibers of the cerebellar nuclei in the cat. *J. Comp. Neurol.* **102**, 607–623.

Jasper, H. H. (1949). Diffuse projection system. The integrative action of the thalamic reticular systems. *Electroenceph. Clin. Neurophysiol.* **1**, 405–420.

Jasper, H. H. (1958). Recent advances in our understanding of ascending activities of the reticular system. *In* "Reticular Formation of the Brain" (H. H. Jasper *et al.*, ed.), pp. 319–331. Little Brown, Boston, Massachusetts.

Jasper, H. H. (1960). Unspecific thalamocortical relations. *In* "Handbook of Physiology, Sec. 1" (J. Field, H. W. Magoun, and V. E. Hall, eds.), pp. 1307–1321. Amer. Physiolog. Soc., Washington, D.C.

Jasper, H. H., and Amjone-Marsan, C. (1952). Thalamocortical integrating mechanisms. *Res. Publ. Ass. Nerv. Ment. Dis.* **30**, 493–512.

Jasper, H. H., and Stefanis, C. (1965). Intracellular oscillatory rhythms in pyramidal tract neurones in the cat. *Electroenceph. Clin. Neurophysiol.* **18**, 541–553.

Jasper, H. H., Hunter, J., and Knighton, R. (1948). Experimental studies of thalamocortical systems. *Trans. Amer. Med. Ass.* **73**, 210–212.

Jasper, H. H., Khan, R. T., and Elliott, K. A. (1965). Amino-acids released from the cerebral cortex in relation to its state of activation. *Science* **147**, 1448–1449.

Jeannerod, M., Mouret, J., and Jouvet, M. (1965). Etude de la motricité oculaire au cours de la phase paradoxale du sommeil chez le chat. *Electroencph. Clin. Neurophysiol.* **18**, 554–566.

Johnson, R., and Armstrong-James, M. (1970). Morphology of superficial postnatal cerebral cortex with special reference to synapses. *Z. Zellforsch.* **110**, 540–558.

Johnson, L., Lubin, A., Naitoh, P., Nute, C., and Autin, M. (1969). Spectral analysis of the EEG of dominant and non-dominant alpha subjects during waking and sleeping. *Electroenceph. Clin. Neurophysiol.* **26**, 361–370.

Jones, B., Bobillier, P., and Jouvet, M. (1969). Effets de la destruction des neurones contenant des catécholamines du mésencéphale sur le cycle veille-sommeil du chat. *C. R. Soc. Biol. (Paris)* **163**, 176–180.

Jones, E. G., and Powell, T. P. S. (1968). The ipsilateral cortical connexions of the somatic sensory areas in the cat. *Brain Res.* **9**, 71–94.

Jones, R., and Oswald, I. (1968). Two cases of healthy insomnia. *Electroenceph. Clin. Neurophysiol.* **24**, 378–380.

Joppich, G., and Michaelis, R. (1967). Über cerebrale aktivitäten bei Neugeborenen und jungen Säuglingen. *Deutsch. Med. Woschr.* **92**, 2295–2315.

Jouvet, M. (1961). Telencephalic and rhombencephalic sleep in the cat. *In* "The Nature of Sleep" (G. E. W. Wolstenholme and M. O'Connor, eds.), p. 188. London, Churchill.

Jouvet, M. (1962a). Sur l'existence d'un système hypnique ponto-limbique, ses rapports avec l'activité onirique. *In* "Physiologie de l'hippocampe," p. 297–330. Centre Nationale de la Recherche Scientifique, Paris.

Jouvet, M. (1962b). Recherches sur les structures nerveuses et les mécanismes responsables des différentes phases du sommeil physiologique. *Arch. Ital. Biol.* **100**, 125–206.

Jouvet, M. (1963). The rhombencephalic phase of sleep. *Progr. Brain. Res.* **1**, 406–424.

Jouvet, M. (1965a). Behavioural and EEG effects of paradoxical sleep deprivation in the cat. *Proc. Int. Congr. Physiolog. Sci. 23rd. Tokyo, 1965* **4**, N° 87, 344–355. Exerpta medica Int. Congr. Ser.

Jouvet, M. (1965b). Paradoxical sleep—A study of its nature and mechanisms. *Progr. Brain Res.* **18**, 20–57, 257.

Jouvet, M. (1965c). Etude de la dualité des états de sommeil et des mécanismes de la phase paradoxale. *In "Aspects anatomo-fonctionnels de la physiologie du sommeil"* (M. Jouvet, ed.), pp. 397–449. Centre National de la Recherche Scientifique, Paris.

Jouvet, M. (1966). Sommeil et monoamines. *Bull. Schweiz. Akad. Med. Wissensch.* **22**, 287–305.

Jouvet, M. (1967a). Neurophysiology of the states of sleep. *Physiolog. Rev.* **47**, 117–177.

Jouvet, M. (1967b). Mechanisms of the states of sleep: a neuropharmacological approach. *In* "Sleep and altered States of Consciousness." *Ass. Res. Nerv. Mental Dis.* **XLV**, 86–126.

Jouvet, M. (1969a). Biogenic amines and the states of sleep. *Science* **163**, 32–41.

Jouvet, M. (1969b). Neurophysiological and biochemical mechanisms of sleep. *In* "Sleep: Physiology and Pathology" (A. Kales, ed.), pp. 89–100. Lippincott, Philadelphia, Pennsylvania.

Jouvet, M. (1970). Neurohumoral basis of sleep. *In* "The Psychodynamic Implications of the Physiological Studies in Dreams" (L. Madow, and L. H. Snow, eds.), pp. 3–23. Springfield, Illinois.

Jouvet, M. (1972). The role of monoamines and acetylcholine containing neurons in the regulation of the sleep-waking cycle. *Ergebnisse Physiolog.* **64**, 166–307.

Jouvet, M., and Delorme, F. (1965). Locus coeruleus et sommeil paradoxal. *C. R. Soc. Biol. (Paris)* **159**, 895–899.

Jouvet, M., and Michel, F. (1959). Corrélations électromyographiques du sommeil chez le chat décortiqué et mésencéphalique chronique. *C. R. Soc. Biol. (Paris)* **153**, 422–425.

Jouvet, M., and Michel, F. (1960). Sur les voies nerveuses responsables de l'activité rapide corticale au cours du sommeil physiologique chez le chat (phase paradoxale). *J. Physiol. (Paris)* **52**, 130–131.

Jouvet, M., Michel, F., and Courjon, J. (1959). Sur un stade d'activité électrique cérébrale rapide au cours du sommeil physiologique. *C. R. Soc. Biol. (Paris)* **153**, 1024–1028.

Jouvet-Mounier, D. (1968). Ontogénèse des états de vigilance chez quelques mammifères. Thèse, Fac. des Sciences, Lyon.

Jouvet-Mounier, D., Astic, L., and Lacote, D. (1970). Ontogenesis of the states of sleep in rat, cat and guinea pig during the first postnatal month. *Develop. Psychobiol.* **2**, 216–239.

Jovanović U. J. (1969). "Der Schlaf, Neurophysiologische Aspekte." p. 252. Barth, München.

Juge, A., Sordet, F., Jouvet, M., and Pujol, J. F. (1972). Modification due métabolisme de la sérotonine cérébrale après 6-Hydroxydopamine chez le rat. *C. R. Acad. Sci. (Paris)* **274**, 3266–3268.

Kaada, B. R. (1951). Somatomotor, autonomic and electroencephalographic responses to electrical stimulation of rhinencephalic and other structures in primates, cat and dog. *Acta Physiol. Scand. suppl.* **24**, 83.

Kahn, E., Fisher, C., and Lieberman, L. (1970). Sleep characteristics of the human aged female. *Comp. Psychiat.* **11**, 274–278.

Kales, A., Heuser, G., Jacobson, A., Kales, J. D., Hanley, J., Zweizig, J. R., and Paulson, M. J. (1967a). All night sleep studies in hypothyroid patients before and after treatment. *J. Clin. Endocrinal.* **27**, 1593–1599.

Kales, A., Jacobson, A., Kales, J., Kun, T., and Weissbuch, R. (1967b). All-night EEG sleep measurements in young adults. *Psychonom. Sci.* **7**, 67–68.

Kales, A., Wilson, T., Kales J., Jacobson, A., Paulson, M., Kollar, E., and Walter, R. (1967c). Measurements of all-night sleep in normal elderly persons: effects of aging. *J. Amer. Geriat. Soc.*, **15**, 405–415.

Kales, A., Malmstrom, E., Scharf, M., and Rubin, R. (1969). Psychophysiological and biochemical changes following use and withdrawal of hypnotics. *In* "Sleep: Physiology and Pathology" (A. Kales, ed.), pp. 331–343. Lippincott, Philadelphia.

Kales, J., Tan, T.-L., Swearingen, C., and Kales, A. (1971). Are over-the-counter sleep medications effective? All-night EEG studies. *Curr. Therapeut. Res.* **13**, 143–151.

Kameda, K., Nagel, R., and Brooks, V. B. (1969). Some quantitative aspects of pyramidal collateral inhibition. *J. Neurophysiol.* **32**, 540–553.

Kaneko, Z., Hishikawa, Y., Ueyama, M., Shimizu, A., and Ida, H. (1962). EEG synchronization induced by electrical stimulation of the hypothalamus. *Proc. Japan EEG Soc., Tokyo.*

Katzman, R., Björklund, A., Owman, Ch., Stenevi, U., and West, K. A. (1971). Evidence for regenerative axon sprouting of central catecholamine neurons in the rat mesencephalon following electrolytic lesion. *Brain Res.* **25**, 579–596.

Kawakami, M., and Sawyer, C. H. (1964). Conditioned induction of paradoxical sleep in the rabbit. *Exp. Neurol.* **9**, 470–482.

Kellaway, P. (1957). Ontogenic evolution of the electrical activity of the brain in man and animals. Proceedings 4th International Meeting of EEG and Clinical Neurophysiology, Bruxelles. *Acta Med. Belg.* 141–154.

Kellaway, P., Gol, A., and Proler, M. (1966). Electrical activity of the isolated cerebral hemisphere and isolated thalamus. *Exp. Neurol.* **17**, 281.

Kennard, M. A. (1943). Electroencephalogram of decorticate monkeys. *J. Neurophysiol.* **6**, 233–242.

Kety, S. S. (1961). Sleep and the energy metabolism of the brain. *In* "The Nature of Sleep" (G. E. W. Wolstenholme and M. O'Connor, eds.), pp. 375–381. London, Churchill.

Kidokoro, Y., Kubota, K., Shuto, S., and Sumino, R. (1968) Reflex organization of cat masticatory muscles. *J. Neurophysiol,* **31**, 695–708.

Kim, C., Choi, H., Kim. J. K., Kim, M. S., Huh, M. K., and Moon, Y. B. (1971). Sleep pattern of hippocampectomized cat. *Brain Res.* **29**, 223–236.

King, D., and Jewett, R. E. (1971). The effects of alpha-methyltyrosine on sleep and brain norepinephrine in cat. *J. Pharmacol. Exp. Ther.* **177**, 188–194.

Klein, M., Michel, F., and Jouvet, M. (1964). Etude polygraphique du sommeil chez les oiseaux. *C. R. Soc. Biol.* **158**, 99–103.

Kleitman, N. (1963). "Sleep and Wakefulness." p. 552. Univ of Chicago Press, Chicago, Illinois.

Kleitman, N. (1967). Phylogenetic, ontogenetic and environmental determinants in the evolution of sleep-wakefulness cycles. *Res. Nerv. Ment. Dis.* **45**, 30–38.

Kleitman, N., and Camille, N. (1932). Studies on the physiology of sleep. VI. The behavior of decorticate dogs. *Amer. J. Physiol.* **100**, 474–480.

Knott, J. R., Ingram, W. R., and Chiles, W. D. (1955). Effects of subcortical lesions on cortical electroencephalogram in cats. *Arch. Neurol. Psychiat,* **73**, 203–215.

Koe, B. K., and Weissman, A. (1966). P-chlorophenylalanine, a specific depletor of brain serotonin. *J. Pharmacol. Exp. Ther.* **154**, 499–516.

Koella, W. P. (1967). "Sleep. Its Nature and Physiological Organization," pp. 118–131. Thomas, Springfield, Illinois.

Koella, W. P. (1970). Serotonin oder Somnotonin. *Schweiz. Med. Woschr.* **100**, 357–364, 424–430.

Koella, W. P., and Czicman, J. S. (1966). Mechanism of the EEG synchronizing action of serotonin. *Amer. J. Physiol.* **211**, 926–934.

Koella, W. P., and Gellhorn, E. (1954). The influence of diencephalic lesions upon the action of nociceptive impulses and hypercapnia on the electrical activity of the cat's brain. *J. Comp. Neurol.* **100**, 243–256.

Koella, W. P., Feldstein, A., and Czicman, J. S. (1968). The effect of parachlorophenylalanine on the sleep of cats. *Electroenceph. Clin. Neurophysiol.* **25**, 481–490.

Koppel, B., Zarcone, V., De La Pena, A., and Dement, W. (1972). Changes in selective attention as measured by the visual averaged evoked potential following REM deprivation in man. *Electroenceph. Clin. Neurophysiol.* **32**, 322–325.

Kostowski, W., Giacalone, E., Garattini, S., and Valzelli, V. (1969). Electrical stimulation of midbrain raphe: biochemical, behavioral and bioelectrical effects. *Eur. J. Pharmacol.* **7**, 170–175.

Krieg, W. J. S. (1946). Connections of the cerebral cortex. I. The albino rat. A topography of the cortical areas. *J. Comp. Neurol.* **84**, 221–275.

Krieger, D. T. (1970). Factors influencing the circadian periodicity of adrenal steroid levels. *Trans. N. Y. Acad. Sci.* **32:3**, 316–329.

Kripke, D. F., Reite, M., Pegram, G., Stephens, L., and Lewis, O. (1968). Nocturnal sleep in rhesus monkeys. *Electroenceph. Clin. Neurophysiol.* **24**, 582–586.

Kripke, D. F., Halberg, F., Crowley, T. J., and Pegram, G. V. (1971). Ultradian rhythms in rhesus monkeys *Psychophysiology* **7:2**, 307–308.

Kristiansen, K., and Courtois, G. (1949). Rhythmic electrical activity from isolated cerebral cortex. *Electroenceph. Clin. Neurophysiol.* **1**, 265–272.

Krnjevic, K., Randic, M., and Straughan, D. W. (1966). An inhibitory process in the cerebral cortex. *J. Neurophysiol.* **184**, 16–48.

Krnjevic, K., Reiffenstein, R. J., and Silver, A. (1970). Chemical sensitivity of neurons in long-isolated slabs of cat cerebral cortex. *Electroenceph. Clin. Neurophysiol.* **29**, 269–282.

Kubota, K., Iwamura, Y., and Niimi, Y. (1965a) Monosynaptic reflex and natural sleep in the cat. *J. Neurophysiol.* **28**, 125–138.

Kubota, K., Sakata, H., Takahashi, K., and Uno, M. (1965b). Location of the recurrent inhibitory synapse on cat pyramidal tract cell. *Proc. Jap. Acad.* **41**, 195–197.

Lamarre, Y., Joffroy, A. J., Filion, M., and Bouchoux, R. (1971a). A stereotaxic method for repeated sessions of central unit recording in the paralyzed or moving animal. *Rev. Can. Biol.* **29**, 371–376.

Lamarre, Y., Filion, M., and Cordeau, J. P. (1971b). Neuronal discharges of the ventrolateral nucleus of the thalamus during sleep and wakefulness in the cat. I. Spontaneous activity. *Exp. Brain. Res.* **12**, 480–498.

Lamarre, Y., Filion, M., and Cordeau, J. P. (1971c). Neuronal discharges of the ventrolateral. nucleus of the thalamus during sleep and wakefulness in the cat. II Evoked activity. *Exp. Brain Res.* **12**, 499–508.

Larroche, J. C. (1962). Quelques aspects anatomiques du développement cérébral. *Biol. Néonat.* **4**, 126–153.

Legrand, J., and Bout, M. C. (1970). Influence de l'hypothyroidisme et de la thyroxine sur le développement des épines dendritiques de cellules de Purkinje dans le cervelet du jeune rat. *C. R. Acad. Sci. (Paris)* **271**, 1199–1202.

Lena, C., and Parmeggiani, P. L. (1964). Hippocampal theta rhythm and activated sleep. *Helv. Physiol. Acta.* **22**, 120–135.

Lenard, H. G. (1970). The development of sleep spindles in the EEG during the first two years of life. *Neuropädiatrie* **1**, 264–270.

Lennox, M., and Coolidge, J. (1949). Electroencephalographic changes after prefrontal lobotomy. *Arch. Neurol. Psychiat.* **62**, 150–161.

Lewis, S. A., and Oswald, I. (1969). Overdose of tricyclic anti-depressants and deductions concerning their cerebral action. *Brit. J. Psychiat.* **115**, 1403–1410.

Lewis, S. A., Oswald, I., Evans, J. I., Akindele, M. O., and Tompsett, S. L. (1970). Heroin and human sleep. *Electroenceph. Clin. Neurophysiol.* **28**, 374–381.

Lewis, S. A., Oswald, I., and Dunleavy, D. L. F. (1971). Chronic fenfluramine administration: some cerebral effects. *Brit. Med. J.* **3**, 67–70.

Lindsley, D., Bowden, J., and Magoun, H. (1949). Effect upon the EEG of acute injury to the brain stem activating system. *Electroenceph. Clin. Neurophysiol.* **1**, 475–486.

Lindsley, D., Schreiner, L., Knowles, W., and Magoun, H. (1950). Behavioral and EEG changes following chronic brain stem lesions in the cat. *Electroenceph. Clin. Neurophysiol.* **2**, 483–498.

Linneweh, F., Ehrlich, M., Graul, E. H., and Hundeshagen, H. (1963). Über den Aminosäuren-Transport bei phenylketonurischer Oligophrenie. *Klin. Woschr.* **41**, 253–255.

Lisch, H. J., and Aigner, A. (1968). Über die Wirkung von L-Thyroxin auf die Aktivität der Mono-aminoxydase (MAO) im Gehirn von Meerschweinchen. *Klin. Woschr.* **46**, 206–209.

Loevenberg, W., Jequier, R., and Sjoerdsma, A. (1967). Tryptophan hydroxylation: measurement in pineal gland, brainstem, and carcinoid tumor. *Science* **155**, 217–219.

Loizou, L. A. (1969). Projections of the nucleus locus coeruleus in the albino rat. *Brain Res.* **15**, 563–566.

Loomis, A., Harvey, E., and Hobart, G. (1937). Cerebral states during sleep as studied by human brain potentials. *J. Exp. Psychol.* **21**, 127–144.

Lubinska, L. (1932). Contributions a l'étude des réflexes non-iteratifs. (Le réflexe linguo-maxillaire). *Ann. Physiol. Physicochim. Biol.* **8**, 668–759.

Lucas, E. A., and Sterman, M. B. (1971). Effects of performance, forebrain lesions and drugs on sleep-wake and rest-activity cycles in the cat. *Proc. Int. Congr. Ist.* p. 211. Ass. for Psychophysiol. Study of Sleep Bruges, Belgium.

Lucas, E. A., and Sterman, M. B. (1972). Effects of performance and forebrain lesions on sleep-wake (SW) and REM cycles in the cat. *Anat. Rec.* **172**, 357.

Lucas, E. A., Sterman, M. B., and McGinty, D. J. (1969). The salamander EEG: A model of primitive sleep and wakefulness. *Psychophysiology* **6**:2, 230.

Lucero, M. A. (1970). Lengthening on REM sleep duration consecutive to learning in the rat. *Brain Res.* **20**, 319–322.

Lund, R. D. (1969). Synaptic patterns of the superficial layers of the superior colliculus of the rat. *J. Comp. Neurol.* **135**, 179–208.

Lynch, G. S. (1970). Separable forebrain mechanisms controlling different manifestations of spontaneous. activity. *J. Comp. Physiol. Psychol.* **70**, 48–59.

Lynch, G. S., Ballantine, P., and Campbell, B. (1969). Potentiation of behavioral arousal following cortical damage and subsequent recovery. *Exp. Neurol.* **23**, 195–206.

MacIllwain, H. (1966). "Biochemistry and the Central Nervous System." Churchill, London.

Madoz, P., and Reinoso-Suarez, F. (1968). Influence of lesions in preoptic region of the states of sleep and wakefulness. *Proc. Int. Un. Physiol. Sci.* **7**, 276.

Maeda, T., and Pin, C. (1971). Topographie des neurones monoaminergiques du pont et de leurs voies ascendantes. *C. R. Soc. Biol.* (*Paris*) **165**, 2137–2141.

Maeda, T., Abe, T., and Shimizu, N. (1960). Histochemical demonstration of aromatic monoamine in the locus coeruleus of the mammalian brain. *Nature* (*London*) **188**, 326–327.

Maekawa, K., and Purpura, D. P. (1967a). Properties of spontaneous and evoked synaptic activities of thalamic ventrobasal neurons. *J. Neurophysiol.* **30**, 360–381.

Maekawa, K., and Purpura, D. P. (1967b). Intracellular study of lemniscal and non-specific synaptic interactions in thalamic ventrobasal neurones. *Brain Res.* **4**, 308–323.

Maekawa, K., and Purpura, D. P. (1967c). Excitatory processes and spike potential variations in reticular neurons. *Fed. Proc.* **26**, 434.

Magnes, J., Moruzzi, G., and Pompeiano, O. (1961a). Synchronization of the EEG produced by low-frequency electrical stimulation of the region of the solitary tract. *Arch. Ital. Biol.* **99**, 33–67.

Magnes, J., Moruzzi, G., and Pompeiano, O. (1961b). Electroencephalogram—synchronizing structures in the lower brain stem. *In* "The Nature of Sleep" (G. E. W. Wolstenholme and M. O'Connor, eds.). Churchill, London.

Magoun, H. W. (1952). An ascending reticular activating system in the brain stem. *Arch. Neurol. Psychiat.* **67**, 145–154.

Magoun, H. W. (1958). "The Waking Brain." Thomas, Springfield, Illinois.

Magoun, H. W. (1963). "The Waking Brain," 2nd ed. Thomas, Springfield, Illinois.

Magoun, H. W., and Rhines, R. (1946). An inhibitory mechanism in the bulbar reticular formation. *J. Neurophysiol.* **9**, 165–171.

Malliani, A., and Purpura, D. P. (1967) Intracellular studies of the corpus striatum. II. Patterns of synaptic activities in lenticular and entopeduncular neurons. *Brain Res.* **6**, 341–354.

Malmfors, T., and Thoenen, H. (eds.) (1971). "6-Hydroxydopamine and Catecholamine Neurons." p. 368. North Holland Publ. Co. Amsterdam.

Mancia, M., (1969). EEG and behavioral changes owing to splitting of the brain stem in cats. *Electroenceph. Clin. Neurophysiol.* **27**, 487–503.

Mantegazzini, P., and Glässer, A. (1960). Action de la DL-3-4-dioxyphenylalanine (dopa) et de la dopamine sur l'activité électrique du chat "cerveau isolé". *Arch. Ital. Biol.* **98**, 367–374.

Mantegazzini, P., Poeck, K., and Santibañez, G. (1959). The action of adrenaline and noradrenaline on the cortical electrical activity of the "encéphale isolé" cat. *Arch. Ital. Biol.* **97**, 222–242.

Marinesco, G., Draganesco, S., Sager, O., and Kreindler, A. (1929). Recherches anatomo-cliniques sur la localisation de la fonction du sommeil. *Rev. neurolog.* **II**, 481–497.

Martin, A. R., and Branch, C. L. (1958). Spontaneous activity of Betz cells in cats with midbrain lesions. *J. Neurophysiol* **21**, 368–379.

Masai, H., Kusunoki, T., and Ishibashi, H. (1965). A histochemical study on the fundamental plan of the central nervous system. *Experientia (Basel)* **21**, 572.

Massion, J. (1968). Etude d'une structure motrice thalamique, le noyau ventro-latéral et de sa régulation par les afférences sensorielles. Thèse, p. 134. Paris.

Matsumoto, J., and Jouvet, M. (1964). Effets de réserpine, DOPA et 5-HTP sur les 2 états de sommeil. *C. R. Soc. Biol. (Paris)* **158**, 2137–2140.

Matsumoto, J., and Watanabe, S. (1967). Paradoxical sleep: Effects of adrenergic blocking agents. *Proc. Jap. Acad.* **43**, 680–683.

Matsuzaki, M., Takagi, H., and Tokizane, T. (1964). Paradoxical phase of sleep: its artificial induction in the cat by sodium butyrate. *Science* **146**, 1328–1329.

Mauthner, L. (1890). Pathologie und physiologie des Schlafes. *Wien. Klin. Woschr.* **3**, 445–446.

McGinty, D. J., and Sterman, M. B. (1968). Sleep suppression after basal forebrain lesions in the cat. *Science* **160**, 1253–1255.

McGinty, D. J., Sterman, M. B., and Iwamuri, Y. (1971) Activity and atonia in the decerebrate cat. *Psychophysiology* **7**, 309.

Meier, G. W., and Berger, R. J. (1965). Development of sleep and wakefulness patterns in the infant rhesus monkey. *Exp. Neurol.* **12**, 257–277.

Metcalf, D. R. (1969). The effect of extrauterine experience on the ontogenesis of EEG sleep spindles. *Psychosom. Med.* **31**, 393–399.

Metcalf, D. R. (1970). EEG sleep spindle ontogenesis. *Neuropädiatrie* **1**, 428–433.

Meyerson, B. J. (1964). Central nervous monoamines and hormone-induced estrus behaviour in the spayed cat. *Acta Physiol. Scand.* **63**, 3–32.

Michel, F., and Roffwarg, H. P. (1967). Chronic split brain stem preparation: effect on the sleep-waking cycle. *Experientia (Basel)* **23**, 126–128.

Mikiten, T., Niebyl, P., and Hendley, C. (1961). EEG desynchronization of behavioral sleep associated with spike discharges from the thalamus of the cat. *Fed. Proc.* **20**, 327.

Minkowski, M. (1965). Discussion M. Jouvet. *In* "Sleep Mechanisms" (K. Akert, C. Bally, and J. P. Schadé, eds.) pp. 60–61. Elsevier, Amsterdam.

Mizuno, N., Clemente, C. D., and Sauerland, K. (1969). Fiber projections from rostral basal forebrain structures in the cat. *J. Comp. Neurol.* **136**, 127–142.

Monnier, M. (1950). Action de la stimulation électrique du centre somnogène sur l'électrocorticogramme chez le chat. *Rev. Neurol.* **83**, 561–563.

Monnier, M., and Tissot, R. (1958). Correlated effects on behavioral and electrical brain activity evoked by stimulation of the reticular system, thalamus and rhinencephalon in the conscious animal. *In* "Neurological Basis of Behavior" (G. E. W. Wolstenholme and M. O'Connor, eds.). Churchill, London.

Monnier, M., Kalbere, M., and Krupp, P. (1960). Functional antagonism between diffuse reticular and intralaminary recruiting projections in the medial thalamus. *Exp. Neurol.* **2**, 271–289.

Monod, N., and Pajot, N. (1965). Le sommeil du nouveau-né et du prématuré. *Biol. Néonat.* **8**, 281–307.

Monroe, L. (1969). Inter-rater reliability and the role of experience in scoring EEG sleep records: Phase I. *Psychophysiology* **5**, 376–384.

Moorcroft, W. H. (1971). Ontogeny of forebrain inhibition of behavioral arousal in the rat. *Brain Res.* **35**, 513–522.

Moore, R. Y., Björklund, A., and Stenevi, U. (1971). Plastic changes in the adrenergic innervation of the rat septal area in response to denervation. *Brain Res.* **33**, 13–35.

Morest, D. K. (1960). A study of the structure of the area postrema with Golgy methods. *Amer. J. Anat.* **107**, 291–303.

Morest, D. K. (1971). Dendrodendritic synapses of cells that have axons: The fine structure of the Golgi type II cell in the medial geniculate body of the cat. *Anat. Entwicklungsges.* **133**, 216–246.

Morest, D. K., and Sutin, J. (1961). Ascending pathways from an osmotically sensitive region of the medulla oblongata. *Exp. Neurol.* **4**, 413–420.

Morgane, P. J. (1969). The function of the limbic and rhinic forebrain-limbic midbrain systems and reticular formation in the regulation of food and water intake. *Ann. N. Y. Acad. Sci.*, **157**, 806–848.

Morgane, P. J., and Stern, W. C. (1972). The neural circuitry of sleep. *In* "The Sleeping Brain" (M. H. Chase, ed.) pp. 85–144. Vol. 1. Perspectives in the Brain Sciences. Brain Information Service, Brain Research Institute, University of California, Los Angeles.

Morison, R. S., and Basset, D. L. (1945). Electrical activity of the thalamus and basal ganglia in the decorticate cats. *J. Neurophysiol.* **8**, 309–314.

Morison, R. S., and Dempsey, E. W. (1942). A study of thalamo-cortical relations. *Amer. J. Physiol.* **135**, 281–292.

Morison, R. S., and Dempsey, E. W. (1943). Mechanism of thalamo-cortical augmentation and repetition. *Amer. J. Physiol.* **138**, 297–308.

Morison, R. S., Finley, K. H., and Lothrop, G. N. (1943). Spontaneous electrical activity of the thalamus and other forebrain structures. *J. Neurophysiol.* **6**, 243–254.

Morrison, A., and Bowker, R. (1972). A lumbar source of cervical and forelimb inhibition during sleep. *Psychophysiology* **9**, 103.

Morrison, A. R., and Pompeiano, O. (1965a). An analysis of the supraspinal influences acting on motoneurons during sleep in the unrestrained cat. Responses of the alpha motoneurons to direct electrical stimulation during sleep. *Arch. Ital. Biol.* **103**, 497–516

Morrison, A. R., and Pompeiano, O. (1965b). Central depolarization of group Ia afferent fibers during desynchronized sleep. *Arch. Ital. Biol.* **103**, 517–537.

Morrison, A. R., and Pompeiano, O. (1965c). Pyramidal discharge from somatosensory cortex and cortical control of primary afferents during sleep. *Arch. Ital. Biol.* **103**, 538–568.

Morrison, A. R., and Pompeiano, O. (1965d). Cortico-spinal influences on primary afferents during sleep and wakefulness. *Experientia* **21**, 660–661.

Morrison, A. R., and Pompeiano, O. (1966), Vestibular influences during sleep. II. Effects of vestibular lesions on the pyramidal discharge during desynchronized sleep. *Arch. Ital. Biol.* **104**, 214–230.

Moruzzi, G. (1954). The physiological properties of the brain stem reticular system. *In* "Brain Mechanisms and Consciousness" (E. D. Adrian, F. Bremer, and H. H. Jasper, eds.), pp. 21–53. Blackwell, Oxford.

Moruzzi, G. (1964). Reticular influences on the EEG. *Electroenceph. Clin. Neurophysiol.* **16**, 2–17.

Moruzzi, G. (1969). Sleep and instinctive behavior. *Arch. Ital. Biol.* **107**, 175–216.

Moruzzi, G. (1971). The sleep-waking cycle. *Ergeb. Physiol.* **64**, 1-165.

Moruzzi, G., and Magoun, H. W. (1949). Brain stem reticular formation and activation of the EEG. *Electroenceph. Clin. Neurophysiol.* **1**, 455–473.

Mountcastle, V. B., Poggio, G. F., and Werner, G. (1963). The relation of thalamic cell response to peripheral stimuli varied over an intensive continuum. *J. Neurophysiol.* **26**, 807–834.

Mouret, J., Jeannerod, M., and Jouvet, M. (1963). L'activité électrique du système visuel au cours de la phase paradoxale du sommeil chez le chat. *J. Physiol.* **55**, 305–306.

Mouret, J., Bobillier, P., and Jouvet, M. (1968). Insomnia following parachlorophenylalanine in the rat. *Eur. J. Pharmacol.* **5**, 17–22.

Mouret, J., Renaud, B., Quenin, P., Michel, O., and Schott, B. (1972). Monoamines et régulation de la vigilance. Apport et interprétation biochimique des données polygraphiques. *In* "Les Médiateurs Chimiques" (P. Girard and P. Courteaux, eds.), pp. 139–155. Masson, Paris.

Murray, M. (1966). Degeneration of some intralaminar thalamic nuclei after cortical removals in the cat. *J. Comp. Neurol.* **127**, 341–367.

Muzio, J. N., Roffwarg, H. P., and Kaufman, E. (1966). Alterations in the nocturnal sleep cycle resulting from LSD. *Electroenceph. Clin. Neurophysiol.* **21**, 313–324.

Nadler, H. L., and Hsia, D. Y. (1961). Epinephrine metabolism in phenylketonuria. *Proc. Soc. Exp. Biol.* (*N.Y.*) **107**, 721–723.

Naito, H., Nakamura, K., Kurosaki, T., and Tamura, Y. (1970). Transcallosal excitatory post-synaptic potentials of fast and slow pyramidal tract cells in cat sensori-motor cortex. *Brain Res.* **19**, 299–301.

Nakamura, Y., and Ohye, Ch. (1964). Delta wave production in neocortical EEG by acute lesions within thalamus or hypothalamus of the cat. *EEG Clin. Neurophysiol.* **17**, 677–684.

Nakamura, Y., Goldberg, L. J., and Clemente, C. D. (1967). Nature of suppression of the masseteric monosynaptic reflex induced by stimulation of the orbital gyrus of the cat. *Brain Res.* **6:1**, 184–198.

Naquet, R., Dénavit, M., Lanoir, J., and Albe-Fessard, D. (1965). Altérations transitoires ou définitives des zones diencéphaliques chez le chat. Leurs effets sur l'activité corticale et le sommeil. *In* "Neurophysiologie des états de sommeil." (M. Jouvet, ed.), p. 107–131. Centre Nationale de la Recherche Scientifique. Paris VII.

Nauta, W. J. H. (1946). Hypothalamic regulation of sleep in rats. An experimental study. *J. Neurophysiol.* **9**, 285–316.

Nauta, W. J. H. (1954). Terminal distribution of some afferent fiber systems in the cerebral cortex. *Anat. Rec.* **118**, 333.

Nauta, W. J. H. (1964). Some efferent connections of the prefrontal cortex in the monkey. *In* "The Frontal Granular Cortex and Behavior" (J. M. Warren and K. Akert, eds.), McGraw-Hill, New York.

Nauta, W. J. H., and Kuypers, H. G. J. M. (1958). Some ascending pathways in the brain stem reticular formation. *In* "Reticular Formation of the Brain" (H. H. Jasper, L. D. Proctor, R. S. Knighton, W. C. Noshay, and R. T. Costello, eds.), pp. 3–30. Little Brown, Boston, Massachusetts.

Neame, K. D. (1961). Phenylalanine as inhibitor of transport of amino acids in brain. *Nature* (*London*) **192**, 173–174.

Nielson, H. C., and Davis, K. B. (1966). Effect of frontal ablation upon conditioned responses. *J. Comp. Physiol. Psychol.* **61**, 380–387.

Niemer, W. T., and Magoun, H. W. (1947). Reticulo-spinal tracts influencing motor activity. *J. Comp. Neurol.* **87**, 367–379.

Nyquist, J. K., and Towe, A. L. (1970) Neuronal activity evoked in cat precruciate cerebral cortex by cutaneous stimulation. *Exp. Neurol.* **29**, 794–512.

O'Leary, J. L. (1940). Structural analysis of the lateral geniculate nucleus of the cat. *J. Comp. Neurol* **73**, 405–430.

Oscarsson, O., and Rosen, I. (1963). Projection to cerebral cortex of large musclespindle afferents in forelimb nerves of the cat. *J. Physiol.* **169**, 924–945.

Oscarsson, O., Rosen, I., and Sulg, I. (1966). Organization of neurones in the cat cerebral cortex that are influenced from group I muscle afferents. *J. Physiol.* **183**, 189–210.

Oswald, I. (1962). Sleep mechanisms: recent advances. *Proc. Roy. Soc. Med.* **55**, 910–912.

Oswald, I. (1969). Human brain protein, drugs and dreams. *Nature (London)* **233**, 893–897.

Oswald, I. (1970). Effects on sleep of amphetamine and its derivatives. *In* "Amphetamine and Related Compounds." *Proc. Mario Negri Inst. Pharmacolog. Res.*, Milan. (E. Costa and S. Garattini, eds.), pp. 865–871. Raven Press, New York.

Oswald, I., and Priest, O. (1965). Five weeks to escape the sleeping pill habit. *Brit. Med. J.* **2**, 1093–1099.

Oswald, I., Lewis, S. A., Dunleavy, D. L. F., Brezinova, V., and Briggs, M. (1971). Drugs of dependence though not of abuse: fenfluramine and imipramine. *Brit. Med. J.* **3**, 70–73.

Othmer, E., Hayden, M. P., and Segelbaum, R. (1969). Encephalic cycles during sleep and wakefulness: a 24-hour pattern. *Science* **164**, 447–449.

Pare, C. M. B., Sandler, M., and Stacey, R. S. (1958). Decreased 5-Hydroxytryptophan decarboxylase activity in phenylketonuria. *Lancet* **2**, 1099–1101.

Parmeggiani, P. L. (1968). Telencephalo-diencephalic aspects of sleep mechanisms. *Brain Res.* **7**, 350–359.

Parmeggiani, P. L., and Zanocco, G. (1963). A study on the bioelectrical rhythms of cortical and subcortical structures during activated sleep. *Arch. Ital. Biol.* **101**, 385–412.

Parmelee, A. J., Jr., and Stern, E. (1972). Development of states in infants. *In* "Sleep and the Maturing Nervous System". (C. D. Clemente, D. P. Purpura, and F. E. Mayer, eds.) pp. 199–228, Academic Press, New York.

Parmelee, A. H., and Wenner, W. H. (1967). Sleep states in premature and full-term newborn infants. *Develop. Med. Child Neurol.* **9**, 70–77.

Parmelee, A. H., Schultz, H. R., and Disbrow, M. A. (1961). Sleep-patterns of the new-born. *J. Pediatr.* **58**, 241–250.

Parmelee, A. H., Bruck, K., and Bruck, M. (1962). Activity and inactivity cycles during the sleep of premature infants exposed to neutral temperatures. *Biol. Néonat.* **4**, 317–339.

Parmelee, A. H., Wenner, W. H., Akiyama, Y., Stern, E., and Flescher, J. (1967). Electroencephalography and brain maturation. *In* "Regional Development of the Brain in Early Life" pp. 459–476. Blackwell, Oxford.

Parmelee, A. H., Akiyama, Y., Schultz, M. A., Wenner, W. H., Schulte, F. J., and Stern, E. (1968). The electroencephalogram in active and quiet sleep in infants. *In* "Clinical Electroencephalography of Children" (P. Kellaway, and I. Petersén, eds.), p. 77. Grune & Stratton, New York.

Patton, H. D., and Amassian, V. E. (1954). Single- and multiple-unit analysis of cortical stage of pyramidal tract activation. *J. Neurophysiol.* **17**, 345–363.

Patton, H. D., Towe, A. L., and Kennedy, T. T. (1962). Activation of pyramidal tract neurons by ipsilateral cutaneous stimuli. *J. Neurophysiol.* **25**, 501–514.

Peiper, A. (1961). "Die Eigenart der kindlichen Hirntätigkeit," 3rd ed. VEB Thieme, Leipzig.

Petitjean, F., and Jouvet, M. (1970). Hypersomnie et augmentation de l'acide 5-hydroxyindolacétique cérébral par lésion isthmique chez le chat. *C. R. Soc. Biol. (Paris)* **164**, 2288–2293.

Petre–Quadens, O. (1965). Etude du sommeil chez le nouveau-né normal. *In* "Le sommeil de nuit normal et pathologique," pp. 149–155. Masson, Paris.

Petre–Quadens, O. (1969). Contribution à l'étude de la phase dite paradoxale du sommeil. *Acta Med. Belg.* **69**, 769–898.

Petre–Quadens, O., and De Lee, C. (1970). Eye-movements during Sleep: a common criterion of learning capacities and endocrine activity. *Develop. Med. Child Neurol.* **12**, 730–740.

Petre–Quadens, O., and Dubois–Dalco, M. (1965). Influence de l'accouchement sur l'électroencéphalogramme du nouveau-né. Note préliminaire. *Bull. Féd. Soc. Gynécol. Obstét. Fr.* **17**, 483–486.

Petre–Quadens, O., and Jouvet, M. (1966). Paradoxical sleep in the mentally retarded. *J. Neurol. Sci.* **3**, 608–612.

Petre–Quadens, O., and Laroche, J. C. (1966). Sommeil du nouveau-né: phases paradoxales spontanées et provoquées. *J. Psychol. Norm. Pathol.* **1**, 19–27.

Petre–Quadens, O., Sfaello, Z., van Bogaert, L., and Moya, G. (1968). Sleep-study in SSPE (First results). *Neurology* **18**, 60–68.

Petre–Quadens, O., Hardy, J. L., and De Lee, C. (1969). Comparative study of sleep in pregnancy and in the newborn. *In* "Brain and Early Behavior" (R. Robinson, ed.), pp. 187–191. Academic Press, New York.

Petre–Quadens, O., De Lec, C., and Remy, M. (1971). Eye movement density during sleep and brain maturation. *Brain. Res.* **26**, 49–56.

Phillips, C. G. (1956). Intracellular records from Betz cells in the cat. *Quart. J. Exp. Physiol.* **41**, 58–69.

Pietrusky, F. (1922). Das Verhalten der Augen im Schlafe. *Klin. Augenheilk.* **68**, 355–360.

Pin, C., Jones, B., and Jouvet, M. (1968). Topographie des neurones monoaminergiques du tronc cérébral du chat: étude par histofluorescence. *C. R. Soc. Biol. (Paris)*, **162**, 2136–2141.

Pivik, T., and Dement, W. (1970). Phasic changes in muscular and reflex activity during NREM sleep. *Exp. Neurol.* **27**, 115–124.

Poley, J. R., and Dummermuth, G. (1968). EEG-findings in patients with phenylketonuria before and during treatment with a low-phenylalanine diet and in patients with some other inborn errors of amino-acid metabolism. *In*: "Some Recent Advances in Inborn Errors of Metabolism" (K. S. Holt and O. Coffey, eds.), pp. 61. Livingstone, Edinburgh and London.

Pompeiano, O. (1965). Supraspinal control reflexes during sleep and wakefulness. *In*: "Aspects Anatomo-Fonctionnels de la Physiologie du Sommeil" (M. Jouvet, ed.) pp. 309–395. Centre National de la Recherche Scientifique, Paris.

Pompeiano, O. (1967a). The neurophysiological mechanisms of the postural and motor events during desynchronized sleep. *In* "Sleep and Altered States of Consciousness" (S. S. Kety, E. V. Evarts, and H. L. Williams, eds.), Ass. Res. Nerv. Ment. Dis. Vol. XLV, pp. 351–423. Williams and Wilkins, Baltimore, Maryland.

Pompeiano, O. (1967b). Sensory inhibition during motor activity in sleep. *In* "Neurophysiological basis of normal and abnormal motor activities" (M. D. Yahr and D. P. Purpura, eds.), pp. 323–375. Raven Press, New York.

Pompeiano, O. (1970). Mechanisms of sensory integration during sleep. *Progr. Physiolog. Psychol.* **3**, 1–179.

Pompeiano, O., and Morrison, A. R. (1966). Vestibular influences during sleep. III. Dissociation of the tonic and phasic inhibition of spinal reflexes during desynchronized sleep following vestibular lesions. *Arch. Ital. Biol.* **104**, 231–246.

Poser, C. M., and van Bogaert, L. (1959). Neuropathologic observations in phenylketonuria. *Brain* **82**, 1–10.

Prechtl, H. F. R. (1965). Problems of behavioral studies in the newborn infant. *Advan. Study Behavior* **1**, 75–98.

Prechtl, H. F. R. (1968). Polygraphic studies of the full-term newborn infant. II. Computer analysis of recorded data. *In* "Studies in infancy" (M. C. O. Bax and R. C. Mac Keith, eds.), Clinics in Develop. Med. N° 27, pp. 26–40. Heinemann, London.

Prechtl, H. F. R., and Beintema, D. J. (1964). "The neurological examination of the full-term newborn infant," pp. 1–72. Little Club Clin. in Develop. Med., N° 12. Heinemann, London.

Prechtl, H. F. R., and Lenard, H. G. (1967). A study of eye movements in sleeping newborn infants. *Brain Res.* **5**, 477–493.

Prechtl, H. F. R., Weinmann, H., and Akiyama, Y. (1969). Organization of physiological parameters in normal and abnormal infants. *Neuropädiatrie* **1**, 101–129.

Puizillout, J., and Ternaux, J. P. (1971). Persistance d'un endormement vagoaortique après destruction chirurgicale et pharmacologique des noyaux du raphé. *J. Physiol. (Paris)* **63**, 272.

Pujol, J. F. (1970). Contribution à l'étude des modifications de la régulation du métabolisme des monoamines centrales pendant le sommeil et la veille, p. 192. Thèse de Doctoratès Sciences. Paris.

Pujol, J. F., Buguet, A., Froment, J. L., Jones, B., and Jouvet, M. (1971). The central metabolism of serotonin in the cat during insomnia: a neurophysiological and biochemical study after p-chlorophenylalanine or destruction of the raphé system. *Brain Res.* **29**, 195–212.

Pujol, J. F., Sordet, F., Petitjean, F., Germain, D., and Jouvet, M. (1972). Insomnie et métabolisme cérébral de la sérotonine chez le chat: étude de la synthèse et de la libération mesurée in vitro 18 heures après destruction du système du raphé. *Brain Res.* **39**, 137–150.

Purpura, D. P. (1959). Nature of electrocortical potentials and synaptic organizations in cerebral and cerebellar cortex. *Int. Rev. Neurobiol.* **1**, 47–163.

Purpura, D. P. (1969). Interneuronal mechanisms in synchronization and desynchronization of thalamic activity. *In* "The Interneuron" (M. A. B. Brazier, ed.), pp. 467–496. UCLA Forum in Med. Sci.

Purpura, D. P. (1970). Operations and processes in thalamic and synaptically related neural subsystems. *In* "The Neurosciences" Vol. II, pp. 458–470. Rockefeller Univ. Press, New York.

Purpura, D. P. Intracellular studies of synaptic organizations in the mammalian brain. *In* "Structure and Function of Synapses" (G. D. Pappas and D. P. Purpura, eds.). Raven Press, New York. (in press).

Purpura, D. P., and Cohen, B. (1962). Intracellular recording from thalamic neurons during recruiting responses. *J. Neurophysiol.* **24**, 621–635.

Purpura, D. P., and Girado, M. (1959). Synaptic mechanisms involved in transcallosal activation of corticospinal neurons. *Arch. Ital. Biol.* **97**, 111–139.

Purpura, D. P., and Malliani, A. (1967). Intracellular studies of the corpus striatum. I. Synaptic potentials and discharge characteristics of caudate neurons activated by thalamic stimulation. *Brain Res.* **6**, 325–340.

Purpura, D. P., and Shofer, R. J. (1963). Intracellular recording from thalamic neurons during reticulocortical activation. *J. Neurophysiol.* **26**, 494–505.

Purpura, D. P., and Shofer, R. J. (1964). Cortical intracellular potentials during augmenting and recruiting responses. I. Effects of injected hyperpolarizing currents on evoked membrane potential changes. *J. Neurophysiol.* **27**, 117–132.

Purpura, D. P., Shofer, R. J., and Musgrave, F. S. (1964). Cortical intracellular potentials during augmenting and recruiting responses. II. Patterns of synaptic activities in pyramidal and nonpyramidal tract neurons *J. Neurophysiol.* **27**, 133–151.

Purpura, D. P., Scarff, T., and McMurtry, J. G. (1965). Intracellular study of internuclear inhibition in ventrolateral thalamic neurons. *J. Neurophysiol.* **28**, 487–496.

Purpura, D. P., Frigyesi, T. L., McMurtry, J. G., and Scarff, T. (1966a). Synaptic mechanisms in thalamic regulation of cerebello cortical projection activity. *In* "The Thalamus" (D. P. Purpura and M. D. Yahr, eds.), pp. 153–170. Columbia Univ. Press, New York.

Purpura, D. P., McMurtry, J. G., and Mackawa, K. (1966b). Synaptic events in ventrolateral thalamic neurons during suppression of recruiting responses by brain stem reticular stimulation. *Brain Res.* **1**, 63–76.

Raiti, S., and Newns, G. H. (1971). Cretinism: Early diagnosis and its relation to mental prognosis. *Arch. Dis. Childhood* **46**, 692–694.

Ralston, K. J. (1971). III. Evidence for presynaptic dendrites and a proposal for the mechanisms of action. *Nature (London)* **230**, 585–587.

Ralston, B., and Ajmone-Marsan, C. (1956). Thalamic control of certain normal and abnormal cortical rhythms. *Electroenceph. Clin. Neurophysiol.* **8**, 559–582.

Ranson, S. W. (1939). Somnolence caused by hypothalamus lesions in the monkey. *Arch. Neurol. Psychiat.* **41**, 1–23.

Rechtschaffen, A., and Chernik, D. (1972). The effect of REM deprivation on periorbital spike activity in NREM sleep. *Psychophysiology* **9**, 128.

Rechtschaffen, A., and Kales, A. (eds.) (1968). "A Manual of Standardized Terminology Techniques, and Scoring System for Sleep Stages of Human Subjects." Public Health Serv., U.S. Gov. Printing Office Washington, D.C.

Rechtschaffen, A., Robinson, T. M., and Wincor, M. Z. (1970). The effect of methaqualone on nocturnal sleep. *Psychophysiology* **7**, 346.

Rechtschaffen, A., Michel, F., and Metz, J. (1972a). Relationship between extra-ocular and PGO activity in the cat. *Psychophysiology* **9**, 128.

Rechtschaffen, A., Watson, R., Wincor, M., Molinari, S., and Barta, S. (1972b). The relationship of phasic and tonic periorbital EMG activity to NREM mentation. Presented at the Ass. for the Psychophysiolog. Study of Sleep, New York, May.

Reite, M., Rhodes, J., Kavan, E., and Adey, W. (1965). Normal sleep patterns in macaque monkey. *Arch. Neurol.* **12**, 133–144.

Renault, J. (1967). Monoamines et sommeils. Rôle du système du raphé et de la sérotonine cérébrale dans l'endormissement (Tixier, ed.), p. 140. Thèse de Médecine, Univ. Lyon.

Rioch, D. Mc. K. (1954). Group discussion. *In* "Brain Mechanisms and Consciousness" (E. D. Adrian, F. Bremer, and H. H. Jasper, eds.), pp. 125–136. Blackwell, Oxford.

Rizzoli, A. A., and Galzigna, L. (1970). Molecular mechanism of unconscious state induced by butyrate. *Biochem. Pharmacol.* **19**, 2727–2736.

Roberts, E., and Eidelberg, E. (1960). Metabolic and neurophysiological roles of gamma-aminobutyric acid. *Rev. Neurobiol.* **2**, 279–332.

Roberts, W. W., and Robinson, T. C. L. (1969). Relaxation and sleep induced by warming of preoptic region and anterior hypothalamus in cats. *Exp. Neurol.* **25**, 282–294.

Roffwarg, H. P., Dement, W. C., and Fischer, C. (1964). Preliminary observations of sleep-dream patterns in neonates, infants, and adults. *In* "Problems of Sleep and Dream in Children" (E. Harms, ed.), Int. Ser. and Monographs on Child Psychiat., vol. 2, pp. 60–72. Pergamon Press, Oxford.

Roffwarg, H., Muzio, J., and Dement, W. (1966). The ontogenetic development of the sleep-dream cycle in the human. *Science* **152**, 604–619.

Roger, A., Rossi, G. F., and Zirondoli, A. (1956). Le rôle des nerfs craniens dans le maintien de l'état vigile de la préparation "encéphale isolé". *Electroenceph. Clin. Neurophysiol.* **8**, 1–13.

Rossi, G. F., and Zanchetti, A. (1957). Brain stem reticular formation. Anatomy and Physiology. *Arch. Ital. Biol.* **95**, 199–438.

Rossi, G. F., Favale, E., Hara, T., Guissani, A., and Sacco, G. (1961). Researches in the nervous mechanism underlying deep sleep in the cat. *Arch. Ital. Biol.* **99**, 270–292.

Rossi, G. F., Palestini, M., Pisano, M., and Rosadini, G. (1965). An experimental study of the cortical reactivity during sleep and wakefulness. *In* "Aspects anatomo-fonctionnels de la physiologie du sommeil." pp. 509–526. C.N.R.S., Paris.

Rothballer, A. B. (1957). The effect of phenylephrine, methamphetamine, cocaine, and serotonin upon the adrenaline sensitive component of the reticular activating system. *Electroenceph. Clin. Neurophysiol.* **9**, 409–417.

Rougeul, A., Le Yaouanc, A., and Buser, P. (1966). Activités neuroniques spontanées dans le tractus pyramidal et certaines structures sous-corticales au cours du sommeil naturel chez le chat libre. *Exp. Brain Res.* **2**, 129–150.

Sabelli, H. C., Giardina, W. J., Alivisatos, S. G., Seth, P. K., and Ungar, F. (1969). Aldehydes of brain amines affect central nervous system. *Nature (London)* **223**, 73–74.

Samson, F. E., and Quinn, D. J. (1967). Na$^+$-K$^+$-activated AT-phase in rat brain development. *J. Neurochem.* **14**, 421–427.

Samson, F. E., Balfour, W. H., and Jacobs, R. J. (1963). Mitochondrial changes in developing rat brain. *Amer. J. Physiol.* **199**, 693–696.

Santini, M., and Purpura, D. P. (1969). Thalamo-striate control of amygdaloid neuron activity. *Anat. Rec.* **163**, 255–256.

Sauerland, E., Knauss, T., Nakamura, Y., and Clemente, C. (1967). Cortically induced inhibition of monosynaptic and polysynaptic reflexes and muscle tone by electrical stimulation of the cerebral cortex. *Exp. Neurol.* **17**, 159–171.

Scheibel, M. E., and Scheibel, A. B. (1958). Structural substrates for integrative patterns in the brain stem reticular core. *In* "Reticular Formation of the Brain" (H. H. Jasper, L. D. Proctor, R. S. Knighton, W. C. Noshay and R. T. Costello, eds.), pp. 31–56. Little, Brown, Boston, Massachusetts.

Scheibel, M. E., and Scheibel, A. B. (1966). The organization of the nucleus reticularis thalami: a Golgi study. *Brain Res.* **1**, 43–62.

Scheibel, M. E., and Scheibel, A. B. (1967). Structural organization of nonspecific thalamic nuclei and their projection toward cortex. *Brain Res.* **6**, 60–94.

Schlag, J., and Balvin, R. (1963). Background activity in the cerebral cortex and reticular formation in relation with the electroencephalogram. *Exp. Neurol.* **8**, 203–219.

Schlag, J. D., and Chaillet, F. (1963). Thalamic mechanisms involved in cortical desynchronization and recruiting responses. *EEG Clin. Neurophysiol.* **15**, 39–62.

Schlag, J., and Villablanca, J. (1968). A quantitative study of temporal and spatial response patterns in a thalamic cell population electrically stimulated. *Brain Res.* **8**, 255–270.

Schlag, J., and Waszak, M. (1971). Electrophysiological properties of units of the thalamic reticular complex. *Exp. Neurol.* **32**, 79–97.

Scholz, W. (1957). Contribution à l'anatomie pathologique du système nerveux central dans l'oligophrénie phénylpyruvique. *Encéphale* **46**, 668–680.

Schrader, M. E. G. (1889). Zur Physiologie des Vogelgehirns. *Pflügers Arch.* **44**, 175–238.

Schulte, F. J., Schrempf, G., and Hinze, G. (1971). Maternal toxemia, fetal malnutrition and bioelectric brain activity of the newborn. *Neuropädiatrie* **2**, 439–446.

Schulte, F. J., Kaiser, H. J., Engelhart, S., Bell, E. F., Castell, R., and Lenard, H. G., Sleep patterns in hyperphenylalaninemia. A lesson on serotonin to be learned from phenylketonuria. *Pediat. Res.* (in press).

Schultz, M. A., Schulte, F. J., Akiyama, Y., Parmelee, A. H. (1968). Development of electro-encephalographic sleep phenomena in hypothyroid infants. *Electroenceph. Clin. Neurophysiol.* **25**, 351–358.

Schwartze, P. (1966). Die Hirnstromkurze in der Ontogenese unter besonderer Berücksichtigung ihrer Veränderung durch Weckreize und Pharmaka. *Acta Univ. Palacianae Olomucensis* **41**, 141–172.

Segundo, J. P., Arana, R., and French, J. D. (1955a). Behavioral arousal by stimulation of the brain in the monkey. *J. Neurosurgery* **12**, 601–613.

Segundo, J. P., Naquet, R., and Buser, P. (1955b). Effects of cortical stimulation on electrocortical activity in monkeys. *J. Neurophysiol.* **18**, 236–245.

Sergio, G., and Longo, V. G. (1959). Action of drugs on the EEG of rabbits after removal of the neocortex. *EEG Clin. Neurophysiol.* **11**, 382.

Sherrington, C. S. (1906). "Integrative Action of the Nervous System." Yale Univ. Press, New Haven, Connecticut.

Sherrington, C. S. (1917). Reflexes elicitable in the cat from pinna, vibrissae and jaws. *J. Physiol* **51**, 404–431.

Shimazono, Y., Horie, T., Yanagisawa, Y., Hori, N., Chikazawa, S., and Shozuka, K. (1960). The correlation of the rhythmic waves of the hippocampus with the behaviors of dogs. *Neurol. Med. Chir.* **2**, 82–88.

Shimizu, A., and Himwich, H. E. (1968). The ontogeny of sleep in kittens and young rabbits. *EEG Clin. Neurophysiol.* **24**, 307–318.

Shimizu, N., Morikawa, N., and Okada, M. (1959). Histochemical studies of monoamine oxydase of the brain of rodents. *Z. Zellforsch.* **49**, 389–400.

Short, R., and Eton, B. (1959). Progesterone in Blood, Part 3. (Progesterone in the peripheral blood of pregnant women). *J. Endocrinol.* **18**, 418–425.

Short, M. J., Hein, P., and Wilson, W. P. (1964). Thyroid hormone and brain function. III. Influence of trijodthyronine on evoked potentials of the cortex and reticular formation and upon the interrelationship of caudate and reticular activity of the cat. *Electroenceph. Clin. Neurophysiol.* **17**, 414–419.

Simon, C., and Emmons, W. (1956). The EEG, consciousness, and sleep. *Science* **124**, 1066–1069.

Sinha, A. K., Smythe, H., Zarcone, V., Barchas, J., and Dement, W. (1972). Human sleep-electroencephalogram: a damped oscillatory phenomenon. *J. Theor. Biol.* **35**, 387–393.

Sinha, A., Henriksen, S., Dement, W., and Barchas, J. (1973). Cat brain amine content during sleep. *Amer. J. Physiol.* **224**, 381–383.

Skillen, R. G., Thienes, C. H., and Strain, L. (1961). Brain 5-hydroxytryptamine, 5-hydroxytryptophan decarboxylase and monoamine oxidase of normal, thyroid-fed and propylthiouracilfed male and female rats. *Endocrinology* **69**, 1099–1102.

Slosarska, M., and Zernicki, B. (1969). Synchronized sleep in the chronic pretrigeminal cat. *Acta Biol. Exp.* **29**, 175–184.

Smith, J. R. (1938). The electroencephalogram during normal infancy and childhood: 1. Rhythmic activities present in the neonate and their subsequent development. 2. The nature of the growth of the alpha-waves. 3. Preliminary observations on the pattern sequence during sleep. *J. Genet. Psychol.* **53**, 431–482.

Smith, J., and Karacan, I. (1971). EEG sleep stage scoring by an automatic hybrid system. *Electroenceph. Clin. Neurophysiol.* **31**, 231–239

Smith, R. D., and Marcarian, H. Q. (1967). The neuromuscular spindles of the lateral pterygoid muscle. *Anat. Anz.* **120**, 47–53.

Smith, J., Cronin, M., and Karacan, I. (1971). A multichannel hybrid system for rapid eye movement detection (REM detection). *Comput. Biomed. Res.* **4**, 275–290.

Snider, R. S., and Niemer, W. T. (1961). "A Stereotaxic Atlas of the Cat Brain." Univ. of Chicago Press, Chicago, Illinois.

Snyder, F. (1966). Toward an evolutionary theory of dreaming. *Amer. J. Psychiat.* **123:2**, 121–142.

Snyder, F. (1967). Autonomic nervous system manifestations during sleep and dreaming. *In* "Sleep and Altered States of Consciousness" (S. Kety, E. Evarts, and H. Williams, eds.), Res. Publ. Ass. nerv. ment. Dis., pp. 469–487. Williams and Wilkins, Baltimore, Maryland.

Snyder, F. (1970). The phenomenology of dreaming. In "The Psychodynamic Implications of the Physiological Studies on Dreams" (L. Madow and L. H. Snow, eds.), pp. 124–151. Thomas, Springfield, Illinois.

Snyder, D., Hobson, J. A., Morrison, D. F., and Goldfrank, F. (1964). Changes in respiration, heart rate and systolic blood pressure in human sleep. J. Appl. Physiol. 19, 417–422.

Sorenson, Ch. A., and Ellison, G. D. (1970). Striatal organization of feeding behavior in the decorticate rat. Exp. Neurol. 29, 162–174.

Soulairac, A., Gottesmann, Cl., and Thangapregassam, M. J. (1965). Etude électrophysiologique des différentes phases de sommeil chez le rat. Arch. Ital. Biol. 103, 469–482.

Sours, J. A. (1963). Narcolepsy and other disturbances in the sleep-waking rhythm: a study of 115 cases with a review of the literature. J. Nerv. Ment. Dis. 137, 525–542.

Starzl, T. E., Taylor, C. W., and Magoun, H. W. (1951). Ascending conduction in the reticular activating system with special reference to the diencephalon. J. Neurophysiol. 14, 461–477.

Spehlmann, R., and Downes, K. (1972). The effects of reticular stimulation on the responses of neurons of the pericruciate cortex of cats to thalamic, transcallosal and pyramidal stimulation. Brain Res. 48, 375–379.

Stefanis, C. (1969). Interneuronal mechanisms in the cortex. In "The Interneuron" (M. A. B. Brazier, ed.), pp. 497–526. Univ. of California Press, Berkeley.

Stefanis, C., and Jasper, H. (1964a). Intracellular microelectrode studies of antidromic responses in cortical pyramidal tract neurons. J. Neurophysiol. 27, 828–854.

Stefanis, C., and Jasper, H. (1964b). Recurrent collateral inhibition in pyramidal tract neurons. J. Neurophysiol. 27, 855–877.

Stein, O., Sordet, F., Jouvet, M., and Pujol, J. F. The effects of alpha-methyl P tyrosine on central 5-HT synthesis and EEG activity in the cat. Brain Res. (in press).

Steriade, M. (1968). The flash-evoked afterdischarge. Brain Res. 9, 169–212.

Steriade, M. (1969). Ascending control of motor cortex responsiveness. Electroenceph. Clin. Neurophysiol. 26, 25–40.

Steriade, M. (1970). Ascending control of thalamic and cortical responsiveness. Int. Rev. Neurobiol. 12, 87–144.

Steriade, M. (1972). Intrathalamic and corticothalamic circuitries underlying the onset of EEG synchronization, with particular emphasis on the genesis of spindle waves. In "The Sleeping Brain" (M. Chase, ed.) pp. 115–121. UCLA Brain Information Service, Los Angeles.

Steriade, M., and Demetrescu, M. (1960). Unspecific systems of inhibition and facilitation of potentials evoked by intermittent light. J. Neurophysiol. 23, 602–617.

Steriade, M., and Demetrescu, M. (1962). Reticular facilitation of responses to acoustic stimuli. Electroenceph. Clin. Neurophysiol. 14, 21–36.

Steriade, M., and Deschênes, M. (1973). Cortical interneurons during sleep and waking in freely moving primates. Brain Res. 50, 192–199.

Steriade, M., and Lamarre, Y. (1969). Réactivité des neurones corticaux moteurs et somatosensoriels pendant l'éveil et le sommeil naturel chez le singe. J. Physiol. (Paris) 61, 411–412.

Steriade, M., and Wyzinski, P. (1972). Cortically elicited activities in thalamic reticularis neurons. Brain Res. 42, 514–520.

Steriade, M., Belekhova, M., and Apostol, V. (1968). Reticular potentiation of cortical flash-evoked afterdischarge. Brain Res. 11, 276–280.

Steriade, M., Constantinescu, E., and Apostol, V. (1969a). Correlations between alterations of the cortical transaminase activity and EEG patterns of sleep and wakefulness induced by brainstem transections. Brain Res. 13, 177–180.

Steriade, M., Iosif, G., and Apostol, V. (1969b). Responsiveness of thalamic and cortical motor relays during arousal and various stages of sleep. *J. Neurophysiol.* **32**, 251–265.

Steriade, M., Apostol, V., and Oakson, G. (1971a). Control of unitary activities in the cerebello-thalamic pathway during wakefulness and synchronized sleep. *J. Neurophysiol.* **34**, 389–413.

Steriade, M., Apostol, V., and Oakson, G. (1971b). Clustered firing in the cerebellothalamic pathway during synchronized sleep. *Brain Res.* **26**, 425–432.

Steriade, M., Wyzinski, P., Deschênes, M., and Guerin, M. (1971c). Disinhibition during waking in motor cortex neuronal chains in cat and monkey. *Brain Res.* **30**, 211–217.

Steriade, M., Wyzinski, P, and Apostol, V. (1972). Corticofugal projections governing rhythmic thalamic activity. *In* "Corticothalamic Pathways and Sensorimotor Activities" (T. Frigyesi, E. Rinvik, and M. D. Yahr, eds.), pp. 221–272. Raven Press, New York.

Steriade, M., Wyzinski, P., and Apostol, V. (1973). Differential synaptic reactivity of simple and complex pyramidal tract neurons at various levels of vigilance. *Exp. Brain Res.* **17**, 87–110.

Sterman, M. B. (1972). The basic rest–activity cycle and sleep: developmental considerations in man and cats. *In* "Sleep and the maturing nervous system" (C. D. Clemente, D. P. Purpura, and F. E. Mayer, eds.), pp. 175–197. Academic Press, New York.

Sterman, M. B., and Clemente, C. D. (1962a). Forebrain inhibitory mechanisms: cortical synchronization induced by basal forebrain stimulation. *Exp. Neurol.* **6**, 91–102.

Sterman, M. B., and Clemente, C. D. (1962b). Forebrain inhibitory mechanisms: sleep patterns induced by basal forebrain stimulation in the behaving cat. *Exp. Neurol.* **6**, 103–117.

Sterman, M. B., and Fairchild, M. D. (1966). Modification of locomotor performance by reticular formation and basal forebrain stimulation in the cat: Evidence for reciprocal systems. *Brain Res.* **2**, 205–217.

Sterman, M. B., and Hoppenbrouwers, T. (1971). The development of sleep-waking and rest-activity patterns from foetus to adult in man. (M. B. Sterman, D. J. McGinty, and A. M. Adinolfi, eds.), "Brain Development and Behavior" pp. 203–227. Academic Press, New York.

Sterman, M. B., Knauss, T. K., Lehmann, D., and Clemente, C. D. (1964). Alteration of sleep patterns following basal forebrain lesions. *Fed. Proc.* **23**, 209.

Sterman, M. B., Knauss, T., Lehmann, D., and Clemente, C. D. (1965). Circadian sleep and waking patterns in the laboratory cat. *Electroenceph. Clin. Neurophysiol.* **19**, 509–517.

Sterman, M. B., Wyrwicka, W., and Roth, S. R. (1969). Electrophysiological correlates and neural substrates of alimentary behavior in the cat. (J. P. Morgane, and M. Wagner, eds.), *Ann. N.Y. Acad. Sci.* **157**, 723–739.

Sterman, M. B., Lucas, E. A., and MacDonald, L. R. (1972) Periodicity within sleep and operant performance in the cat. *Brain Res.* **38**, 327–341.

Stern, W. C. (1970). The D state, dreaming and memory. *Int. Psychiat. Clin.* **7**, 249–257.

Stern, E., Parmelee, A. H., Akiyama, Y., Schultz, M. A., and Wenner, W. H. (1969). Sleep cycle characteristics in infants. *Pediatrics* **43**, 65–70.

Suzuki, H., and Tukahara, Y. (1963). Recurrent inhibition of the Betz cell. *Jap. J. Physiol.* **13**, 386–398.

Szabo, I., Kellenyi, L., and Karmos, G. (1965). A simple device for recording movements of unrestrained animals. *Acta Physiol. Acad. Sci. Hung.* **26**, 343–349.

Szentagothai, J. (1948). Anatomical considerations of monosynaptic reflex arcs. *J. Neurophysiol.* **11**, 445–454.

Szentagothai, J. (1949). Functional representation in the motor trigeminal nucleus. *J. comp. Neurol.*, **90**, 111–120.

Tabushi, K., and Himwich, E. H. (1970). 5-Hydroxytryptophan and the sleep-wakefulness cycle in rabbits. *Biolog. Psychiat.* **2**, 183–188.

Takahashi, K. (1965). Slow and fast groups of pyramidal tract cells and their respective membrane properties. *J. Neurophysiol.* **28**, 908–924.

Tauber, E. S., Rojas-Ramirez, J., and Hernández-Peón, R. (1968). Electrophysiological and behavioral correlates of wakefulness and sleep in the lizard, ctenosaura pectinata. *Electroenceph. Clin. Neurophysiol.* **24**, 424–433.

Taylor, P. M. (1960). Oxygen consumption in newborn rats. *J. Physiol.* **154**, 153–168.

Taylor, A. N., and Branch, B. J. (1971). Inhibition of ACTH release by a central inhibitory mechanism in the basal forebrain. *Exp. Neurol.* **31**, 391–401.

Tcheng, F. C., and Laroche, J. L. (1965). Phases de sommeil et sourires spontanés. *Acta Psychol.* **24**, 1–28.

Teitelbaum, H. A. (1954). Spontaneous rhythmic ocular movements: their possible relation with mental activity. *Neurology* **4**, 350–353.

Thauer, R., and Peters, G. (1938). Sensibilitä und Motorik bei lange überlebenden Zwischen-Mittelhirntauben. *Pflügers Arch.* **240**, 503–526.

Thompson, W. D., Stoney, S. D., Jr., and Asanuma, H. (1970). Characteristics of projections from primary sensory cortex to motorsensory cortex in cats. *Brain Res.* **22**, 15–27.

Tilney, F., and Kubie, S. S. (1931). Behavior in its relation to the development of the brain. *Bull. Neurol. Inst. N.Y.* **1**, 229–313.

Timiras, P. S., and Woodbury, D. M. (1965). Effect of thyroid activity on brain function and brain electrolyte distribution in rats. *Endocrinology* **58**, 181–184.

Timo-Iaria, C., Negrao, N., Schmidek, W. R., Hoshino, K., Lobato de Menezes, C. E., and Leme da Rocha T. (1970). Phases and states of sleep in the rat. *Physiol. Behav.* **5**, 1057–1062.

Tirri, R., Pantio, M., and Tarkkonen, H. (1968). Metabolic effects of thyroxine in infant rats. *Experientia* **24**, 365–367.

Tissot, R., and Monnier, M. (1959). Dualité des systèmes thalamiques de projection diffuse. *EEG Clin. Neurophysiol.* **11**, 675–686.

Tömbol, T. (1967). Short neurons and their synaptic relations in the specific thalamic nuclei. *Brain Res.* **3**, 307–326.

Tönnies, J. F. (1969). Automatische EEG-Intervall-Spektrumanalyse (EISA) zur Langzeitdarstellung der Schlafperiodik und Narkose. *Arch. Psychiat. Nervenkrankheiten* **212**, 423–445.

Torda, C. (1967). Effect of brain serotonin depletion on sleep in rats. *Brain Res.* **6**, 375–377.

Towe, A. L., Patton, H. D., and Kennedy, T. T. (1963). Properties of the pyramidal system in the cat. *Exp. Neurol.* **8**, 220–238.

Ungerstedt, U. (1971). Stereotaxic mapping of the noradrenaline pathways in the rat brain. *Acta Physiol. Scand., Suppl.* **367**, 1–48.

Uno, M., Yoshida, M., and Hirota, I. (1970). The mode of cerebello-thalamic relay transmission investigated with intracellular recording from cells of the ventrolateral nucleus of the cat's thalamus. *Exp. Brain Res.* **10**, 121–139.

Ursin, R. (1968). The two stages of slow wave sleep in the cat and their relation to REM sleep. *Brain Res.* **11**, 347–356.

Ursin, R. (1970). Sleep stage relations within the sleep cycles of the cat. *Brain Res.* **20**, 91–97.

Valatx, J. L., Jouvet-Mounier, D., and Jouvet M. (1964). Evolution électro-encéphalographique des différents états de sommeil chez le chaton. *Electroenceph. Clin. Neurophysiol.* **17**, 218–232.

Valverde, F. (1967). Apical dendritic spines of the visual cortex and light deprivation in the mouse. *Exp. Brain Res.* **3**, 337–352.

Van Twyver, H., and Allison, T. (1969). EEG studies of the shrew (blarina brevicauda): a preliminary report. *Psychophysiology* **6**, 231.

Van Twyver, H., and Allison, T. (1970). Sleep in the opossum didelphis marsupialis. *EEG Clin. Neurophysiol.* **29**, 181–189.

Velasco, M., and Lindsley, D. B. (1965). Role of orbital cortex in regulation of thalamo-cortical electrical activity. *Science* **149**, 1375–1377.

Verley, R., and Mourek, J. (1962). Evolution postnatale de l'amplitude de l'activité électrocorticale. *J. Physiol. (Paris)* **54**, 427–428.

Villablanca, J. (1962). Electroencephalogram in the permanently isolated forebrain of the cat. *Science* **138**, 44–46.

Villablanca, J. (1965). The electrocorticogram in the chronic "cerveau isolé" cat. *Electroenceph. Clin. Neurophysiol.* **19**, 576–586.

Villablanca, J. (1966a). Behavioral and polygraphic study of "sleep" and "wakefulness" in chronic decerebrate cats. *Electroenceph. Clin. Neurophysiol.* **21**, 562–577.

Villablanca, J. (1966b). Ocular behavior in the chronic "cerveau isolé" cat. *Brain Res.* **2**, 99–102.

Villablanca, J. (1966c). Electrocorticogram in the chronic "isolated hemisphere" of the cat. Effect of atropine and eserine. *Brain Res.* **3**, 287–291.

Villablanca, J., and Marcus, R. (1972). Sleep–wakefulness, EEG, and behavioral studies of chronic cats without the neocortex and striatum: The "diencephalic" cat. *Arch. Ital. Biol.* **110**, 348–382.

Villablanca, J., and Salinas-Zeballos, M. E. (1972). Sleep–wakefulness, EEG, and behavioral studies of chronic cats without the thalamas: The "athalamic cat." *Arch. Ital. Biol.* **110**, 338–411.

Villablanca, J., and Schlag, J. (1968). Cortical control of thalamic spindle waves. *Exp. Neurol.* **20**, 432–442.

Vital-Durand, F., and Michel, F. (1971). Effets de la déafférentation périphérique sur le cycle veille-sommeil chez le chat. *Arch. Ital. Biol.* **109**, 166–186.

von Baumgarten, R., Mollica, A., and Moruzzi, G. (1954). Modulierung der Entladungsfrequenz einzelner Zellen der Substantia reticularis durch corticofugale und cerebelläre Impulse. *Pflüg. Arch. Ges. Physiol. Menschen Tiere* **259**, 56–78.

von Economo, C. (1929). Schlaftheorie. *Ergeb. Physiol.* **28**, 312–339.

von Holst, E., and von Saint Paul, U. (1960). Vom Wirkungsgefüge der Triebe. *Naturwissenschaften* **47**, 409–422.

von Holst, E., and von Saint Paul, U. (1962). Electrically controlled behavior. *Scient. Amer.* **206**, 50–59.

Wada, J. A., and Terao, A. (1970). Effect of parachlorophenylalanine on basal forebrain stimulation. *Exp. Neurol.* **28**, 501–506.

Wagner, I. F. (1939). Curves of sleep depth in newborn infants. *J. Genet. Psychol.* **55**, 121–135.

Walker, A. E. (1938). "The Primate Thalamus," p. 321. Univ. of Chicago Press, Chicago, Illinois.

Wall., P. D. (1958). Excitability changes in afferent fibre terminations and their relation to slow potentials. *J. Physiol.* **142**, 1–21.

Walsh, J. T., and Cordeau, J. P. (1965). Responsiveness in the visual system during various phases of sleep and waking. *Exp. Neurol.* **11**, 90–103.

Walshe, F. M. R. (1961). Contributions of John Hughlings Jackson to neurology. *Arch. Neurol.* **5**, 17–29.

Wang, G. H., and Akert, K. (1962). Behavior and reflexes of chronic striatal cats. *Arch. Ital. Biol.* **100**, 48–85.

Watson, R. (1972). Mental correlates of periorbital PIPs during REM sleep. Presented at the Ass. for the Psychophysiolog. Study of Sleep, New York, May.

Weil-Malherbe, H., Whitby, L. G., and Axelrod, J. (1961). The uptake of circulating (^{3}H)-norepinephrine by the pituitary gland and various areas of the brain. *J. Neurochem.* **8**, 55–64.

Weiss, T., and Roldan, E. (1964). Comparative study of sleep cycle in rodents. *Experientia (Basel)* **29**, 280–282.

Weitzman, E., Kripke, D., Pollak, C., and Dominguez, J. (1965). Cyclic activity in sleep of macaca mulatta. *Arch. Neurol.* **12**, 463–467.

Weitzman, E. D., Schaumburg, H., Fishbein, W. (1966). Plasma 17-hydroxycorticosteroid levels during sleep in man. *J. Clin. Endocrin.* **26:2**, 121–127.

Weitzman, E., Rapport, M. M., McGregor, P., and Jacobi, J. (1968). Sleep patterns of the monkey and brain serotonin concentration: Effect of p-chlorophenylalanine. *Science* **160**, 1361–1363.

Whitlock, D. G., Arduini, A., and Moruzzi, G. (1953). Microelectrode analysis of pyramidal system during transition from sleep to wakefulness. *J. Neurophysiol.* **16**, 414–429.

Williams, R. L., Agnew, H. W., and Webb, W. B. (1964). Sleep patterns in young adults: an EEG study. *EEG Clin. Neurophysiol.* **17**, 376–381.

Wikler, A. (1952). Pharmacologic dissociation of behavior and EEG "sleep patterns" in dogs: morphine, N-allylnormorphine, and atropine. *Proc. Soc. Exp. Biol. Med.* **79**, 261–265.

Wilsocki, G. B., and Putnam, T. J. (1920). Note on the anatomy of the areae postremae. *Anat. Rec.* **19**, 281–287.

Wilson, C. W. M., and Brodie, B. B. (1961). The absence of bloodbrain barrier from certain areas of the central nervous system. *J. Pharmacol. Exp. Therap.* **133**, 332–334.

Wolff, P. H. (1959). Observation on new-born infants. *Psychom. Med.* **21**, 110–118.

Wolff, P. H. (1965). The development of attention in young infants. *Ann. N.Y. Acad. Sci.* **118**, 815–830.

Wolff, P. H. (1966). The causes, controls and organization of behavior in the neonate. *Psychol. Issues* **17**, 1–105.

Woods, J. W., Bard, P., and Bleier, A. (1966). Functional capacity of the deafferented hypothalamus: Water balance and responses to osmotic stimuli in the decerebrate cat and rat. *J. Neurophysiol.* **29**, 751–768.

Wyatt, R. J., Fram, D. H., Kupfer, D. J., and Snyder, F. (1971a). Total prolonged drug-induced REM sleep suppression in anxious-depressed patients. *Arch. Gen. Psychiat.* **24**, 145–155.

Wyatt, R. J., Zarcone, V., Engelman, K., Dement, W. C., Snyder, F., and Sjoerdsma, A. (1971b). Effects of 5-hydroxytryptophan on the sleep of normal human subjects. *Electroencephal. Clin. Neurophysiol.* **30**, 505–509.

Wyrwicka, W., and Chase, M. H. (1969). Projections from the inferior dental nerve to the dien- and mesencephalic areas related to feeding. *Physiologist* **12**, 401.

Yamaguchi, N., Marczinski, T. J., and Ling, M. (1963). The effects of electrical and chemical stimulation of the preoptic region and some non-specific thalamic nuclei in unrestrained, waking animals. *Electroenceph. Clin. Neurophysiol.* **15**, 145–166.

Yoshida, M., Yajima, K., and Uno, M. (1966). Different activation of the two types of the pyramidal tract neurons through the cerebello-thalamocortical pathway. *Experientia (Basel)* **22**, 331–332.

Zander, J. (1955). Progesterone in menschlichen Blut and Geweben, Part 1. (Progesterone im peripheren venösen Blut der Frau). *Klin. Woschr* **33**, 697–701.

Zbrozyna, A., and Bonvallet, M. (1963). Influence tonique inhibitrice du bulbe sur l'activité du noyau d'Edinger-Westphal. *Arch. Ital. Biol.* **101**, 208–222.

Zernicki, B., Dreher, B., Krzywosinski, L., and Sychowa, B. (1967). Some properties of the acute midpontine pretrigeminal cat. *Acta Biol. Exp. (Warsaw)* **27**(1), 123–139.

Zile, M. H. (1960). Effect of thyroxine and related compounds on monoamine oxidase activity. *Endocrinology* **66**, 311–315.

Zipperling, W. (1913). Über eine besondere Form motorischer Reizzustände beim Neugeborenen (Sog. "Stäupchen") *Z. Kinderheilk.* **5**, 31–40.

Index